D0892064

Human Risk Assessment —
The Role of Animal Selection and Extrapolation

Human Risk Assessment — The Role of Animal Selection and Extrapolation

Editor in chief
M. V. Roloff

Assistant editor
A. G. E. Wilson

Associate editors
W. E. Ribelin, W. P. Ridley and F. A. Ruecker

Environmental Health Laboratory,
Monsanto Company
St. Louis, Missouri, U S A

Taylor & Francis
London – Philadelphia – New York
1987

UK   Taylor & Francis Ltd, 4 John St., London WC1N 2ET

USA   Taylor & Francis Inc., 242 Cherry St., Philadelphia,
PA 19106-1906

Copyright © Taylor & Francis Ltd 1987

British Library Cataloguing in Publication Data

Human risk assessment: the role of animal
   selection and extrapolation.
   1. Toxicology—Technique   2. Laboratory
   animals.
   I. Roloff, M.V.
   615.9'00724   RA1199

   ISBN 0-85066-368-7

Library of Congress Cataloging in Publication Data

Human risk assessment.

   Includes bibliographies and index.
   1. Toxicology—Animal models.   2. Health risk
assessment. I. Roloff, M. V. (M. Val) II. Wilson,
A. G. E. [DNLM: 1. Animals, Laboratory. 2. Disease
Models, Animal. 3. Toxicology—methods. 4. Toxicology
—standards.   QV 600 H918]
RA1199.4.A54H86 1987   619   87-10067
ISBN 0-85066-368-7

*Typeset by Mathematical Compositon Setters Ltd.,
Salisbury, Wilts
Printed and bound by Taylor & Francis (Printers) Ltd.,
Rankine Road, Basingstoke, Hants*

Contents

Preface

An integral factor in any meaningful assessment of risk and safety is the difficulty of extrapolating the data obtained in animal toxicity studies to man. Before meaningful extrapolations between species can be attempted, a significant amount of information is required on the effects of the chemical substance in the test species, the similarities and differences in effects as expressed in the test species to man, and those in man that are relevant to the toxic effect observed in the test species.

The need to develop suitable animal models for extrapolation purposes is apparent since human experimentation is largely precluded or, when available, yields limited data. The realization of the need to develop animal models capable of predicting human response has been apparent for many years. However, relatively little progress has been made in unifying the scientific basis on which an appropriate animal species is selected. Rather, we still largely select animals on the basis of historical precedent or convenience, with little regard to the appropriateness of the selected animal model to man.

The objective of this book is to explore our current understanding of the factors which are critical in the selection of an appropriate animal species for toxicology studies and the subsequent extrapolation of the data to man. The chapters in this book have been written by experts in the fields of metabolism, pharmacokinetics, risk assessment, carcinogenesis, genetic toxicology, reproductive toxicology, pharmacogenetics, physiology, pathology, nutrition, industrial and regulatory toxicology. These authors have provided excellent guidance on the factors that constitute a scientific basis for species selection. It is our hope that consideration of the factors discussed in this book by toxicologists from academia, industry and regulatory agencies will significantly reduce the uncertainties that currently exist in the extrapolation of animal toxicity data to man.

R. M. Folk
M. V. Roloff
A. G. E. Wilson

St Louis, September, 1986

Acknowledgements

The symposium on which this volume is based was held on 28–31 October 1985, at the Doubletree Hotel and Conference Center, St Louis, Missouri.

The following are acknowledged for their participation in the symposium – Organizing Committee: William E. Ribelin, William P. Ridley, M. Val Roloff, Frederick A. Ruecker and Alan G. E. Wilson (Chairman); World Headquarters Administration Meeting and Planning: June Nienaber and F. Eugene McCoskey; accounting and administration: Jack G. Cooper, Laurel B. Cook and Janet Angelica.

A note of appreciation is extended to Larry D. Kier and George Levinskas for their expert chairmanship of two of the scientific sessions. In addition, thanks are due to Linda Kraus for her excellent graphics work for this publication.

A special word of thanks is due to Dr Leon Golberg for his invaluable guidance in establishing the focus and content of the scientific programme.

Contributors

Melvin E. Andersen
Biochemical Toxicology Branch
Toxic Hazards Division
Armstrong Aerospace Medical
  Research Laboratory
Wright-Patterson AFB,
Ohio, 45433-6573

James S. Bus
Pathology/Toxicology Research
Upjohn Company
Kalamazoo, MI 49007

Mitchell N. Cayen
Drug Metabolism Section
Ayerst Laboratories Research Inc.
CN 8000
Princeton, NJ 08540

Harvey J. Clewell III
Biochemical Toxicology Branch
Toxic Hazards Division
Armstrong Aerospace Medical
  Research Laboratory
Wright-Patterson AFB,
Ohio, 45433-6573

Michael W. Conner
Mallory Institute of Pathology
Department of Pathology
Boston University School of
  Medicine
784 Massachusetts Avenue
Boston, MA 02118

Vera C. Glocklin
Center for Drugs and Biologics
Food and Drug Administration
Public Health Service
Department of Health and Human
  Services
Rockville, MD 20857

Ronald W. Hart
National Center for Toxicological
  Research
Jefferson, AR 72079

Richard N. Hill
Office of Pesticides and Toxic
  Substances
Environmental Protection Agency
Washington, DC 20460

Michael D. Hogan
Biometry and Risk Assessment
National Institute of Environmental
  Health Sciences
National Institutes of Health
Research Triangle Park, NC 27709

G. H. Hottendorf
Medical University of South
  Carolina
171 Ashley Avenue
Charleston, SC 29425-2216

Kenneth S. Korach
Developmental Endocrinology and
  Pharmacology Section
Laboratory of Reproductive and
  Developmental Toxicology
National Institute of Environmental
  Health Sciences
National Institutes of Health
Research Triangle Park, NC 27709

Walter F. Loeb
Director of Veterinary Services
Metpath Inc.
5516 Nicholson Lane
Kensington,
MD 20895

Donald R. Mattison
Division of Reproductive
  Pharmacology and Toxicology
Department of Obstetrics and
  Gynecology
University of Arkansas for Medical
  Sciences
4301 West Markham, Slot 518
Little Rock, AR 72205

Michael J. McKenna
Department of Pathology and
  Experimental Toxicology
Warner-Lambert/Parke-Davis
2800 Plymouth Road
Ann Arbor, MI 48105

John A. McLachlan
Developmental Endocrinology and
  Pharmacology Section
Laboratory of Reproductive and
  Developmental Toxicology
National Institute of Environmental
  Health Sciences
National Institutes of Health
Research Triangle Park, NC 27709

I. C. Munro
Canadian Centre for Toxicology
645 Gordon Street
Guelph, Ontario
Canada, N1G 2W1

Paul M. Newberne
Mallory Institute of Pathology
Department of Pathology
Boston University School of
Medicine
784 Massachusetts Avenue
Boston, MA 02118

Retha R. Newbold
Developmental Endocrinology and
Pharmacology Section
Laboratory of Reproductive and
Developmental Toxicology
National Institute of Environmental
Health Sciences
National Institutes of Health
Research Triangle Park, NC 27709

Frederick W. Oehme
Comparative Toxicology
Laboratories
Veterinary Medical Center
Kansas State University
Manhattan, KS 66506

G. Edward Paget
Monsanto Company
G. D. Searle
4901 Searle Parkway
Skokie, IL 60077

Richard H. Reitz
Toxicology Research Laboratory
Dow Chemical Company
1803 Building
Midland, MI 48674

James H. Resau
Department of Pathology
University of Maryland School of
Medicine
10 South Pine Street
Baltimore, MD 21201

F. J. C. Roe
19 Marryat Road
Wimbledon Common
London, SW19 5BB, UK

Andrew J. Sivak
Life Sciences Section
Arthur D. Little Inc.
Cambridge, MA 02140

Stephen P. Spielberg
Division of Clinical Pharmacology
The Hospital for Sick Children
University of Toronto
555 University Avenue
Toronto, Ontario
Canada, M5G 1X8

Thomas B. Starr
Department of Epidemiology
Chemical Industry Institute of
Toxicology
Research Triangle Park, NC 27709

Peter J. Thomford
Division of Reproductive
  Pharmacology and Toxicology
Department of Obstetrics and
  Gynecology
University of Arkansas for Medical
  Sciences
4301 West Markham, Slot 518
Little Rock, AR 72205

Benjamin F. Trump
Department of Pathology
University of Maryland School of
  Medicine
10 South Pine Street
Baltimore, MD 21201

Angelo Turturro
National Center for Toxicological
  Research
Jefferson, AR 72079

Elliot S. Vesell
Milton S. Hershey Medical Center
Pennsylvania State University
Hershey, PA 17033

John H. Weisburger
Naylor Dana Institute for Disease
  Prevention
American Health Foundation
Dana Road
Valhalla, NY 10595-1599

Gary M. Williams
Naylor Dana Institute for Disease
  Prevention
American Health Foundation
Dana Road
Valhalla, NY 10595-1599

Animal selection and extrapolation – the problem defined

G. Edward Paget

Monsanto Company, G. D. Searle, 4901 Searle Parkway, Skokie, IL 60077, USA

It is not perhaps surprising that the very first symposium on a toxicological subject to which I contributed some 30 years ago included a paper, by Dr Weston Hurst, on species differences in toxicity testing – the central issue in this volume. Dr Hurst discussed a range of examples of striking species differences in response to toxins, leading to the conclusion that species selection was important and to a great extent arbitrary. His paper exemplified what could be called the natural history or phenomenological approach to this problem. This approach has characterized much of what has been said on this subject in the intervening period, culminating in Dr Calabrese's compendious book that he has called, I think optimistically, *Principles of Animal Extrapolation*. By saying optimistically I do not intend to decry this book, which is both important and useful – it contains many analyses of the basis of species differences and derives some rules from which more valid extrapolations can be made in particular situations. However, I do not believe that general principles governing such extrapolations exist, that is if one means by "principles" a general set of universally valid operating rules which can be applied to all of a class of problems.

This nihilism is forced upon us partly because we are confronted by not one but several only distantly related problems that, because they can be described in the same type of phrases and discussed in the same type of symposium and even examined in the same type of experiment, we perceive as being the same problem. (Parenthetically I would insert the thought that this confusion arises to a degree from the current obsession of working toxicologists with what they do and how they do it, rather than concern with what they think and how they express those thoughts.)

The whole issue is further clouded by the different purposes that have to be addressed by our ultimate evaluation. Unless one is concerned with Simon pure toxicology for its own sake, using it as a tool, as Claude Bernard suggested, to dissect the most intimate processes of physiology, we are usually trying to estimate the likelihood that a human population will suffer ill from exposure to a particular chemical. However, within that general problem there are two very different situations: on the one hand, drugs and environmental chemicals in a catastrophe situation are given in high doses to relatively small populations (even with very successful drugs, the worldwide exposure of individuals to any one agent may number only a small number of millions), while on the other hand, environmental chemicals in their ordinary use may affect significant fractions of the total population of a country, or even of the whole world, at low or very low levels. These intrinsic differences in ultimate use should, and do, condition not only our approach to extrapolation, but also our approach to the design and scale of experiments. The high-dose exposure situation would seem to offer the best chance for the successful exercise of extrapolative toxicology, and its numerous failures must give us all cause for concern about the infinitely more difficult task of the environmental toxicologist. It is a sad fact that despite all the development in toxicological testing and interpretation, the toxicology of drugs appears to be no more successful in predicting serious use-limiting toxic effects than it was a generation ago.

The toxicologists' task can be broken down into several separate and only distantly related activities, as I said earlier. These are the detection of a problem experimentally, the analysis of the mechanism at the basis of the problem by relevant techniques with investigation of the unknowns involved in attempts at extrapolation, and finally the intellectual integration of all that has been learned, and interpretative extrapolation to the relevant human situation.

I would like to offer some probably simplistic thoughts in each of these areas. The first problem is to detect and to delineate the possible problems of toxicity experimentally, especially in relation to the choice of appropriate species. In discussing the design of appropriate experiments, all toxicologists have to consider 'the choice of appropriate species'. Underlying such discussion is the (never expressed) slightly wistful feeling among toxicologists that nature in her wisdom ought to have provided some sort of mini-man that would as a species always be predictive of all (or even one!) human toxic response. Even to state this perception makes it appear absurd, but few of us would swear that we have never harboured such a thought. At the other extreme is the toxicologist who regards all species as being generally equivalent – after all mice and elephants are grey, have four feet, twitching noses and tails; what more points of similarity does one need? Nevertheless, mice are not elephants, as certain would-be investigators of LSD and the luckless Rajah found out to their cost. This is not merely a flippancy—it makes two points relating to selection of animal species: (1) in initial toxicity experiments one has no basis for choosing mice rather than elephants (in principle), and (2) one species of animal does not predict for another species more closely related than is man to the investigated species. Mice are not predictive of effects in rats, let alone elephants. In view of the enormous diversity of potential biological response, I have always believed that well-performed and observed experiments on numerous small groups of animals from diverse species are likely to be of more guidance to further experiment than are the usual highly organized experiments on very large numbers of individuals of two or rarely three species. In the future, I believe that evolutionary molecular biology will provide important insights into the evolutionary relationships not only of species and genera to one another but possibly also of different enzyme systems to one another. I am not enough of an evolutionist to know if it necessarily follows that because many systems in two species show a close evolutionary relationship, all molecular systems would show the same relationship. I suspect that would be too simple a circumstance. A recent article in *Scientific American* (Wilson, 1985) should be read by everyone concerned with this subject. To my mind, evolutionary molecular biology is one of the most intriguing and unexpected developments of the new biology.

Of course from the perspective of molecular biology it is clear that our molecular structure, as well as our gross anatomy, and even behaviour, link us most closely to the great apes, and after them to other primates. As I contemplate the implications of these findings – now exemplified but I suppose always there for the perceptive to see – I must confess that in the past I have been quite wrong to state that experiments in dogs are likely to be as illuminating as experiments in apes or monkeys. Now I think there are compelling reasons at a molecular level to consider the use of primates in toxicity testing. Of course, molecular biology is not the only input here, as cost, availability and ethical considerations all play a role. I am not happy to consider experiments on chimpanzees, not only for cost reasons, but also because these creatures are plainly to a major degree self-aware, a touchstone in my mind for ethical animal experiment. I pose the question whether, if populations of *Homo habilis* or *Homo erectus*, our immediate ancestors, were available for experiment, we would use them in view of the possibly more predictive results relating to *Homo sapiens* that such experiments might produce?

This is perhaps an appropriate point at which to address an increasingly important concern – the question of animal rights. By this I do not mean that lunatic fringe of ill-informed hooligans who are prepared to attack any individual or organization that uses animals experimentally for any purpose, just because of that fact. I do mean the increasing body of thoughtful and responsible people who are concerned with the human assumption that we have a right to do anything to our environment or its inhabitants without further question. As toxicologists concerned with animals, and with choosing species of animals for experiment, we must be sensitive to that concern, and be sure that the magnitude of the problem is related to the magnitude of the ethical questions that are posed by approaches to its resolution. To return to a thought I expressed in the last paragraph, what would our ethical position be if populations of *Homo habilis* were available for experiment? If we concede we might use this species in toxicology, can we exclude using populations of *Homo sapiens*? And if we say we would not use *Homo habilis*, how can we justify using *Pan pan*, where in fact does the ethical line get drawn? I have formulated and expressed my own views on this difficult problem elsewhere (Paget, 1975) but it is one that all experimental toxicologists must face and resolve and certainly bears on our choice of species. In the same vein, however, I have to say that we must also have no hesitation in stating plainly that now, and for the foreseeable future, it will be necessary to use whole animals in toxicological research and often animals such as cats and dogs that evoke particular sentimental reactions in humans. We have to say too that even the LD_{50} test – now so much derided and decried – still has a useful place in toxicology, as somewhat temerariously I have pointed out elsewhere (Paget, 1983). Finally, on this aspect of my subject, I would like to make a more than semantic point and stress that species for experiment should always be selected as a matter of choice, not solely because of tradition, availability or bureaucratic decree, although all these considerations must be borne in mind.

Plainly, the choice of species is intimately linked to the question of how thoughtfully the experiment is performed. For some purposes, a careful experiment on a growing bean shoot will be more useful than a mindless experiment on a hecatomb of mice or monkeys.

Presumably, the toxicologist is most vulnerable because of his general inability to explain at any level of molecular function the sort of changes that are encountered in initial toxicity experiments. There are several reasons for this, of which the least is the lack of sufficiently powerful techniques (although this is still a major factor). An important factor is what I might call the unexplored positive. We will all recall bizarre toxic effects, that, because of their extremely serious nature or wide distribution across dose levels and species, inhibit any further use or interest in the chemical concerned, whether as a drug or for some potentially environment contaminating purpose. The vast majority of these positive effects are neither published nor further investigated, but are relegated to the files of the laboratory concerned to gather dust. In my view such bizarre phenomena merit investigation, if only to clarify mechanisms of toxicity for further study. This is especially important in the not-infrequent cases of qualitative differences in species sensitivity.

A further reason for inadequate investigational toxicology is the sheer weight of effort and cost arising from the prescribed 'conventional' toxicity tests. This persuades industrial administrators to rest content with what *has* to be done rather than allowing for what *should* be done in addition for explanatory toxicology. The idea that extrapolation from animals to man would be greatly facilitated if we understood the metabolism of the compound in sensitive species and could describe in biochemical and pharmacokinetic terms the mechanisms by which a particular effect is produced remains the only possible resolution of an otherwise impenetrable problem. Only comprehensive fundamental knowledge will in the end permit sensible choice of species and ultimately sensible extrapolation by means other than rules of thumb.

Of course progress is being made. At one time, the most difficult problem seemed to be the estimate of the likely carcinogenic effect of compounds in man. While we are still a very long way from that complete understanding of carcinogenesis that would permit us to predict human effects with confidence, we are certainly emerging from the shadows of prejudice and mysticism that have hitherto shrouded this particularly difficult area, and I foresee with some certainty that within a decade we will be more confident in predicting whether a particular chemical at a particular dose level will be carcinogenic in man than in predicting whether it will be hepatotoxic. The new knowledge, that is accumulating so rapidly and enables one to make that sort of statement, is due to advances in molecular biology and powerful unifying concepts to which it gives rise, and not at all from toxicology.

Another force for obscurantism and formalism in toxicology, as opposed to open investigation and enlightenment, is the fear among administrators and research managers that to undertake any investigations not specifically required by regulatory agencies is to risk opening Pandora's box, with incalculable consequences. There are indeed examples of laboratories set up with the intent that they should pursue what I might term explicative toxicology, only to be diverted to routine test performance, as much from fear of what unconstrained research might disclose as from consideration of the cost of undertaking it. Nevertheless, sponsors of toxicology and evaluators alike must appreciate that problems of species differences and extrapolation to man can only be resolved by meaningful non-routine, exploratory toxicology of a kind not readily prescribed in some code of rules or evaluated by some Good Laboratory Practice check-list.

It is in the final episode of the toxicological drama that the working toxicologist finds his most exciting activity and justifies his employment. This is, of course, the process for which all the preliminary data gathering has been a preliminary – the culmination of the whole toxicological process, the assessment of human risk and, more importantly, risk–benefit analysis. Here we depart from any possible science and enter a world where the elements of judgment and philosophy are exposed to the pressures of commerce and politics in some not wholly rational process. In the area of drug toxicology the assessment is perhaps somewhat easier than in environmental toxicology, since some physicians at least are accustomed to the notion that there are no no-risk situations, that any intervention, just as any non-intervention, carries a risk, and risk assessment can at least in principle be a relatively quantitative procedure. Even in this relatively easy field where analysis of biological activity and concepts of risk assessment are common ground to toxicologist and physician, unexpected problems and disagreeable surprises abound, and there is no dearth of unprincipled lawyers and irrationally aggrieved patients to pursue those phenomena in court.

How much more difficult then in the process of risk assessment is the vastly more important field of the toxicology of environmental chemicals. Indeed, even retrospectively when all is said and done with a particular assessment, the true balance of risk and benefit can remain obscure. We, in the Western World, can view complacently the final risk–benefit balance in the withdrawal of chlorinated insecticides such as DDT and be happy that our eagle eggs are fertile again. But how about those untold millions in Third World tropical countries ravaged by malaria and other insect-borne diseases? Can they be so comfortable as their disease-induced lethargy drags their struggling country into yet further morasses of poverty and hunger?

The problem of risk assessment would be easier if one could realistically recommend open informed debate of the issues of major risk–benefit analyses. Unfortunately, this is not a feasible course of action except on rare occasions. There are just too many ill-informed special-interest groups ready to plunge into such a debate with unrealistic demands and nonfactual analyses, pandering for their own self-interested and often sinister reasons to the hysterical 'toxicophobia' that passes for discussion in public debate of these matters. In the state of Missouri in particular, one only has to say "dioxin" to someone who would not recognize a dioxin if they were presented with one to complete the ritual phrase "the most toxic substance known to man". In this respect, the hysteria became so severe that a proposal to transport supposedly dioxin-contaminated dirt in a sealed container through a community had to be abandoned because of the hysterical outcry against it, including many who should have known better. Dioxins are, of course, a clear example of toxins where species differences appear to be of enormous importance in evaluating likely risk, where orders of magnitude differences in sensitivity are encountered and where humans appear to be very much less sensitive than might have been supposed from animal experiment.

In such circumstances, rational public debate of issues of risk assessment and–risk benefit analysis simply cannot be conducted. Nevertheless, risk assessment is intimately linked to risk–benefit analysis, and this is a societal rather than a technical matter. What can the toxicologist contribute to such a discussion? In my view it would be wrong for us to give the impression that our evaluation of risk is to any real degree quantitative, except in very special cases, and it is disconcerting to read that such and such an action or inaction may lead to 50 new cases of cancer a year – in the absence of epidemiological data, such quantitative statements are wholly misleading (and in that particular case even epidemiology cannot help us make such a statement). Since we must, if we are honest, admit that all risk analysis is beset with uncertainties, we should try to educate our colleagues, our regulators, the media and, most of all, the general public to accept that uncertainty, and to make assessments based upon a complex analysis of probabilities. Unfortunately, uncertainty is one element that is equally unacceptable to commercial colleagues, regulators, lawyers, and the general public alike. All of them would prefer a confidently stated certainty, however inaccurate, to a guarded probability statement, however close to reality it may be. Therefore, an important function of the toxicologist is to educate our colleagues in the acceptance and manipulation of uncertainty and of avoiding stating probabilities or possibilities as established facts.

References

Paget, E., 1983, The LD50 test. *Acta Pharmac. Tox.*, **2**, Suppl. 2, 6–19.
Paget, G. E., 1975, The ethics of vivisection. *Theology*, **78** (661), 355–361.
Wilson, A. C., 1985, The molecular basis of evolution. *Scient. Am.*, **253**, 164–173.

PART 1

Current industrial practices and regulatory status of animal selection and extrapolation

Section editor:
F. A. Ruecker

Current EPA perspectives on animal selection and extrapolation

Richard N. Hill

Office of Pesticides and Toxic Substances, Environmental Protection Agency,
Washington, DC 20460, USA

Certain Federal regulatory agencies, including the Environmental Protection Agency (EPA), are charged with the evaluation of chemical safety. Under two of the statutes at the EPA – the pesticides and toxic substances acts – companies are required to submit data on chemical substances for review. The bulk of toxicity information is generated in experimental animals, and then used to assess risks from exposure to humans.

A number of considerations arise as to the selection of animals for testing and the nature of test protocols, as well as the way the data will be analysed to estimate the consequences of potential human exposure. This chapter will briefly review these topics and indicate some future directions for risk-assessment activities at EPA.

Testing guidelines

Industrial groups that provide data to the EPA have for a long time requested that the Agency develop testing guidelines for evaluating chemical toxicity. As a consequence, the Agency proposed guidelines in the late 1970s, and following extensive public hearings and written comments, final protocols were published in 1982 (EPA, 1982 a, b). Testing guidelines are not viewed as being static; instead, modifications and additions are made from time to time. For instance, in 1984 the pesticides and toxic substances programmes announced changes in the acute toxicity testing protocols that would help minimize the use of experimental animals, yet maximize the amount of information gained from them. In future years it is expected that many more changes of this nature will occur that will reduce or obviate animal usage.

Each EPA guideline names the animal species for consideration and often gives a preferred species. Critics have claimed that the Agency is too limited in its specification of animals for testing; let us investigate this claim.

Choice of animal species in the guidelines has been based on numerous factors, among them purchase cost, husbandry requirements, size, lifespan, characterized genetic and developmental history, and knowledge of historical control records. As an example, in the 90 d subchronic study, our guidelines specify testing in a rodent and non-rodent species, preferably the rat and the dog. In fact the opportunity exists to select among a variety of species, as long as one chooses among commonly used laboratory strains. Selection of a given species is further illustrated by the metabolism guideline. Although the rat is identified as the preferred species, it states that preliminary testing in several species may be attempted to get some idea of comparative metabolic patterns which, upon occasion, may aid in selection of species for subsequent toxicity testing.

The EPA's general policy is that alternative animal selection is possible. Guidance and preference are provided in the guidelines without specification of the animals to be used. The protocols state that various mammals may be chosen for testing as long as there is justification for selecting that species. People are encouraged to come to the Agency before testing to discuss issues of animal selection and test design.

A few examples help to illustrate that animal selection can be based on scientific appropriateness:

1. In the pesticide programme a chemical was shown to produce adverse effects in a rat reproduction study. Metabolism information on this agent indicated that the rat did not metabolize the compound as did humans. Therefore, we asked for testing in a mammalian species that handled the chemical like humans did.
2. In the toxic substances programme, the teratology test rule for acetonitrile called for the hamster instead of the rat or rabbit – the preferred species in our test guideline – because other nitriles had demonstrated adverse effects in the hamster.
3. In the EPA testing programmes, in-depth evaluation of existing chemicals frequently results in requesting tests that are not part of our existing guidelines. In these cases, animal selection and test protocol development need to be determined on a case-by-case basis.

In summary, then, the EPA has developed test guidelines that identify mammalian species and often name those that are preferred. Modifications in animal selection can and should be considered; we ask that any deviations be accompanied by a scientific rationale. Agency practice demonstrates that modifications occur, and we encourage companies to confer with Agency scientists about such changes before testing commences.

Risk assessment

The EPA has proposed a set of risk-assessment guidelines for cancer, the evaluation of chemical exposure, mutagenicity, developmental toxicity, and complex mixtures (EPA, 1984 a, b, c, d, 1985). The guidelines indicate the methods the Agency will take to assess data for potential toxicity to humans, potential human exposure and the potential risks from exposure to such agents.

The guidelines stress the appropriateness of the animal model to the human condition. For a fall-back strategy, when we lack such information, we use the most sensitive animal. In a similar manner, in the absence of data on inter-species differences we scale carcinogenic effects among species on a weight per body surface area basis.

Future directions

Progress has been made over the past few years in the area of risk assessment, and the future looks even brighter. There are many exciting developments to-day that will greatly enhance our ability to make judgements about chemical safety. We are moving from a stage of phenomenology — chemical in and toxic effects out — to one where there is much more regard for mechanism of toxic action. Many current discussions revolve around topics of peroxisome pro-liferation, free-radical formation and the like. The Agency is currently embarking on a review of carcinogenic effects that seem to result from inhibi-tion of a physiological endocrine-feedback loop; the knowledge about mechanism of action may lead us to re-evaluate the way we evaluate cancer risks produced by these chemicals.

Metabolic considerations represent another important area that will in-fluence risk assessment. Species differences in the handling of chemical agents are being investigated. Specific pharmacokinetic profiles are being developed for a number of chemicals such as methylene chloride and formaldehyde. These investigations point out similarities and differences among species in their metabolism of agents and also direct attention to the delivered dose at the target site instead of focusing on the dose administered to the organism.

In all, these advancements will contribute significantly to the risk-assessment process: they will allow us to make better predictions about chemical hazards and risks; they will reduce some of the uncertainty that now abounds; and they will set the stage for more reasonable regulatory decisions.

References

EPA, 1982 a, *Pesticide Assessment Guidelines. Subdivision F. Hazard Evaluation: Human and Domestic Animals*, Office of Pesticide Programs. NTIS Publication PB83-153916 (Springfield, VA: National Technical Information Service Publications).

EPA, 1982 b, *Health Effects Test Guidelines*, Office of Toxic Substances. NTIS Publication PB82-232984 (Springfield, VA: National Technical Information Service Publications).

EPA, 1984 a, Proposed guidelines for carcinogen risk assessment. *Fed. Reg., 49,* 46294–46301.

EPA, 1984 b, Proposed guidelines for exposure assessment. *Fed. Reg.,* **49,** 46304–46312.

EPA, 1984 c, Proposed guidelines for mutagenicity risk assessment. *Fed. Reg.,* **49,** 46314–46321.

EPA, 1984 d, Proposed guidelines for the health assessment of suspect developmental toxicants. *Fed. Reg.,* **49,** 46324–46331.

EPA, 1985, Proposed guidelines for the health risk assessment of chemical mixtures. *Fed. Reg.,* **50,** 1170–1176.

Current FDA perspectives on animal selection and extrapolation

Vera C. Glocklin

Food and Drug Administration, Center for Drugs and Biologics, Office of Drug Research and Review, Public Health Service, Department of Health and Human Services, Rockville, MD 20857, USA

Introduction

To what extent and degree of assurance is it possible to use animal studies to forecast and prevent toxicity from the chemicals to which humans are exposed? Retrospective toxicological research has shown that, with rare exceptions, almost all types of serious human toxicity can be replicated in animals, but that this correlation does not necessarily apply to all species and strains. How, then, can appropriate animals be chosen prospectively for reliable prediction of unknown toxicity in humans? Despite such uncertainty, terms such as 'animal model', 'predict', 'extrapolate', 'validate' in current risk-assessment arguments are often used in an absolute literal sense that goes far beyond their original specific intent or biological implications. Because of this, there are people who seem to believe that somewhere there exists the ideal mouse, rat, *in vitro* system or computer program that will predict any or all human toxicity with exact stoichiometric precision. Their zeal frequently mimics the alchemists' search for the Philosophers' Stone to turn lead into gold. As unrealistic is the opposite view (Anonymous, 1974), that "*Rufus herringus*" is the likely animal species for human extrapolation.

By contrast, the Food and Drug Administration has long appreciated that there is no 'quick fix' to toxicological predictions or disclaimers. Useful application of animal data to human risk decisions is necessary and possible, but it is a remarkably complex process that involves separating red herrings from valid concerns.

For risk-assessment purposes, the FDA currently requires a variety of studies in rodent and non-rodent species as prerequisites for the clinical investigation and eventual marketing of new drugs, and for marketing approval of new food additives. Short- and long-term toxicity is usually assessed in rats and dogs, teratogenicity in rats and rabbits and carcinogenicity in rats and mice. Sometimes another rodent such as the hamster, or another non-rodent such as the monkey is used as an alternative or additional species. Occasionally, as with the systemic contraceptives, carcinogenicity is also assessed in non-rodents.

15

Evolution of FDA toxicology guidelines

How did the need for such extensive animal testing evolve? What determines species selection? How are the data from the studies used for human risk decisions?

FDA-regulated products are ingested or otherwise applied directly to the body, and thus pose risks of toxicity that may be unavoidable in the case of food additives or unwarranted in the case of drugs. In addition to having to assess presumptive human risks, the FDA throughout its long regulatory history has also had to respond to periodic episodes of totally unexpected new types of human toxicity. This has resulted in progressive strengthening of its scientific as well as its regulatory objectives. For this reason, the FDA's pioneering role in applied toxicology goes back many years, as does its active involvement in guideline development and innumerable extramural discussions related to the topic of this volume. Indeed, my own first speaking assignment for the FDA, at a 1969 symposium on the Long Evans rat, was entitled "Selection of Laboratory Animals for Drug Safety Evaluation" (Glocklin, 1969).

Under the first Food and Drug Act, at the beginning of this century, the initially recognized regulatory problem pertained to widespread adulteration of food by toxic chemicals intended to reduce or mask spoilage, or merely added weight for increased profit. To identify and emphasize these problems, Dr Harvey Wiley conducted the first toxicology studies for regulatory purposes, on substances such as benzoic and boric acids, using government employee volunteers as "test animals" in his laboratory at the Department of Agriculture. However, one could not go on exposing human subjects, even devoted civil servants, to unknown toxic hazards. It became increasingly apparent that there were insidious, even life-threatening, toxicities lurking in adulterated foodstuffs and patent medicines, that went far beyond the transient gastro-intestinal upsets or general malaise than Dr Wiley's so-called "Poison Squad" would have been willing to accept.

The Bureau of Chemistry evolved into the Food and Drug Administration which, in 1933, began to revise its regulatory process. By 1935, there was a Division of Pharmacology staffed by an interdisciplinary group of highly qualified scientists brought in from various universities at mid-depression salaries of about $3000 per year. An alumnus of this period recently recalled that this was "a really excited group of people working in exciting new areas – there was no such thing as toxicology before we started doing this kind of work" (Woodard, 1980).

After the enactment of the Food, Drug and Cosmetics Act in 1938, this innovative and well co-ordinated group, which expanded further under the direction of Dr Arnold Lehman, developed and articulated many of the fundamental principles that apply to toxicological assessment today. These included the concepts of dose–response, use of non-treated controls, the importance of what is now called toxicokinetics, and use of uniform stock of different species for toxicological comparisons. They applied techniques of diagnostic medicine and statistical analysis for identifying toxicity and they attempted wherever possible to interpret toxicological mechanisms and notable species differences.

These toxicology assessment principles were published during the 1950s (Lehman *et al.*, 1955) and served for several years as the Agency's primary guideline. They became the fundamental basis for most of the subsequent guidelines developed by other agencies as well as the FDA, including the expanded guidelines for drug testing that became necessary after the thalidomide catastrophe and the enactment of the 1962 Drug Amendments, upon which this paper focuses.

Between 1938 and the mid-1960s the type and amount of toxicology testing for human drug development had expanded in a continuing effort to avert the unacceptable episodes of human toxicity that were experienced during this period. First there had been acute poisoning from elixir of sulphanilamide, then cataract or retinopathy from certain chronically used drugs, and then thalidomide teratogenicity. More recently, concern about drug-induced carcinogenicity has become important because of the increasing number of drugs that are used chronically or repeatedly, and knowledge of induced human neoplasia from drugs such as diethystilboestrol, conjugated oestrogens and phenacetin.

Toxicologic evaluation of new human drugs

We regard as still relevant the principle that more than one species should be used for toxicologic evaluations. This approach continues, not because of tradition or sentiment, but because this still provides the most practical and comprehensive way of assessing the toxic potential of new chemicals intended for direct human exposure. Chronic exposure can be maximized in the rodent, whereas the larger non-rodent species permit more frequent blood-letting and diagnostic procedures, as well as terminal pathological examination. In addition, there is a prudent logic that similar toxicity in different types of animals means that similar toxicity is more likely in humans.

Although the principles of toxicological evaluation are the same for drugs as for other types of compounds, the use of animal data for human drug risk decisions differs in some important ways from their application to decisions for food additives and environmental chemicals. First, drugs make up the only group of chemicals that are deliberately used or are administered at doses intended to have an effect on the body. By definition, a drug is biologically active and, therefore, can be expected to be toxic at some dose. Ideally, the toxic dose is separable by an adequate margin of safety from its beneficial effect, but this is not always the case. For example, warfarin, first used as a rat poison, has life-saving and relatively safe use as an anticoagulant at lower controlled dosage in humans, whereas the therapeutically effective dose of an anti-cancer drug may be only marginally sublethal. Acceptable toxicity for drugs is not based on a mathematically derived upper limit of acceptable exposure, but rather on an acceptable separation of toxic and beneficial doses that vary according to the particular disorder being treated, the therapeutic benefit sought, and the extent to which the particular type of toxicity can be detected early and reversed in humans. For this reason, it is the clinician and not the toxicologist who is usually responsible for risk-assessment decisions for human drugs.

In new drug evaluation, animal data are developed in a sequential fashion for basically three major types of clinical risk decisions. Initial short-term administration to humans, usually normal males or sometimes patients, followed by limited investigation in patients, must be preceded by dose–response characterization of the drug's pharmacology, acute toxicity and subchronic toxicity in animals, usually by the proposed human route of exposure. Second, administration of the drug to women who may become pregnant must be preceded by reproductive toxicology and teratology studies. Third, marketing approval of drugs intended for chronic or widespread repeated use is dependent upon satisfactory results of long-term animal studies. Chronic toxicity and carcinogenicity studies are usually initiated when prolonged clinical investigation is proposed, and are continued to completion during these clinical trials.

Pharmacological screening tests in a variety of animal models have been in use for many years. Of particular importance to drug risk decisions are cardiovascular effects, usually determined in dogs, and anaphylactic responses, usually determined in guinea-pigs.

Rabbits are usually used for skin, muscle or eye irritation studies for topical and parenteral drugs because they provide a greater area of exposure than the rat and have more delicate, human-like tissue than do dogs or monkeys.

The rabbit has been shown to be particularly susceptible to teratogens such as thalidomide, and so is considered to be an appropriate species, along with rats, for assessment of this effect. Mice, hamsters, monkeys and other types of animals are also occasionally used for this purpose.

As was said earlier, subchronic and chronic toxicity studies are usually done in rats and dogs. Monkeys are used occasionally instead of dogs, particularly for drugs that cause unremitting emesis in dogs, or for drugs that may have neurotoxic effects that can be observed better in primates. Sometimes, monkeys are also used as an additional species for further characterization of toxicity important to benefit–risk considerations for drugs of therapeutic significance.

The selection of rats and mice for carcinogenicity studies is in keeping with current, generally accepted principles of the carcinogenicity bioassay.

Comparison of drug disposition in animals and humans during the early stages of clinical investigation was recommended by the FDA in 1968 (Goldenthal, 1968), so that the most comparable species or strains could be selected for the chronic toxicity studies. Although this has occasionally been used to exclude a particular species that shows major qualitative differences from humans in drug metabolism, generally this approach has not proven to be particularly useful. There is almost always some type or degree of difference in drug pharmacokinetics and metabolism between humans and animals, and the variety of available species and strains is necessarily limited by practical considerations. Therefore, usual selection of the rodent strains and the non-rodent species remains largely dependent on consistent supply, good health, proven experimental use and reliable background information.

Although these animal studies are sometimes referred to as 'safety studies' to 'establish human safety', the use of these terms can be misleading. Animal studies are intended to provide a full characterization of the drug's toxicity, and not to prove that no adverse effects occur. Therefore, all types of studies are conducted with at least three drug dose levels and concurrent control. In subchronic and chronic toxicity studies, the highest dose should be sufficient to elicit overt, but sublethal, toxicity. The lowest dose should ideally show no important toxicity at a comfortable multiple, at least 5–10 times, the proposed human dose, although this may not be possible with certain drug classes that have narrow safety margins. If there is no evidence whatever of toxicity, or exaggerated pharmacological activity, even at high doses of a drug, this does not necessarily mean that the drug is 'safe'; it may only mean that it is not being absorbed effectively.

In reproduction and carcinogenicity studies, the highest dose is usually the maximum tolerated dose identified by subchronic studies in those species, with the lowest dose ideally higher than what is anticipated in humans.

The purpose of these animal studies is to provoke and exaggerate the drug's effects and to determine their dose and time relationships under the various experimental conditions. These data may identify certain types of toxicity or narrow safety margins that suggest unacceptable risk for the proposed patient population, or for humans in general. Otherwise, these animal data serve to direct attention to potential adverse effects that warrant rigorous clinical monitoring or patient exclusion during clinical investigation, and full disclosure in the post-approval package insert, until sufficient knowledge about the drug's actual effects in humans have rendered these animal data academic.

By these criteria, human investigation or marketing approval of a drug for a trivial disorder would not be permitted if there is prohibitive toxicity even in one species of animal. For example, drugs with teratogenic potential would not be permitted investigation in women of childbearing potential, nor permitted eventual marketing, unless the clinical disorder in the patient is important and the expected therapeutic benefit is substantial. If marketed, such a drug would be contra-indicated for use in pregnancy unless teratogenicity is characteristic of the entire drug category, such as is the case with the anti-epileptic drugs. In this case the package insert would warn the physician about this toxic potential. Benefit–risk decisions for drugs with neoplastic potential are particularly conservative because of an almost total lack of prevailing knowledge about the interpretation and extrapolation of carcinogenicity data in general, and the lack of known exclusion criteria for particularly susceptible individuals. Dose–response characteristics, and identification and reversibility of pre-neoplastic changes are still debatable or unknown. Furthermore, low-dose extrapolations to permissible levels are not feasible for drugs that must be used at substantial doses for therapeutic effect. For this reason, marketing approval for drugs with evidence of tumourigenic potential, even in one species, is permitted only when there is important therapeutic potential for a life-threatening or incapacitating disorder.

For reasons described earlier, one must accept practical limitations in the use of comparative drug disposition data for species selection. On the other hand, knowledge of inter-species similarities and differences in pharmacokinetics and metabolic pathways may contribute to elucidating toxic mechanisms. Regardless of the particular species or number of species studied, the predictive usefulness of the pre-clinical data, and the degree of conservatism or caution necessary to assume human safety, will be influenced by how well the results of the animal studies can be interpreted. Information about drug disposition and related mechanisms of toxicity may contribute to this.

Even in the absence of human data for comparison, as is the case in the initial investigational drug application (IND) submission, correlation of drug disposition data with the dose responses of pharmacological and toxic effects in the pre-clinical studies may not only be useful in identifying or interpreting apparent or observed species differences, but may also be of value in identifying drug-absorption or drug-accumulation problems that might be of concern in human use.

While all of these considerations are clearly relevant to the investigation of a new drug entity, they have generally not been explored effectively. Drug disposition studies have paid little attention to dose-dependent and duration-dependent considerations, suggesting lack of effective interdisciplinary communication and co-operation to co-ordinate and integrate all comparative or otherwise related data (Glocklin, 1982, 1984).

In a survey of drug disposition studies in 36 INDs for new oral drugs submitted to the FDA by 18 different companies during 1982 and 1983, I found that all had some type of pre-clinical drug disposition data submitted in the original submission or in an early subsequent amendment. These data showed reasonable within-company consistency, but varied appreciably from company to company in the types and extent of testing done, with no apparent relationship to the particular class of drug.

All of these 36 INDs had blood-level data and some identification of major metabolites in at least one species, primarily in rats, and about half also had biliary excretion studies in rats. About half of the INDs had pharmacokinetic and metabolite data in two species and four had such data in more than two species. However, sometimes these were not the same species or strains as were used in the toxicity studies. For example, one IND had pharmacokinetic and metabolite data only in Fisher rats and dogs, whereas toxicology studies were done in Sprague–Dawley rats and monkeys.

Organ distribution studies in rats were submitted to about half of the INDs but seldom included data to account for all of the drug administered. Only one company provided data to compare the relative tissue concentration after single and sequential dosing. Furthermore, apart from this diversity in types and extent of testing, there was a consistent lack of stated rationale for the doses selected for these studies. There was only one company that explored the steady-state levels at all dosage levels used in the subchronic toxicity studies.

Otherwise, the few other sequential dosing studies, and most of the acute dosing studies, employed only one dose. Acute dose-ranging studies, when done, were very limited. The doses used in about half of the single-dose studies were generally comparable to the middle to high dose range used in the subchronic studies. The rest used doses lower than these, often lower than the subchronic low dose level, and sometimes even considerably lower than the pharmacologically effective dose. Mention of pharmacologic or toxic signs was never included in the drug disposition study reports. In none of these INDs was drug disposition explored over the full range of pharmacologic and toxic doses that were identified in other pre-clinical studies.

There is obviously great room for improvement, and great potential usefulness, in developing toxicokinetics–toxicology correlates. On the other hand, one must not be too quick to use such data to reach conclusions that are based on false assumptions about cause and effect. The fact that an increase in a detected metabolite is parallel to a toxic response may not necessarily mean that the two are directly related. These two findings could be coincidental, or they could represent unrelated endpoints of an unknown distant mechanism. For this reason, directed research, instead of a routine screening programme, would be necessary to yield convincing conclusions about the lack of human relevance of a particular animal finding.

Also one should not be misled into believing that toxicokinetic differences will provide the sole and total explanation of all species differences in toxicity. This might result in substituting the arcane for the obvious. I once reviewed a pre-publication paper that reported anaemia in rats treated subchronically with high doses of a long-marketed CNS stimulant. The rats showed a physiologically important, as well as statistically significant, decrease in haemoglobin and red cell count. The authors concluded that this suggested covalent binding to the red cell and posed a great risk to mankind (even though anaemia was not a recognized adverse effect of this drug in humans). Further studies in rats were proposed to study erythrocyte ultrastructure and covalent binding. Noted in the report without any further mention was the fact that the animals were group-caged and had massive bleeding wounds from fighting throughout the entire experiment. No wonder they were anaemic! This was certainly a drug-induced effect in these rats, but any relationship to covalent binding, or to human risk, was doubtful.

In conclusion, the FDA's regulation of drugs and other potentially toxic compounds is dependent on good science. Good science in toxicology depends on interdisciplinary co-operation and communication for better understanding of the physiological and chemical mechanisms that lead to toxic endpoints within and between species. Only in this way can human risk extrapolation be improved.

References

Anonymous, 1974, Animal models in cancer research. *Lancet*, **2**, 1506.

Glocklin, V. C., 1969, Selection of laboratory animals for drug safety evaluation. *Lab. Anim. Care*, **19**, 700–701.

Glocklin, V. C., 1982, General considerations for studies of the metabolism of drugs and other chemicals. *Drug Metab. Rev.*, **13**, 929–939.

Glocklin, V. C., 1984, Correlation of drug disposition and toxicity studies. In *Experimental and Clinical Toxicokinetics*, edited by A. Yacobi and H. Barry III (Washington, DC: American Pharmaceuticals Association), pp. 75–85.

Goldenthal, E. I., 1968, Current views on safety evaluation of drugs. *FDA Papers*, pp. 13–18. (May).

Lehman, A. J., Patterson, W. I., Davidow, B., Hagan, E. C., Woodard, G., Laug, E, P., Frawley, J. P., Fitzhugh, O. G., Bourke, A. R., Draize, J. H., Nelson, A. A. and Vos, B. J., 1955, Procedures for the appraisal of the toxicity of chemicals in foods, drugs and cosmetics. *Fd. Drug Cosmet. Law J.*, **10**, 679–748.

Woodard, G., 1980, Interview. In *Transcription of Oral History of the U.S. Food and Drug Administration: Pharmacology*, edited by J. H. Young, F. L. Loftsvold, W. F. Janssen and R. G. Porter (Bethesda: National Library of Medicine), p. 15.

International perspectives on animal selection and extrapolation

I.C. Munro

Canadian Centre for Toxicology, 645 Gordon Street, Guelph, Ontario,
Canada, N1G 2W1

Introduction

Public perception of risk may differ significantly between nations and cultures depending upon political, social and religious beliefs and the economic forces that set the tone of domestic and international commerce. These factors, more than any others, account for the differences between countries in the development and application of regulatory statutes.

On the other hand, toxicologists in various industrialized nations approach the evaluation and assessment of human risk, based on laboratory animal epidemiological studies, in a remarkably similar fashion which, in part, reflects the important role that international agencies such as the OECD (Organization for Economic Co-operation and Development) and WHO (World Health Organization) play in harmonizing scientific views. But it is also a reflection of the fact that the thrust of national legislation pertaining to foods, drugs and other chemicals tends to be somewhat similar among developed countries. In addition, the international community of regulatory toxicologists comprised a surprisingly small number of individuals possessing similar experience and training. It is often said in the USA that the Delaney Clause represents the epitome of regressive legislation aimed at controlling potentially hazardous substances in that it leaves no latitude for judgement regarding risk acceptability. What is often not recognized in that country is that the principle behind the Delaney Clause pervades regulatory policies regarding carcinogens in most industrialized countries, and indeed these same principles were embodied in policy statements made by WHO (1961) when the Food and Agriculture Organization (FAO)/WHO Joint Expert Committee on Food Additives in their fifth report noted that known carcinogenic substances should not be used as food additives. The fundamental dilemma here is not that the legislation or basic principles are wrong or ill-intended but that the methodology available for risk assessment does not permit us to assess human risks with a degree of reliability and accuracy that is acceptable to all segments of the scientific community.

The legislative instrument found in most acts respecting, for example, food safety, making reference to the fact that "no person shall sell any article of food that contains in or upon it any poisonous or deleterious substance", obviously requires that judgements be made regarding risk acceptability. Thus it is incumbent upon regulatory and industrial toxicologists to fulfil this requirement, Delaney notwithstanding.

Risk assessment of animal carcinogens

Remarks in this paper in respect to the safety evaluation will concentrate on the question of carcinogenesis because this area of regulatory science occupies, at present, a predominant status on the international stage in the overall concern regarding chemical toxicity. Most toxicologists would agree that the risk assessment of carcinogens and, in particular, the facet that deals with the extrapolation of animal findings to humans is fraught with great uncertainty. While we can disguise the difficulty inherent in this process, as some conveniently do, by the use of over-simplified models of hazard assessment, there can be no doubt that the development of point estimation of human risk based on animal studies is a highly subjective process, subject to substantial and biological error.

The National Academy of Sciences (1978) in their report on saccharin drew attention to this problem when they pointed out that the estimates of human risk of bladder cancer based upon quantitative extrapolation of studies in rodents ranged from 0·2 to 1 144 000 cases of cancer in the US population over the next 70 years. This problem is not unique to the saccharin molecule because similar discrepancies have been noted in risk estimates for DDT, dimethylnitrosamine and ethylenethiourea (Van Ryzin, 1980). Because all of the available mathematical models for quantitative risk assessment fit these data sets equally well in the observable dose range, it is not surprising that the estimates of risk diverge considerably when the data are extrapolated to, say, a risk of one in one million. Some have argued that linear extrapolation, the most conservative of the mathematical procedures, should be used at all times for downward extrapolation of data. This position discounts the value of knowledge regarding time of onset, the pattern and types of tumours developed (i.e. degree of malignancy), the extent to which the tumours are associated with toxicity or other physiological perturbation, the biochemical activity and other biological actions of the compound in question, nor does it permit the consideration of apparent thresholds which may be observed and documented with some substances. The growing tendency to base critical regulatory decisions solely on the outcome of mathematical extrapolation on animal bioassay data, rather than on the cumulative weight of scientific evidence, deviates from the traditional practice of strict adherence to scientific principles in regulatory decision-making.

A cardinal principle of regulatory toxicology requires that animal data generated for risk-assessment purposes be biologically credible in terms of observed dose–effect relationships and relevant to the human setting. There are now numerous examples of substances which clearly produce tumours in rodents, although their action in this regard is of questionable relevance to humans. Well-accepted examples of this phenomenon include the injection-site tumours induced by food colours, the production of forestomach tumours by BHA, acrylates and related substances, the development of bladder tumours by the detergent builder NTA and the plastic component terephthalic acid and the apparent induction of pheochromocytoma by xylitol. The typical reaction of agencies to conduct a risk assessment on every substance found to induce tumours in animals needs to be tempered by a thoughtful evaluation, in the first instance, of the relevance of such findings for humans. Indeed, rather than concentrating, as we do, on risk-assessment criteria and arguing over methodology for extrapolation, we might be better served to concentrate more energies on the development of appropriate criteria to assess the relevance of animal studies for humans. Priority needs to be given to a critical examination of the existing database on chemical carcinogenesis in the light of contemporary knowledge of mechanisms in carcinogens and dose–effect/response relationships, taking into consideration the suitability of genetically cancer-prone animal strains which demonstrate high background tumour rates as surrogates for the human populations.

In assessing risks from carcinogenic substances it is possible to gain a feeling for the potency of a substance without introducing the kind of uncertainty inherent in the commonly employed mathematical models. Clayson *et al.* (1983) developed a procedure for ranking carcinogens in terms of their potency which involves estimation of the ED_{50}. Such estimates usually involve extrapolation of data over a very narrow dose range and are not subject to the same uncertainty associated with extrapolation of data well beyond the observable range. Other refinements of this procedure for ranking carcinogens have now been published by others and include estimation of the ED_{10}, and the incorporation into the model of background responses. A range of carcinogen potencies for selected chemicals in the report by Clayson *et al.* (1983) demonstrates that the most potent, aflatoxin B_1, is several million times as active as the least potent, trichloroethylene. These data demonstrate the wide range of potencies we are dealing with in the hazard evaluation of carcinogenic substances.

However, the use of information on potency *per se*, as observed in animal studies, provides no special advantage in gaining a perspective on quantitative risk assessment in man because of the uncertainty associated with the extrapolation of such data to humans. Nevertheless, it is certainly possible to make greater use of the potency information in ranking 'concern levels' over carcinogens, provided data relative to trans-species extrapolation are used in categorizing the level of concern. For example, comparative studies of DNA binding and adduct formation *in vitro* in animal and human tissue slices demonstrate species differences which appear to correlate with carcinogen potency. Booth *et al.* (1981) and Stoner *et al.* (1982) showed that the extent of DNA adduct formation with aflatoxin in liver slices taken from rats, hamsters and mice correlated with the magnitude of carcinogenic response to aflatoxin in these species. Human liver adducts formed at roughly the same level as those in the hamster liver, giving the impression that humans may not be as sensitive to aflatoxin as are rats. Likewise, methods now exist for detecting DNA adducts in human urine, and Pereira & Chang (1981) have recently observed a higher degree of binding of carcinogens to haemoglobin than was observed with non-carcinogens. Also, methods may be used *in vivo* to assess the effectiveness and efficiency of repair processes and to measure thresholds for DNA binding in animal systems. Of particular importance is the need to gain a better understanding of the relationship between the ad-ministered dose and dose of active intermediates delivered to the target site for a range of carcinogens of varying potency. Initial attempts along these lines have demonstrated that the relationship between the administered dose (e.g., formaldehyde) and the dose delivered to the target site, the nasal epithelium, is highly curvilinear, strongly suggesting a metabolic threshold for DNA binding (Casanova-Schmitz & Heck, 1983; Casanova-Schmitz *et al.*, 1984). Collectively these methods may be exploited to advantage in sharpening the risk-assessment process because they provide biochemical and pharmaco-kinetic information which can be used to gain a better appreciation of the quantitative relationships between dose and effect. The development of accept-able exposure limits for human exposure to chemicals requires the integration of these various endpoints in a way that permits the development of a biologically credible basis for extrapolation. Subsequent steps in the risk-assessment process, including the selection of appropriate statistical and mathematical methods for risk estimation, must take into consideration the biological profile of the compound in question.

Modulation of carcinogenesis

Modulation may result in enhanced tumour development as in the case of promoters or a host of other factors, or it may result in an inhibition of or reduction in tumour development. It is generally recognized that cancer development is a multi-stage process involving, among other steps, 'initiation' and 'promotion'. Initiation usually involves a complex series of biochemical events, including activation of the carcinogen to its electrophilic form (or other reactive species such as superoxides) and reaction with the target molecule, nuclear DNA, resulting in expression of an altered cell genotype which presumably acts as the nidus for tumour development. The concept of tumour promotion arose out of studies conducted by Rous & Kidd (1941), and subsequent investigations by Berenblum & Shubik (1947 a, b), which demonstrated that application of weakly carcinogenic amounts of the potent initiating agents dimethylbenzanthracene (DMBA) or 3-methylcholanthrene (MCA) to the skin of mice followed, after an appropriate period, by several applications of the non-carcinogenic irritant, croton oil, gave rise to a larger number of tumours at the site of treatment than if the croton oil was not used. In these classic experiments careful attention was focused on the order and timing of the administration of the two substances. The authors noted, for example, that if the carcinogen was given after croton oil treatment, substantially fewer tumours developed than if it was administered before. The term promotion was used to describe the operational characteristics of the carcinogen/croton oil model, in which croton oil was thought to stimulate the growth and development of initiated latent tumour cells.

Subsequent to this early work several chemicals have been reported to act as 'promoters' or enhancers of carcinogenesis. Hicks *et al.* (1975) and Cohen *et al.* (1979) reported promotion by saccharin in the bladder of rats initiated by low doses of methylnitrosourea and *N*-[4-(5-nitro-2-furyl)-2-thiazolyl] formamide (FANFT) respectively, while others observed the promoting action of phenobarbital in the liver of rats initiated with carcinogens. Many other studies of 'promotion', too numerous to mention here, are reported in the literature. In recent years, the term promotion has unfortunately been used by some authors to describe any tumour-enhancing effect that results when two chemicals are administered to animals sequentially, whether or not the first chemical does induce tumours when given at initiating doses and whether or not the promoter is itself carcinogenic. This is a marked departure from the original strict criteria which described the promoter as non-carcinogenic. At present, there is no universally accepted definition of promotion.

While promotion represents one form of modulation of chemically-induced cancer, other enhancing (or inhibitory) actions of chemicals, operating by different mechanisms, have been described. Modulation may result from the effect the modifying agent has on the metabolism, pharmacokinetics or metabolic action of the carcinogen at the target site, or it may occur as a result of alterations in hormonal status or effects on the immune system, to name but a few possible courses of action (Williams, 1985).

Given the fact that the populace is usually exposed simultaneously to low levels of an array of chemicals, it is important to recognize that modulating factors may represent a potential hazard to consumers depending upon the nature and level of previous or concurrent exposure to carcinogens. It has been suggested, for example, that induction of human cancer in the lung, prostate, bowel, breast and several other tissues by exogenous substances may depend as much on promoting and/or enhancing effects of chemicals as it does on initiating agents (Wynder & Hoffman, 1976; Reddy *et al.*, 1980).

The distinction in level of public health concern over modulating agents as opposed to carcinogens becomes important in the evolution of regulatory policy, because it is believed, but not proven, that these substances may possess quantitatively different risks from carcinogens. Many so-called promoting agents do not possess genotoxic properties and are hence considered to lack the ability to initiate cellular transformation through mutagenic mechanisms (Williams, 1985). It is sometimes stated, admittedly on the basis of very limited data, that they display thresholds in terms of their promoting action. Assessing risk from these agents, however, poses a unique set of problems. Promoting agents tend to show specificity in terms of target sites, hence their detection could require testing in a wide variety of organs and tissues, a task that could be prohibitively expensive. In addition, the extrapolation of data on tumour promotion from animals to man is infinitely more difficult than for carcinogens *per se* because of overwhelming uncertainties associated with the predictive value of currently employed model systems. This is further compounded by the problems inherent in estimating the added risk from modulating agents in sub-populations of humans who, as Knudson (1985) points out, may already be 'at risk' because of predisposing factors in their environment or because of their genetic constitution. These points were highlighted recently in the National Academy of Sciences Report on Carcinogenicity of Cyclamate (1985), which noted that the relevance for humans of animals systems to detect promoting or enhancing effects is yet to be determined and that research to identify relevant models is required. The answer to the regulatory dilemma concerning modulating agents lies in research to identify cellular mechanisms involved in enhancement. Unfortunately, at this time, these mechanisms are so little understood and are potentially so varied that risk from these agents is difficult to specify in any general sense.

Conclusions

Traditionally, regulatory agencies have placed great emphasis and reliance on the carcinogen bioassay as means of assessing potential human cancer risks from chemicals. In the early days of carcinogen regulation, this was fraught with numerous difficulties, partly because of the relative insensitivity of animal studies done at the time which precluded the development of conclusions regarding potency and partly because of a woefully poor understanding of mechanistic aspects of cancer induction. Until quite recently, animal bioassays did not often possess sufficient sensitivity or statistical resolving power to define differences in potency between carcinogens. This is becoming less and less the case as more chemicals are subjected to standardized large-scale testing procedures which permit comparisons to be made between various carcinogens. As our ability to distinguish differences in potency increases, so will our ability to assess human health hazards from reported animal carcinogens. Thus, in each case, information regarding numerical potency must be supplemented with knowledge regarding toxicity, DNA binding, pharmacokinetic behaviour and metabolism, all of which assist in defining the level of potency and consequently the level of risk associated with human exposure of the substance in question.

Future policies on carcinogen regulation need to reflect the fact that chemicals of low carcinogenic potency which appear to induce tumours by virtue of their ability to cause physiological, toxicological or biochemical perturbations at high doses should possibly not be considered as hazardous as those that are clear-cut carcinogens which produce an abundance of tumours at low doses.

While modulation and promotion represent interesting laboratory observations in experimental chemical carcinogenesis, at the present state of our knowledge it is difficult to define any generally acceptable approach to the regulation of these substances.

The prevailing evidence clearly points to the fact that mechanistic considerations taken together with data on carcinogen potency, dose–response relationships and biochemical reactivity will, in the future, lead to an increased ability to refine risk estimates. Approaching the regulation of carcinogens within such a conceptual framework makes it possible to exercise scientific judgement regarding the magnitude of risk. This is essential if we are to base decisions on sound scientific principles.

References

Berenblum, I. and Shubik, P., 1947 a, The role of croton oil applications, associated with a single painting of a carcinogen in tumour induction in the mouse's skin. *Br. J. Cancer*, **1**, 379–382.

Berenblum, I. and Shubik, P., 1947 b, A new quantitative approach to the study of the stages of chemical carcinogenesis in the mouse's skin. *Br. J. Cancer*, **1**, 383–391.

Booth, S. C., Bosenburg, H., Garner, R. C., Hertzog, P. J. and Norpoth, K., 1981, The activation of aflatoxin B1 in liver slices and bacterial mutagenicity assays using livers from different species including man. *Carcinogenesis*, **2**, 1063–1068.

Casanova-Schmitz, M. and Heck, H. D'A., 1983, DNA–protein cross-linking induced by formaldehyde. In *Formaldehyde Toxicity*, edited by J. E. Gibson (Washington, DC: Hemisphere), pp. 154–156.

Casanova-Schmitz, M., Starr, T. B. and Heck, H. D.'A., 1984, Differentiation between metabolic incorporation and covalent binding in the labeling of macromolecules in the rat nasal mucosa and bone marrow by inhaled [^{14}C]- and [^{3}H]-formaldehyde. *Toxic. Appl. Pharmac.*, **76**, 26–44.

Clayson, D., Krewski, D. and Munro, I. C., 1983, The power and interpretation of the carcinogenicity bioassay. *Regul. Toxic. Pharmacol.*, **3**, 329–348.

Cohen, S. M., Arai, M., Jacobs, J. B. and Friedall, G. H., 1979, Promoting effect of saccharin and DL-tryptophan in urinary bladder carcinogenesis. *Cancer Res.*, **39**, 1207–1217.

Hicks, R. M., Wakefield, J. and Chowaniec, J., 1975), Evaluation of a new model to detect bladder carcinogens or co-carcinogens; results obtained with saccharin, cyclamate and cyclophosphamide. *Chem. Biol. Interact.*, **11**, 225–233.

Knudson, A. G., 1985, Hereditary cancer, oncogenes, and antioncogenes. *Cancer Res.*, **45**, 1437–1443.

National Academy of Sciences, 1978, *Committee for a Study on Saccharin and Food Safety Policy. Part 1. Saccharin: Technical Assessment of Risk and Benefits* (Washington, DC: National Academy Press).

National Academy of Sciences, 1985, *Evaluation of Cyclamate for Carcinogenicity* (Washington, DC: National Academy Press).

Pereira, M. A. and Chang, L. W., 1981, Binding of chemical carcinogens and mutagens to rat hemoglobin. *Chem. Biol. Interact.*, **33**, 301–305.

Reddy, B. S., Cohen, L. A., McCoy, D. G., Hill, P., Weisburger, J. H. and Wynder, E. L., 1980, Nutrition and its relationship to cancer. *Adv. Cancer Res.*, **32**, 238–345.

Rous, P. and Kidd, J. G., 1941, Conditional neoplasms and subthreshold neoplastic states: a study of the tar tumors of rabbits. *J. exp. Med.*, **73**, 365–389.

Stoner, G. D., Daniel, F. B., Schenck, K. M., Schut, H. A. J., Goldblatt, P. J. and Sandwisch, D. W., 1982, Metabolism and DNA binding of benzo(*a*)pyrene in cultured human bladder and bronchus. *Carcinogenesis*, **3**, 195–201.

Van Ryzin, J., 1980, Quantitative risk assessment. *J. occup. Med.*, **22**, 321–326.

Williams, G. M., 1985, Types of enhancement of carcinogenesis and influences on human cancer. In *Cancer of the Respiratory Tract: Predisposing Factors*, edited by M. J. Mass, D. G. Kaufman, J. M. Siegfried, V. E. Steele and S. Nesow (New York: Raven Press), pp. 447–457.

World Health Organization, 1961, Food and Agriculture Organization/World Health Organization Expert Committee on Food Additives. Fifth Report. Evaluation of carcinogenic hazards of food additives. World Health Organization Tech. Rep. Series 220.

Wynder, E. L. and Hoffman, D., 1976, Tobacco and tobacco smoke. *Semin. Oncol.*, **3**, 5–15.

Opinions on animal selection for the assessment of carcinogenicity

F. J. C. Roe

19 Marryat Road, Wimbledon Common, London SW19 5BB, UK

I had a bad dream. I dreamed that I was dead. But that wasn't really the bad part. The obituary notices were really quite good. They said such things as "He was industrious", "He was thoughtful and imaginative in his opinions", "He was a prolific contributor to the scientific literature but arguably contributed too much to conference proceedings which no one read", and so on. No, it wasn't the being dead or the obituaries that were the bad aspect of the dream, it was the following interview with Himself-up-Above (HUA) that was so disturbing!

HUA. So you practised as a toxicologist?

ME. Yes Sir.

HUA. In the process you took some of My creatures out of the wild. You confined them to small boxes and you deliberately encouraged them to mate in such a way that diseases which had not been eliminated by My masterly 'Evolution–Natural Selection Scheme' were not only perpetuated but actually fostered. Can you tell Me – why did you do these things?

ME. Please Sir, I thought that the main object of your 'Evolutionary–Natural Selection Scheme' was to evolve Man (in the image of your Goodself). The aim of we toxicologists was to try to prevent disease in Man, and we thought You would like this.

HUA. It was presumptuous of you to think you knew the object of My Scheme. But why were you so unbelievably naive and stupid in what you actually did?

ME. Please Sir, may I sit down, I feel a bit faint?

HUA. In your experience as a toxicologist did you ever encounter a rat or mouse who felt faint?

ME. I do not know, Sir. They can't speak – only squeak.

HUA. If that is a criticism of one of My Creations, don't be impertinent! I'll ask you a related question. Did you ever encounter a rat or mouse that died from coronary thrombosis?

ME. No Sir.

HUA. You knew very well that your fellow Men were committing suicide in large numbers by eating some of My other Creations in excess and developing cardiovascular disease. You knew that this was the most common cause of premature death among your fellow Men. Nevertheless, you quite deliberately chose two species, rats and mice, for testing new chemicals to see if they might endanger man's health.

ME. But our main objective was to try to prevent man from developing cancers.

HUA. If that was your aim, why did you conduct your experiments under conditions that were so unnatural and which actually predisposed them to develop cancers in high incidence? Why did you deprive My poor creatures of exercise and of the possibility to consort with the opposite sex? Why did you feed them on diets which led them to develop all manner of diseases to which Man is not prone? Why did you make them into endocrinological cripples?

ME. Please Sir, I did try from 1973 onwards to draw attention to the points which You are making. I can give You the references (Roe & Tucker, 1973; Roe, 1981).

HUA. Nevertheless, you still went along with the system. You sat silently through meetings where data from toxicity studies conducted under unphysiological conditions were discussed. You didn't walk out in protest. Before you go, I'm going to show you just two tables. Table 1 lists side by side the diseases from which men in your country most commonly die and those which are most common in the laboratory rat. When you look at this table, can you really defend the use of the rat for predicting disease risk in man? The second table (Table 2) contrasts My view of the aims and

Table 1. Percentage causes of death and incidence of endocrine neoplasia in humans and rats.

	Humans†		Rats‡	
	Male	Female	Male	Female
Nephritis/nephrosis				
Fatal	0·7	—	—	—
Debilitating/fatal	—	—	60	65
Heart disease				
Fatal	31·9	20·6	0	0
Endocrine/nutritional/metabolic disease				
Fatal	0·2	0·5	—	—
Debilitating/fatal				
pituitary neoplasia	—	—	15	30–80
all endocrine neoplasia	—	—	20	40–90
Mammary gland neoplasia				
Fatal	—	7·1	1	5
Debilitating/fatal	—	—	5	40–90

† Mortality data for England and Wales 1970–72 (ages 15–74 years).
‡ Typical data for untreated Sprague–Dawley rats.

Table 2. Overview of aims and achievements of toxicology.

	Illusion	*Reality*

Aim	Prevent human diseases from chemicals	Provide living for:
		  Contract laboratories
		  Civil servants
		  Lawyers
		  Statisticians
		  Consultants
		  Conference organizers

Achievements	Public reassured that chemicals are properly tested for carcinogenic activity	Public worried to 'death' (or indifference) by:
		  Politicians
		  Sensational press statements

achievements of toxicology with the illusion under which you seem to have been labouring.

ME. But Sir, I have been saying just these things at lectures and in articles in learned journals for many years.

HUA. That's the trouble with you. You are nothing more than a didactic academic. If you had made the effort to master politics you might have got the message across! This interview is at an end! Go to Hell!

It was in the wake of this dreadful dream that I had to sit down to prepare this paper. Although I remain full of remorse, I cannot help feeling that there have been mistakes on both sides. For instance, it might have been better if God had arranged for biologists and biochemists to evolve *before* statisticians, and for statisticians to evolve *before* politicians and journalists. Indeed, I suspect that the problems are still so complex at the scientific level that the optimal time for the evolution of politicians and journalists still lies in the future! But that is not the way it is. We are in a situation where we cannot, as toxicologists, pursue our enquiries on the basis of our own list of priorities. We are pressurized into continuing to use standard and sometimes old-fashioned laboratory methods and into devoting most of the resources available to us to the unachievable task of trying to prove a negative, that is, to show that chemicals are *not* toxins and are *not* carcinogens. Meanwhile, the scourge of cancer as a common disease of humans continues more or less unchanged, and experts in the field of epidemiology are shouting to us that we are looking for carcinogens in the wrong places.

The two main themes of this volume are *Animal selection* and *extrapolation* in toxicity testing. It is my view that one cannot meaningfully discuss either of these topics unless one has a clear understanding of the purpose of the testing and the constraints.

The purpose of testing

As to the purpose, I do not dispute that there is a need to evaluate new chemicals for possible toxic and carcinogenic hazard to man. However, resources spent in this way cannot affect the existing incidence of environmentally induced toxicity or cancer in man. At most, careful testing might hold the level steady. If we want to reduce the existing burden of cancer we must first make sure that we are looking for carcinogens in the right place and are using the best methods.

How much cancer can the present programme of testing prevent?

Sir Richard Doll and Richard Peto (1981), from a broadly based survey of data of many different kinds derived from many different sources, concluded that diet (not food additives), tobacco, alcohol, reproductive and sexual behaviour,

Table 3. Proportions of cancer deaths attributed to various different factors.

Factor or class of factors	Percentage of all cancer deaths	
	Best estimate	Range of acceptable estimates
Tobacco	30	25–40
Alcohol	3	2–4
Diet	35	10–70
Food additives	<1	−5†–2
Reproductive and sexual behaviour	7	1–13
Occupation	4	2–8
Pollution	2	<1–5
Industrial products	<1	<1–2
Medicines and medical procedures	1	0·5–3
Geophysical factors	3	2–4
Infection	10?	1–?
Unknown	?	?

From Doll & Peto (1981).
† Allowing for a possibly protective effect of antioxidants and other preservatives.

geophysical factors and infection probably account for nearly 9 out of every 10 deaths from cancer among humans (Table 3). By contrast, they estimated that fewer than 1% are attributable to food additives (indeed, the addition of some chemicals to food may actually reduce cancer risk). Their best estimate for the contribution of occupational factors was 4% and for that of medicines and medical procedures, 1%. Industrial products chipped in with less than 1% and pollution with 2%.

Of course, one may argue that the low estimates for food additives and medicines, etc., reflect the effectiveness of existing test requirements. Even so, we are left with 30% of human cancer attributable to smoking, for which there is no obvious animal model, and the huge total of 35% for general dietary factors which remains largely ill-defined and uninvestigated. Until we have a much better idea of which dietary factors are important determinants of cancer risk in man, we have no basis for believing that one animal model is superior to any other.

Selection of species for carcinogenicity testing

At many meetings someone or other expresses the view that the ideal animal for use for the carcinogenicity testing of a compound is the one that metabolizes it in the same way as man. Whatever the theoretical merits of this view, in practice it rarely has much value. First, it assumes that there actually exists a species which mimics man in the way it metabolizes the particular compound. Secondly, it ignores the possibility that although the metabolism may be similar, the distribution of some important receptor site may be different. Thirdly, it overlooks the fact that it could be more expensive to identify a species that mimics man than to carry out a carcinogenicity test in a rodent. Finally, it ignores the very serious constraint that, for a carcinogenicity test to be meaningful, it must be conducted in a sufficiently large number of animals to permit a statistically significant effect on cancer risk to be seen. Also, before carcinogenicity activity can be excluded with any degree of confidence, animals must have been exposed to the test agent for the majority of their natural lifespan. If, by chance, the Marion's tortoise (*Testudo sumeirii*) turned out to be the one species that handled a chemical in the same way as man, it would be for toxicologists in one's grandchildren's generation to evaluate the results of a study started now. From the viewpoint of timing, it would be easier to assess whether a chemical is safe for giant tortoises by testing it in man, than vice versa!

In practice, therefore, for logistic reasons, only a very limited number of species (rats, mice, hamsters and possibly dogs) can be used for routine carcinogenicity testing irrespective of whether they metabolize compounds in the same way man does.

Which strain? Inbred or outbred?

The choice of strain for a carcinogenicity test is heavily dependent on the precise aim of the study. If the main aim is simply to obtain reproducible results irrespective of what they may mean, then unquestionably one should choose an inbred strain or an F_1 hybrid. However, even if one does this, reproducibility is not always very good, particularly between laboratories. Environmental variables, particularly diet, but also other variables that have not been clearly defined, influence the incidence of spontaneously arising neoplasms to a major extent.

Alternatively, if the main aim of a carcinogenicity test is, as it should surely be, to provide data which is useful in the prediction of *possible cancer risk in man* or, equally importantly, *likely freedom from cancer risk in man*, then the emphasis of choice should be on avoiding the use of strains of animals which are genetically flawed in such a way that they develop 'spontaneously' very high incidences of tumours of kinds which are rare, or do not occur at all, in man. The high incidences of testicular, pituitary and mammary tumours in many strains of rats and the high incidences of liver, lung and lympho-reticular neoplasms in many strains of mice are, in my view, serious handicaps to meaningful predictive carcinogenicity testing. The extent to which these

Table 4. Reported incidence of adrenal medullary tumours in three different strains of male and female rats

Strain	Tumour development (%) in untreated rats		Reference
	Males	Females	
Wistar-derived	81	56	Gillman *et al.* (1953)
	0	2	Boorman & Hollander (1972)
Sprague–Dawley	51	8	Kociba *et al.* (1979)
	16	4	Thompson & Hunt (1963)
Fischer 344	37	12	Jacobs & Huseby (1967)
	4	0·5	Sass *et al.* (1975)

characteristics represent genetic flaws and the extent to which they reflect overfeeding and inappropriate environmental conditions is presently uncertain, although it is already clear that background tumour incidence in the long-term rodent studies can be greatly reduced by the avoidance of overfeeding.

When considering the reality of the present situation, I am far from happy that either the Fischer 344 rat or the B6C3F1 hybrid mouse are really suitable for predicting cancer risk or lack of cancer risk for man. However, I know of no other strains, either inbred or outbred, that are more suitable.

Table 4 illustrates the variation in incidence of adrenal medullary tumours in three strains of rats – two random-bred (Wistar and Sprague–Dawley) and one inbred (Fischer 344) – in long-term studies. Clearly, it would be meaningless to regard any of these strains as especially prone or especially resistant to the 'spontaneous' development of adrenal medullary tumours. On the other hand, it is clear that dietary composition may greatly influence the incidence of these tumours in rats (see Table 5).

During recent years, I have come to realize that apparent differences in response between different strains of rats (or different strains of mice) to the same chemical agent are more likely to be due to differences between the diets fed to the animals or to other differences in laboratory environments than to

Table 5. Effect of composition of diet on incidence of adrenal medullary tumours in rats.

Diet composition (%)			Life-time incidence of adrenal medullary tumour (%)	
Carbohydrate	Protein	Fat	Males	Females
60	15	11	63	47
4	82	10	13	15

From Gilbert *et al.* (1958).

Table 6. Endocrine tumour incidence in control rats (%) and significant effects of exposure (↑ or ↓) to the same neuroleptic drug in three separate two year studies of similar design.

| | Strain of rat | | | | | |
| | Wistar I | | Wistar II | | Sprague–Dawley II | |
Endocrine tumour	Male	Female	Male	Female	Male	Female
Pituitary	22(↑)	62	17	53	41	46
Mammary						
Benign	0	86	2	11	8	77
Malignant	0(↑)	10(↑)	0	0	2(↑)	22
Adrenal						
Medulla	18(↑)	22	0	0	2	0
Cortex	10	10	0	0	0	3
Thymoma (endocrine type)	4(↑)	10(↑)	0	0	0	0
Thyroid						
Follicular	26(↓)	18	0	0	0	0
C-cell	0	6	9	5	1	0
Pancreas						
Islet cell	4(↑)	0(↑)	4(↑)	3(↑)	4	5

I and II, indicates laboratory experiment carried out in.

genetic differences between the strains. A striking example of this is illustrated in Table 6, in which the results of three very similar two-year studies on the same neuroleptic drug gave rise to three very different results. In Sprague–Dawley rats, the only statistically significant effect was an increased incidence of mammary tumours. In one study in Wistar rats at the same laboratory, the only effect was an increased incidence of insulinomas in both sexes. But in another study in Wistar rats in a different laboratory, increased incidences of mammary, pancreatic islet cell and thymic (endocrine-type) tumours were seen in both sexes, and increased adrenal medullary and pituitary tumours and decreased thyroid follicular tumours were seen in males. In the light of such variation in response, between nominally the same strain of rat under different conditions and between different strains of rat under the same conditions, I feel that great caution is necessary in attributing apparent differences in response solely to genetic constitution.

Extrapolation to man

Extrapolation is a mathematical term referring to the calculation from known terms of a series of other terms. Its use by toxicologists to bridge the gap between rodent and man is, to say the least, etymologically dubious. Indeed, it is almost beyond belief that toxicologists uncomplainingly allowed, under the

Table 7. Gaps to be bridged in extrapolating results from laboratory rodents to man.

Differences in

1. Body size, basic metabolic rate and longevity
2. Extent of inbreeding
3. Composition of, and day-to-day variation in diet; Coprophagia.
4. Indulgence in alcohol, tobacco, contraceptive pill and drugs
5. Exercise
6. Opportunity for sexual fulfilment.
7. Spectra of commonly occuring diseases and common causes of death
8. Speech: ability to describe symptoms and availability of surgery and other forms of therapy
9. Information available on morbidity
10. Information available on cause of death and incidental findings at death

umbrella term 'extrapolation', their findings in carefully conducted laboratory studies to be manipulated by statisticians and translated into risk assessments for man. Table 7 lists some of the gaps which such extrapolations ignore. Surely common sense dictates that if one cannot predict from the results in one strain of rat what will happen in another strain, or even in the same strain in another laboratory (Table 6), how can one hope to predict across the rodent–man species gap and across the other gaps listed in Table 7?

Effects of overfeeding on non-neoplastic disease in rats

Although several decades have passed since Tannenbaum and Silverstone began to report the effects of caloric intake and dietary composition on tumour incidence in rats and mice (for review see Clayson, 1975), and despite

Table 8. The effects of overfeeding on the incidence of certain non-neoplastic diseases in untreated male Sprague–Dawley rats

Disease	Percentage of sample developing disease
Moderate to severe glomeronephritis	67
Parathyroid hyperplasia	67
Calcification of aorta	34
Adrenal medullary	
hyperplasia/neoplasia	32
neoplasia	20
Chronic fibrosing myocarditis	83

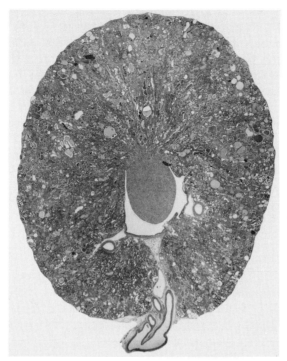

Figure 1. Photomicrograph of chronic progressive nephropathy in untreated male Wistar rats given free access 24 h each day to a standard laboratory diet for a period of 2 years.

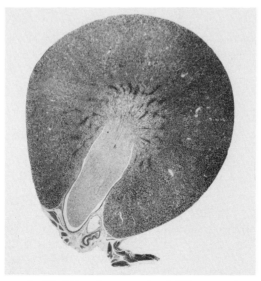

Figure 2. Photomicrograph of the kidney in untreated male Wistar rats given access to a standard laboratory diet for six hours per day for two years.

numerous publications by myself and others during more recent years (Roe & Tucker, 1973; Tucker, 1979; Conybeare, 1980; Roe, 1981), the folly of overfeeding animals during the conduct of carcinogenicity studies persists. Table 8 illustrates some of the dire consequences in terms of the incidences of certain non-neoplastic diseases resulting from overfeeding in untreated male Sprague–Dawley rats which I encountered in a recent study. Figures 1 and 2 illustrate how overfeeding affects the severity of chronic progressive nephropathy in untreated male Wistar rats. Figure 1 was prepared from an animal given free access throughout the 24 h of each day to a standard laboratory diet for a period of 2 years. By comparison, Figure 2 was prepared from an exactly comparable rat that was given access to the same diet but for only 6 h per day for 2 years. Chronic progressive nephropathy may lead to a severe disturbance of calcium homeostasis, with consequent parathyroid hyperplasia, and cortical nephrocalcinosis which parathyroid hyperplasia gives rise to in kidneys already severely affected by progressive nephropathy.

Table 9. Association of metastatic calcification of aorta, lung and kidney with adrenal medullary hyperplasia and/or neoplasia in animals in a two year carcinogenic study.

	Adrenal medullary hyperplasia/neoplasia	
	−	+
Metastatic calcification (aorta, kidney, lung, etc.)		
−	55	26
+	14	24

Significance of positive association: $P = 0.01$.

Figure 3. Effects of overfeeding on adrenal medullary tumour incidence.

OVERFEEDING ⟶ CHRONIC PROGRESSIVE NEPHROPATHY (CPN)

CPN ⟶ PARATHYROID HYPERPLASIA AND NEOPLASIA

EXCESS PARATHORMONE ⟶ 1. HYPERCALCAEMIA
2. METASTATIC CALCIFICATION (AORTA/KIDNEY)

HYPERCALCAEMIA ⟶ ADRENAL MEDULLARY HYPERPLASIA AND NEOPLASIA

Table 9 shows the statistically significant ($P < 0 \cdot 01$) association that occurs between metastatic calcification of the aorta, kidney, lung, etc. and adrenal medullary hyperplasia and/or neoplasia in the two-year carcinogenicity study illustrated in Table 8. Figure 3 illustrates a sequence of effects linking overfeeding to increased adrenal medullary tumour incidence.

Effects of high concentration of polyols or lactose in the diet of rats

During recent years, there has been concern that certain polyols, including sorbitol, xylitol and lactitol, when fed in high dietary concentrations to rats, predispose to adrenal medullary hyperplasia and neoplasia (Roe & Baer, 1985). The clue to the mechanism involved came from observations on the long-term effects of high dietary concentrations of lactose. Like the polyols, lactose increases the absorption of calcium from the gut of rats. This increased calcium absorption is associated with pelvic nephrocalcinosis and with adrenal medullary hyperplasia and neoplasia. Table 10 summarizes the data in terms of the effect of 20% dietary lactose on the incidence of adrenal proliferative changes.

Table 10. Effect of 20% dietary lactose on adrenal medulla in rats.

	Rats with tumours (%)			
	Males		Females	
Adrenal medullary tumours	Control	20% Lactose	Control	20% Lactose
Hyperplasia or phaeochromocytoma	41	71	16	26
Phaeochromocytoma	23	44	2	4
Malignant phaeochromocytoma	7	20	0	2

Effects of overfeeding on incidence of neoplastic disease

Previously, much attention (Roe, 1981) has been drawn to the outrageously high incidence of neoplasia which has come to be accepted as the norm for control groups in carcinogenicity studies on rats. To illustrate this, Table 11 depicts the incidences of certain kinds of neoplasia in the untreated Sprague–Dawley rats which constituted the controls in a definitive carcinogenicity study on 2,4,5-T (Kociba *et al.*, 1979). Table 12 illustrates how simple dietary restriction can dramatically reduce two of the kinds of tumour listed in the previous tables, namely, tumours of the pituitary and mammary gland. Table 13 illustrates how dietary restriction can reduce the incidence of tumours of many kinds in mice, including lung, liver and lympho-reticular.

Table 11. Hormone-associated neoplasms (%) in *ad libitum* fed untreated control Sprague–Dawley rats observed for up to 26 months (86 rats of each sex).

	Rats with neoplasms (%)	
Site/type of neoplasm	Males	Females
Pituitary	31	63
Adrenal		
Cortex	2	7
Medulla	51	8
Thyroid		
C-cell	8	8
Parathyroid	0	1
Pancreas		
Exocrine	33	0
Endocrine	16	9
Testis	7	—
Ovary	—	5
Mammary gland	—	
Fibroadenoma		76
Adenoma	5	12
Other	—	29

From Kociba *et al.* (1979).

Table 12. Effect of dietary restriction on incidence of pituitary and mammary tumours in rats.

	% Rats with tumours under different feeding regimens			
	Males		Females	
Tumour	*Ad lib.*	Restricted	*Ad lib.*	Restricted
Pituitary	3^2	0^{***}	66	39^{**}
Mammary	0	0	34	6^{***}

From Tucker (1979).
$**P < 0.01$, $***P < 0.001$.

Concluding remarks

For many years I have been drawing attention to the need for basic research designed to define the conditions needed for the maintenance of laboratory rats and mice in good health until they are old. So far, my pleas have seemingly fallen mainly on deaf ears, although some research in this area has now been started or is planned. In rats, overfeeding predisposes to all manner of endo-

Table 13. Effect of simple dietary restriction on tumour incidence in mice.

Tumour	Males		Females	
	Ad. lib	Restricted to 75% of ad lib.	Ad. lib.	Restricted to 75% of ad lib.
Lung	30	19*	24	8**
Liver	47	12***	7	1*
Lymphoma	4	1	11	4*
Other	8	4	12	4*
Any tumour at any site	71	36***	50	17**
Any malignant tumour	17	7*	23	7**

Header note: Mice (no.) developing tumours at any time during study†

From Conybeare (1980).
† n = 160 males, 160 females.
*P < 0·05, **P < 0·01, ***P < 0·001.

crine disturbances and these are bound to distort the response of animals exposed to chemicals in carcinogenicity tests. There can be no sense in testing chemicals for carcinogenicity in rats maintained under conditions such that 50–100% of them develop pituitary and mammary tumours, etc. There is no identifiable population of humans for which such rats could constitute a model.

I have no doubt that many of the findings in carcinogenicity studies carried out in overfed rats and mice are no more than nonsensical gobbledygook. The problem is that where these effects suggest a beneficial effect of treatment on the incidence of a particular type of tumour, Regulatory Authorities ignore them, whereas adverse effects are regarded as evidence of carcinogenicity. Elsewhere (Roe, 1983), I have proposed the term 'pseudocarcinogenicity' to describe the enhancement of tumour risk by a non-genotoxic mechanism in animals plagued with abnormalities because of overfeeding and laboratory-associated artefacts.

References

Boorman, G. A. and Hollander, C. F. 1972, Occurrence of spontaneous cancer with aging in an inbred strain of rats. *TNO-nieuws*, **27**, 692–695.

Clayson, D. B., 1975, Nutrition and experimental carcinogenesis: a review. *Cancer Res.*, **35**, 3292–3300.

Conybeare, G., 1980, Effect of quality and quantity of diet on survival and tumour incidence in outbred Swiss mice. *Fd Cosmet. Tox.*, **18**, 65–72.

Doll, R. and Peto, R., 1981, The causes of cancer. *J. Natn. Cancer Inst.*, **66**, 1191–1308.

Gilbert, G., Gillman, J., Loustalot, P. and Lutz, W., 1958, The modifying influence of diet and the physical environment on spontaneous tumour frequency in rats. *Br. J. Cancer*, **12**, 565–593.

Gillman, J., Gilbert, C. and Spence, I., 1953, Pheochromocytoma in the rat. Pathogenesis and collateral reactions and its relation to comparable tumours in man. *Cancer*, **6**, 494–511.

Jacobs, B. B. and Huseby, R. A., 1967, Neoplasms occurring in aged Fischer rats, with special reference to testicular, uterine, and thyroid tumours. *J. Natn. Cancer Inst.*, **39**, 303–309

Kociba, R. J., Keyes, D. G., Lisowe, R. W., Kalnins, R. P., Dittenber, D. D., Wade, C. E., Gorzinski, S. J., Mahle, N. H. and Schetz, B. A., 1979, Results of a 2-year chronic toxicity and oncogenic study of rats ingesting diets containing 2,4,5-trichlorophenoxyacetic acid (2,4,5-T). *Fd Cosmet. Tox.*, **17**, 205–221.

Roe, F. J. C., 1981, Are nutritionists worried about the epidemic of tumours in laboratory animals? *Proc. Nutr. Soc.*, **40**, 57–65.

Roe, F. J. C., 1983, Testing for carcinogenicity and the problem of pseudocarcinogenicity. *Nature*, **303**, 657–658.

Roe, F. J. C. and Baer, A., 1985, Enzootic and epizootic adrenal medullary proliferative diseases of rats: influence of dietary factors which affect calcium absorption. *Human. Tox.*, **4**, 27–52.

Roe, F. J. C. and Tucker, M., 1973, Recent developments in the design of carcinogenicity tests on laboratory animals. *Proc. Eur. Soc. Study of Drug Tox.*, **XV**, June 1973, *Excerpta Med. Int. Congr. Ser.*, **311**, 171–177.

Sass, B., Rabstein, L. S., Madison, R., Nims, R. H., Peters, R. L. and Kelloff, G. J., 1975, Incidence of spontaneous neoplasms in F344 rats throughout the natural life span. *J. Natn. Cancer Inst.*, **54**, 1449–1456.

Thomson, S. W. and Hunt, R. D., 1963, Spontaneous tumours in the Sprague–Dawley rat: incidence rates of some types of neoplasms as determined by serial section versus single section techniques. *Ann. N.Y. Acad. Sci.*, **108**, 832–845.

Tucker, M. J., 1979, The effect of long-term food restriction on tumours in rodents. *Int. J. Cancer*, **23**, 803–807.

PART 2

Use of physiological and toxicological data from man and animals as aids in animal selection and extrapolation

Section editor:
M. V. Roloff

Anatomical and physiological considerations in species selections – animal comparisons

Frederick W. Oehme

Comparative Toxicology Laboratories, Kansas State University, Manhattan, KS 66506, USA

Human beings and animals may be equally exposed to hazardous chemicals by the oral and the dermal route of exposure, but their biological responses are not necessarily similar. Indeed, variations in biological response are seen among all species of animal, even though the routes of exposure, and frequently the dosages used, are identical. This variability in response to chemical exposure is related to numerous factors that are qualitatively and quantitatively unique for each animal species – and even within species, these factors account for individual variation between members of that species.

The researcher utilizes species variations when designing protocols for specific objectives. Also, species variations may be employed to explain away unusual experimental results or to justify extrapolation to higher animals or human beings. It is likely that all scientists recognize the existence of the species differences phenomenon, and that we probably subconsciously react to this variable in our research designs, interpretations of experimental results, and in recommendations for the next step in the research and development process. Therefore, it may be useful to have an overview of the basic factors that affect biological response to chemicals, to review the anatomical and physiological considerations in animals species selections, and to give several examples of species variations in biological response and the reasons for those variations.

Factors affecting biological response

Route of exposure

Although several animals may be exposed to chemicals via the oral route, and occasionally dermally in our experimental studies, the effects seen from those exposures relate to a variety of factors, listed in Table 1. All of these factors, and even others, will have an impact upon what animal species are selected for particular studies. Each factor is worthy of its own chapter and in fact several,

Table 1. Factors affecting the biological response
to chemicals.

---

1. Amount of chemical received
2. Physical and chemical properties of chemical
3. Route of exposure
4. Absorption of chemical
5. Biotransformation of chemical
      a, Distribution
      b, Metabolism
      c, Accumulation
      d, Elimination
6. Species involved
7. Size, age and sex of exposed animal
8. Health of animal
9. Individual variations

---

such as the variations that occur due to sex differences (Calabrese, 1985) have
had books written about them. All these factors produce variables that are
dependent on the species involved.

Physiological response

Once the chemical enters the body, the animal responds by a variety of
detoxication systems to handle that compound (Table 2). The degree of success
these systems have will determine what expression of toxicity results.
Physiologically, vomiting and some digestive tract response may occur. The
chemical may be binding to proteins, stored in tissues, or may have variable
amounts excreted as the unchanged compound in breath, different body secretions, and in bile and urine.

Table 2. Biological detoxication of chemicals.

---

1. Physiological detoxication
      (*a*) Vomiting, diarrhoea
      (*b*) Bind to protein, store in tissues
      (*c*) Excrete in breath, secretions, bile, urine
2. Biological detoxication
      (*a*) Enzymatic attack to increase excretion
      (*b*) Liver, kidney, intestinal mucosa
      (*c*) Make easier to detoxify further, make more
          water-soluble, split or destroy
      (*d*) Most detoxications decrease toxicity or inactivate

---

Biochemical response

Superimposed on all the above responses are the biochemical factors involved
with detoxication (Table 2). When considering all responses, the species

biochemical variations are probably responsible for more species variation than the anatomical and physiological factors. Here we are concerned about differences in enzyme activities and their effects, activities that occur predominantly in selected tissues such as liver, kidney, intestinal tract, mucosa and some others. These biochemical reactions allow animals to modify, detoxicate and excrete chemicals that are insulting their biological systems. Most of these detoxications produce a compound that is less toxic; however, some 10% or so of these reactions activate the foreign chemical and produce a compound that is more reactive and more toxic than the parent structure was.

Variations in biological response

Considering those variables, a significant variation in response to chemicals is observed between animals, as well as between species. Figure 1 illustrates how individual animal variation (in this case between three dogs) can affect therapeutic and toxic biological responses. The effective toxic dose, as well as the effective therapeutic dose, fluctuates with the animal and can vary considerably depending upon the degree of fluctuation. This is the reason why significant numbers of animals are used and why statistical evaluation is employed – in order to reduce the influence of variations between individual animals. Also, there are important individual species variations that must be considered, for these variations will determine to a large degree which particular species are selected for a particular study.

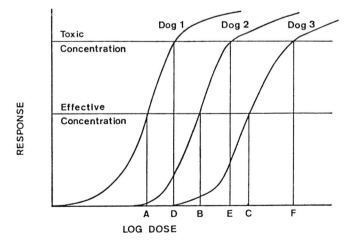

Figure 1. Responses observed in three dogs of differing sensitivity to a drug.

Variations in the biological response

Occurrence of spontaneous poisonings in domestic animals

Variability in species response is seen typically in the incidence of clinical field cases (Oehme, 1975). The most common poisonings in dogs and cats, in order of frequency, are those induced by rodenticides, followed by insecticides, various environmental toxins, heavy metals and, to a lesser degree, animal-origin toxins and plant poisons (Oehme, 1975). When the range and priority of those toxicities are compared with the types of poisonings seen in cattle, considerable differences are noted. Heavy metals, predominantly lead, are the most common poisoning agents in cattle, and these are followed by organophosphates. Insecticide-induced problems, agricultural chemicals, nitrate–nitrite toxicities, and poisonous plants are a common concern (Oehme, 1975). Mycotoxins and a variety of other chemicals are of less importance in causing toxicity in cattle.

These observations suggest that species variations, in addition to management factors, play an important role in determining what type of toxicities various animal species will commonly exhibit and also how severely affected one species will be compared to another. Why are cattle so highly sensitive to lead toxicity, while dogs and humans do not demonstrate toxicity to that same degree? If blood and tissue concentrations are examined, one finds that the blood level of lead in the cow showing clinical signs of lead toxicity is approximately half that associated with similar clinical toxicity in humans or dogs. Why is that? I suggest there is a biochemical basis for that unique response and that it emphasizes the importance of biochemical understanding for rationalizing how one species is selected over another for a toxicity evaluation.

Species differences, then, occur at two major levels: (1) variations in anatomical structure and physiological functioning, and (2) differences in the biochemical activity of various tissues (Oehme, 1970; Clarke, 1976).

Anatomical/physiological differences between species

The anatomical/physiological differences between species (Table 3) are due to the absorptive fluctuations of the digestive tract, the pH changes in the digestive tract, the length of the digestive tract, the individual variations in ability to excrete foreign compounds, available mechanisms of excretions, the urine volume and pH, and the amount of body fat, to name a few such factors. If a researcher were concerned with a fat-soluble compound and the effect a particular mechanism of storage might have on the expressions of toxicity, the amount of fat present in a pig's body compared to that of a rat or a dog would be highly important in species selection.

Researchers also select animals for studies on an anatomical basis, perhaps more for convenience than for a specific species effect upon the chemical of

Table 3. Anatomical/physiological species differences.

1. Absorptivity in various regions of the digestive tract
2. Length of the digestive tract
3. Presence of bacteria, enzymes in digestive tract
4. Excretory ability
5. Methods of excretion possible
6. Urine volume and pH
7. Amount of fat in body
8. Constituents of diet
9. Physical activity and other stresses

concern. Because convenience translates to economics, many mice and rats rather than pigs are employed because of the practical aspects. Yet there are many advantages, from the viewpoint of the cardiovascular system and dermatology, for the use of swine as opposed to rats for some studies. A larger animal is selected for some studies because frequent collection of large amounts of blood is required.

Biochemical differences between species

Probably more important than structural and functional differences is the biochemistry of the species. It is in this area that major decisions and progress in toxicology are being made to understand better the biochemical differences between species, and therefore select the most biochemically appropriate species for the particular compound being investigated. The general areas in which biochemical variations between species arise are: (1) digestive tract enzymes; (2) the level of circulating enzymes; (3) the liver enzymes; (4) other degradative processes, or the detoxification processes that are present in these enzyme systems that help animal to handle or deal efficiently with the test compound, to a greater or lesser extent. Details of individual cellular and subcellular biochemical processes are being explained on a daily basis in a greater and more directly applicable way; and this is where a good deal of research energy is directed.

Ultimately, however, it is the total effect of the toxic compound that needs to be understood. What clinical response will the animal show to a particular chemical? This requires classical whole-animal studies, that end up finally with man. This is the bottom-line of species differences in response to chemicals. Figure 2 depicts the result of intravenously administering radioactive phenol in four species of animals, therefore bypassing the anatomical/physiological differences and establishing the half-life based upon the plasma disappearance of the radioactive phenol. A tremendous variation is seen between those four species, with the cat showing a very long half-life, based upon now recognized deficient biochemical mechanisms. The bottom-line is that phenolic products

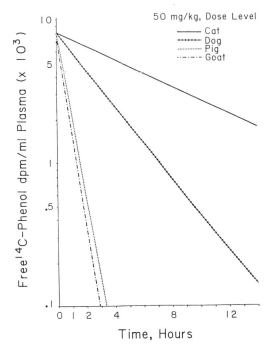

Figure 2. Disappearance of intravenously injected ^{14}C-phenol (dose level 50 mg/kg body weight) from the plasma of dogs (···········), cats (————), pigs (··············) and goats (·—·—·—·). Disappearance rates in each species were adjusted slightly to a similar concentration at time zero.

and cats do not mix, a fact that has been widely recognized once the underlying biochemical basis was identified.

Biotransformation

The entire process of anatomical, physiological and biochemical factors inter-acting in the intact animal body can be summarized by a biotransformation model (Figure 3). The absorption characteristics, the biochemical metabolism efforts, and the excretion possibilities are evident in the influence they each have on the animal's response. The variations that occur between animal species in the ability of chemicals to move across membranes, to interact with target organs and cell organelles, and to be, to a greater or lesser degree, excreted are what account for all the differing responses toxicologists con-tinually try to understand and study.

Clinical expressions of species variations

Clinical expressions of these species variations in response to chemical exposure between and within animal species are the practical end-product of

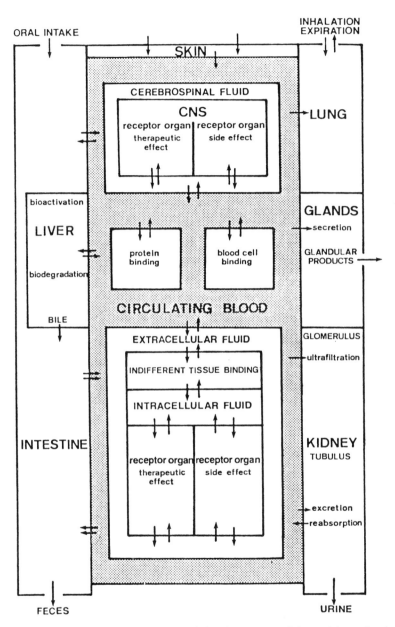

Figure 3. Biotransformation model depicting the exposure of the model to a chemical by various routes, absorption, distribution possibilities, potential organ and subcellular receptors, biodegradation, and excretion/compartmental movement options for the parent compound or metabolites.

these differences (Oehme, 1970; Clarke, 1976; Davis, 1979). The amount of strychnine that will kill rabbits is usually safe for humans, even when dosed on a per kilogram basis. Cyanide sufficient to kill dogs will be safe for humans, and the per kilogram dose of cyanide that is usually responsible for killing a cow is frequently safe for a horse or a sheep. Penicillin is routinely toxic for birds, guinea-pigs, and hamsters, and yet it is used, often in overdose, as an important therapeutic drug in other animals. Frogs are resistant to the effects of Compound 1080 (monofluoroacetic acid), and yet children and most domestic animals are potently poisoned by the pesticide. Alpha-naphthylthiourea (ANTU) does not affect guinea-pigs, but it is one of the more potent rodenticides available. Dogs and cats are resistant to zinc phosphide toxicity due to the vomiting capability of those species. Aspirin, phenol and morphine are some 10 times more toxic for feline species than for other animals. Is it any wonder that toxicology is a comparative science? (Oehme, 1970).

Examples of species uniqueness

With this background, let us review some of the variations in toxic response as seen in various animal species.

Phenols

Cats show extreme reactions to phenolic compounds, as well as to some other chemicals. We studied the comparative toxicity and excretion in dogs and cats of a common phenolic disinfectant, *ortho*-phenylphenol (OPP) (Oehme, 1971). Figure 4 shows the plasma concentrations of OPP when identical doses on a mg/kg basis were given orally to similar groups of cats and dogs. The OPP plasma concentration in the cat increased until death occurred within a few hours after dosing, while in dogs the OPP plasma concentration rose considerably above that which caused death in the cat, but had no clinical effect in the dog, and then slowly declined as the OPP was eliminated in the urine. When we looked at the urinary excretion of radioactive (^{14}C-labelled) OPP using two different dosages of OPP in cats and dogs, the minimal ability of the cat to excrete phenolic chemicals was obvious (Figure 5). At a high OPP dose the cats died before much excretion could occur, while at the low OPP dose, the cats survived, but urinary OPP excretion was very small over the three days after dosing. When dogs were given doses of OPP identical to those the cats received, the dog's excretion of OPP in the urine was rapid and efficient at both dose levels, suggesting that there are biochemical differences in the species' abilities to conjugate and excrete this phenolic chemical. The cat does have a deficiency in glucuronide formation ability, with the result being limited excretion of phenolic chemicals (Davis, 1979).

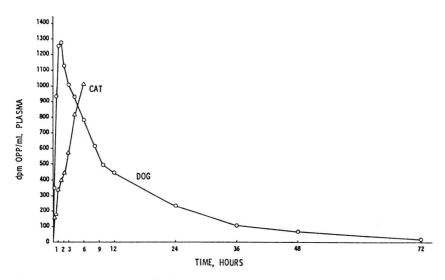

Figure 4. *Ortho*-phenylphenol (OPP) plasma concentrations in groups of six cats and six dogs, each receiving identical OPP doses orally on a per weight basis.

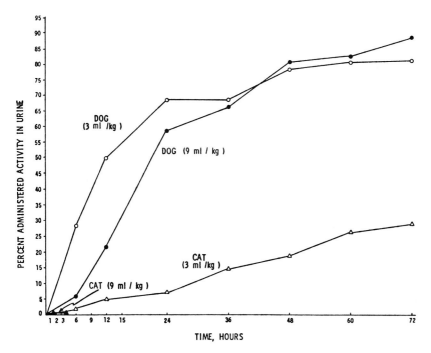

Figure 5. Urinary excretion of ^{14}C-labelled *ortho*-phenylphenol (OPP) in groups of six cats and six dogs after oral administration of two dosage levels to each species.

Acetaminophen

Acetaminophen has a biotransformation scheme in which an active intermediate metabolite is formed (Figure 6). Glutathione is utilized to bind that activated metabolite, but if the glutathione is exhausted, then macromolecules within the target cells are bound until cell death results in toxicity (Savides & Oehme, 1983). Interestingly, liver toxicity is the common expression of that effect in humans and in dogs, but in cats a different form of clinical effect is expressed (Savides *et al.*, 1984).

Acetaminophen produces a unique facial oedema in the cat. In addition, about 8–12 h after the toxic insult, cats develop cyanosis, with gums and tissues becoming brownish/blue in colour. Methaemoglobinaemia is promi-

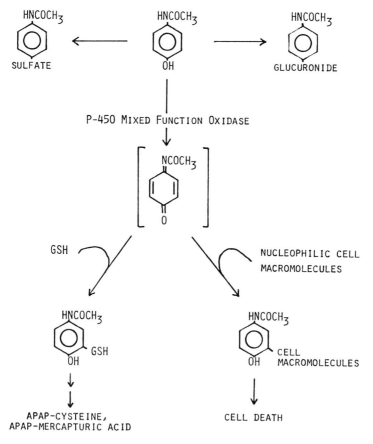

Figure 6. Biotransformation of acetaminophen (APAP) with active intermediate and glutathione (GSH) conjugate and cell macromolecule binding indicated. Note the alternate pathways to sulphate and glucuronide formations.

nent (Savides *et al.*, 1984). This is not routinely seen in dogs or humans, and yet it is a dramatic expression of toxicity in cats. Cats with acetaminophen toxicity die of the methaemoglobinaemia and do not die from liver damage as is seen in humans and dogs. Histopathological study of the livers of cats recovered from acetaminophen toxicity 7–10 d after poisoning showed that the degree of injury present in the liver was not significant (Savides *et al.*, 1984); yet this same chemical in at least two other species produces severe and frequently fatal liver destruction.

This uniqueness of the cat is also demonstrated when plasma half-lives were determined for acetaminophen after the oral administration of increasing dosages (Figure 7). At a dose of 20 mg acetaminophen/kg the half-life was about 0·5 h. Following a dose of 60 mg acetaminophen/kg, the half-life was 2·5 h, and at a dose of 120 mg acetaminophen/kg, the half-life was almost 5 h. As the dose was increased, the half-life increased accordingly, suggesting that saturation of one or more excretion pathways had occurred (Savides *et al.*, 1984).

Understanding the biochemistry of cats in detoxifying acetaminophen suggested some possibilities for therapy. Recognizing the decreased ability of

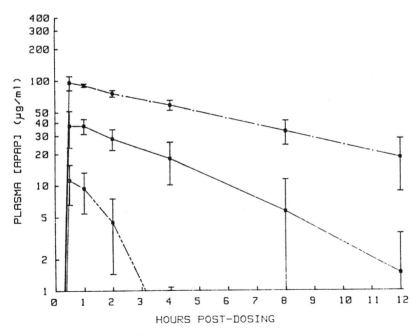

Figure 7. Plasma half-lives for cats receiving 20, 60 or 120 mg acetaminophen/kg of body weight. The half-life of acetaminophen (APAP) at 20 mg/kg (-------) was 0·63 h, at 60 mg/kg (————) was 2·38 h, and at 120 mg/kg (-·————·) was 4·86 h (Savides *et al.*, 1984).

Table 4. Acetaminophen (APAP) and metabolites excreted in the urine (percentage of total) after single oral APAP administrations and subsequent various antidotal treatments (Savides et al., 1985).

Treatment	Metabolites detected in urine (% of total excreted)					
	APAP-glucuronide	APAP-cysteine	APAP	APAP-sulphate	APAP-mercapturic acid	Unknown metabolite
None	16·1 ± 6·8[a]	9·6 ± 3·6[a]	15·3 ± 7·3[a]	57·0 ± 13·3[b]	2·3 ± 2·1[b]	2·8 ± 0·7[a]
N-Acetylcysteine (oral)	6·0 ± 1·5[b]	7·2 ± 2·3[a,b]	8·0 ± 2·0[b]	74·9 ± 3·3[a]	3·9 ± 1·7[a,b]	2·1 ± 1·0[a]
N-Acetylcysteine (i.v.)	6·4 ± 1·7[b]	7·8 ± 2·0[a,b]	8·5 ± 3·0[b]	72·4 ± 4·7[a]	5·0 ± 1·7[a]	2·5 ± 1·2[a]
Sodium sulphate (i.v.)	6·2 ± 2·1[b]	6·2 ± 1·4[b]	8·0 ± 2·3[b]	76·3 ± 3·7[a]	3·3 ± 1·0[a,b]	2·4 ± 0·9[a]

Values represent mean ± s.d. for six cats.
[a,b] Means for a given metabolite with the same letter are not significantly different from each other ($P > 0·05$).

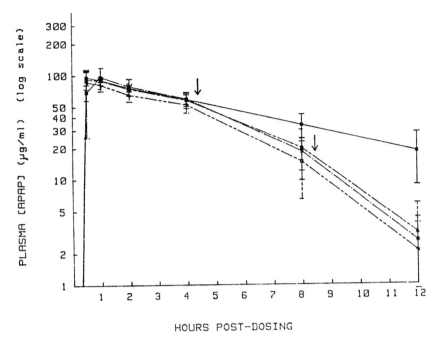

Figure 8. Effect of various antidotal treatments on acetaminophen (APAP) half-live in cats. Plasma acetaminophen concentrations in groups of six cats each given 120 mg acetaminophen/kg and treated at 4·5, 8·5 and 12·5 h after dosing (arrows) with one of the following therapies: no treatment (————); oral *N*-acetylcysteine (— — — — —); i.v. *N*-acetylcysteine (— — — — —); i.v. sodium sulphate (— · — — — · —) (Savides *et al.*, 1985)

the cat to conjugate acetaminophen with glucose because of its deficient glucuronidation pathways, the sulphate conjugate pathway becomes very vital in cats. Providing exogenous sources of sulphate would give benefit for increased excretion of acetaminophen as the sulphate metabolite before cellular damage occurred (Savides *et al.*, 1985). Figure 8 shows the results of treatment with three different sulphate donors. All three treatments effectively reduced the plasma acetaminophen concentrations and produced clinical recovery in the treated cats. Table 4 demonstrates the effect of the sulphate donors on urinary excretion of the acetaminophen and its metabolites (Savides *et al.*, 1985). The sulphate conjugate excretion was increased from 57% to approximately 75% in the treatment groups, and the unchanged acetaminophen available for urinary excretion was reduced to almost one-half the control value. This confirmed that the ability of the cat to conjugate with sulphate may be increased if exogenous sulphate is provided to increase excretion and recovery. By understanding the biochemistry of the poisoning, therapy can be designed that will modulate the clinical effects of toxicity and increase the pattern of patient recovery.

Propylene glycol

As a species, cats are uniquely sensitive to oxidizing agents. This sensitivity manifests itself as a Heinz body anaemia in cats exposed to such chemicals. While most animals rarely have observable Heinz bodies in their circulating red blood cells, cats usually have between 2 and 5% Heinz bodies in their red blood cells. If cats are receiving semi-moist foods that contain propylene glycol, it is suggested that the incidence of Heinz bodies in the red blood cells of those cats increases in some cases to as high 20–30% of the total red cells. Wright's stain for blood smears is commonly used for blood counts, and with this stain Heinz bodies do not stain well; hence they are difficult to observe with the routine use of Wright's stain. It has been suggested that the presence of Heinz bodies in the circulating blood of cats on propylene diets has gone undetected as most practitioners utilize Wright's stain for blood smear examination. If new methylene blue stain is used as the blood stain, the Heinz bodies are much more obvious. Are Heinz bodies more significant than has been reported? What is the biochemistry of Heinz body formation? Does propylene glycol induce increased Heinz body formation? Is this a significant health risk in our pets? The results of continuing research are needed to help answer these questions, but the unique biochemistry of cats is critical to understanding the basis for this concern.

Ethylene glycol

Antifreeze or ethylene glycol produces significant problems in dogs and cats, especially when automobile antifreeze is being changed, and a cat or dog may drink some of it. The toxic dose for dogs is approximately 4.5 ml of ethylene glycol per kilogram of body weight, but it requires only 1.5 ml/kg to cause toxicity in the cat (Oehme, 1983). Why is the cat only able to tolerate about one third the dose that the dog can take? Differences in species biochemistry seem to be the answer. The parent glycol is toxic in its own right and causes acute death within several hours. The glycol is also metabolized through a series of acids to oxalic acid, with the oxalic acid combining with calcium to form calcium oxalate crystals that precipitate in the kidney. Most dogs die from the resulting uraemia (Sanyer *et al.*, 1973). The acidosis from the conversion of glycol to oxalic acid is responsible for other deaths. Most cats die from the depressant effects of the slowly metabolized ethylene glycol or from the acidosis (Penumarthy & Oehme, 1975). The biochemical differences between dogs and cats are shown in this difference in toxicity to ethylene glycol.

Lead

Lead toxicity is very common in cattle, and when blood smears from cattle affected showing signs of lead toxicity are examined, the red blood cells appear normal. However, nucleated red blood cells and basophilic stippling are commonly seen in humans and dogs affected with lead poisoning (Green *et al.*, 1978). The anaemia accompanying the red blood cell changes is also observed in human beings and dogs, but is not seen commonly in cattle (Osweiler *et al.*, 1978; Scharding & Oehme, 1978). However, there is a similarity between human beings, dogs and cattle in the presence of a radiopaque lead line in the bones of growing individuals exposed to excess dietary lead. The increased density is in the growth plates of the long bones and appears very similar in growing children, puppies or calves exposed to lead. Children may have gum lead lines also, but these are rarely seen in cattle and less so in dogs (Green *et al.*,1978; Osweiler *et al.*, 1978). These differing responses may be difficult to explain currently, but a more thorough understanding of biochemical differences between species will help greatly to put these variations in proper perspective.

Carbamate insecticides

The carbamate insecticide, carbaryl, is a cholinesterase inhibitor and produces its lethal effect upon brain cholinesterase (Mount & Oehme, 1981). A good correlation exists between brain cholinesterase depression and the presence of carbaryl in brain; as the concentration of carbaryl increases in the brain, cholinesterase depression became more significant (Figure 9, Mount *et al.*, 1981). Organophosphate insecticides continue to be an experimental problem and a real-life problem. Why in some individuals does death occur without a significant reduction in cholinesterase activity, while in others a dramatic

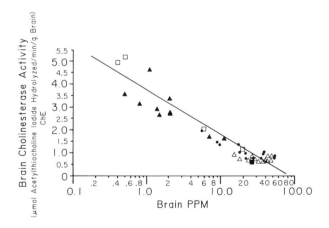

Figure 9. Relationship of brain carbaryl residues (expressed as logarithm) and brain cholinesterase activities in 10 rats receiving 800 mg carbaryl/kg and killed at 28 h (▲) 29 rats receiving 800 mg carbaryl/kg (●) or 1200 mg carbaryl/kg (△) and dying at various times, and moribund rats receiving 800 mg (□) carbaryl/kg or 1200 mg carbaryl/kg (■) (Mount *et al.*, 1981).

reduction in cholesterase activity causes no effect? Why does a patient develop toxicity three to four days after exposure, with small or minimal response to the specific antidotal therapy? There is much remaining to be understood in order to assist in selecting appropriate animal models and to utilize them knowledgeably.

Organophosphates and delayed neurotoxicity

Delayed neurotoxicity induced by organophosphates occurs in man and all domestic animals (Barrett & Oehme, 1985). Its occurrence has been related to neurotoxic esterase inhibition in the central nervous system. The chicken is the animal model for man because of its responsiveness to organophosphate-induced delayed neurotoxicity. Why do we not use other models, or better, why do other species not respond to the delayed neurotoxicity effects of organophosphates? There may be value in looking at the pig as another model for this delayed neurotoxic reaction. The pig responds with typical spinal cord demyelinization 17 d after exposure to tri-*ortho*-tolyl phosphate (TOPC), a known delayed-neurotoxicity inducer in humans and in hens (D. S. Barrett, unpublished data). The pig eats, it feels well, but it has complete paralysis of the hind parts from this dermal exposure. Lymphocyte neurotoxic esterase is altered in activity the first 24 h after TOCP exposure, from which could follow the prediction that a neurotoxic spinal cord effect will occur some 17 d later. The pig seems to be a fruitful animal for organophosphate-induced neurotoxicity studies, and as more is learned of the physiological and biochemical factors that are unique to this species, its usefulness as a model for other species and man increases.

Conclusion

Biological and biochemical factors modify toxicity and must be considered in the selection of species to be used for toxicity studies. Biochemical factors are probably the most critical in determining which species are more or less sensitive to chemicals. Metabolism, kinetics, the presence of chemicals in tissues, and biotransformation must be studied increasingly for a better understanding of species differences. The variables that affect the target cell, the presence of target organelles within the cell, the ratio of strong versus weak binding sites within cells, the location of receptor sites, the presence of other chemicals as promoters, and the structure and properties of target enzymes are necessary details. This knowledge is needed and will assist in evaluating why one species is more or less sensitive to a specific chemical group. From this all, more appropriate selection and use of various research animal species will be possible.

References

Barrett, D. S. and Oehme, F. W., 1985, A review of organophosphorous ester-induced delayed neurotoxicity. *Vet. Human. Tox.*, **27**, 22–37.

Calabrese, E. J., 1985, *Toxic Susceptibility, Male/Female Differences* (New York: John Wiley).

Clarke, E. G. C., 1976, Species differences in toxicology. *Vet. Rec.*, **98**, 215–218.

Davis, L. E., 1979, Species differences as a consideration in drug therapy. *J. Am. vet. med. Assoc.*, **175**, 1014–1015.

Green, V. A., Wise, G. W. and Callenbach, J. C., 1978, Lead poisoning. In *Toxicity of Heavy Metals in the Environment, Part 1.*, edited by F. W. Oehme (New York: Marcel Dekker), pp. 123–142.

Mount, M. E. and Oehme, F. W., 1981, Brain cholinesterase activity in healthy cattle, swine and sheep and in cattle and sheep exposed to cholinesterase-inhibiting insecticides. *Am. J. vet. Res.*, **42**, 1345–1350.

Mount, M. E., Dayton, A. D. and Oehme, F. W., 1981, Carbaryl residues in tissues and cholinesterase activities in brain and blood of rats receiving carbaryl. *Toxic. appl. Pharmac.*, **58**, 282–296.

Oehme, F. W., 1970, Species differences: the basis for and importance of comparative toxicology. *Clin. Tox.*, **3**, 5–10.

Oehme, F. W., 1971, New information on the toxicity of phenolic compounds in small animals. In *Gaines Newer Knowledge about Dogs, 21st Veterinary Symposium, October 20, 1971* (White Plains, NY: Gaines Dog Research Center), pp. 8–15.

Oehme, F. W., 1975, This is veterinary toxicology. In *Toxicology Annual, 1974*, edited by C. L. Winek and S. P. Shanor (New York: Marcel Dekker), pp. 11–26.

Oehme, F. W., 1983, Ethylene glycol (antifreeze) poisoning. In *Current Veterinary Therapy VIII, Small Animal Practice*, edited by R. W. Kirk (Philadelphia: Saunders), pp. 114–116.

Osweiler, G. D., Van Gelder, G. A. and Buck, W. B., 1978., Epidemiology of lead poisoning in animals. In *Toxicity of Heavy Metals in the Environment, Part 1*, edited by F. W. Oehme (New York: Marcel Dekker), pp. 143–172.

Penumarthy, L. and Oehme, F. W., 1975, Treatment of ethylene glycol toxicosis in cats. *Am. J. vet. Res.*, **36**, 209–212.

Sanyer, J. L., Oehme, F. W. and McGavin, M. D., 1973, Systematic treatment of ethylene glycol toxicosis in dogs. *Am. J. vet. Res.*, **34**, 527–534.

Savides, M. C. and Oehme, F. W., 1983, Acetaminophen and its toxicity. *J. appl. Tox.*, **3**, 96–111.

Savides, M. C., Oehme, F. W., Nash, S. L. and Leipold, H. W., 1984, The toxicity and biotransformation of single doses of acetaminophen in dogs and cats. *Toxic. appl. Pharmac.*, **74**, 26–34.

Savides, M. C., Oehme, F. W. and leipold, H. W., 1985, Effects of various antidotal treatments on acetaminophen toxicosis and biotransformation in cats. *Am. J. vet. Res.*, **46**, 1485–1489.

Scharding, N. N. and Oehme, F. W., 1978, The use of animal models for comparative studies of lead poisoning. In *Toxicity of Heavy Metals in the Environment, Part 1*, edited by F. W. Oehme (New York: Marcel Dekker), pp. 191–198.

The role of diet and nutrition in safety evaluation of drugs and other chemicals

Paul M. Newberne and Michael W. Conner†

Department of Applied Biological Sciences, Massachusetts Institute of Technology, Cambridge, MA 02139 USA

Introduction

The role of diet and nutrition in safety evaluations of drugs and chemicals has been accorded scant attention over the past two to three decades, during the time when bioassays have grown in numbers on little less than a logarithmic scale. The concept that laboratory animals are biological systems with all the complexities typical of mammalian organisms has somehow been lost in the shuffle. The headlong plunge towards developing bigger and more complex methods to extract statistically significant results from biologically insignificant data has obscured our views and muddled the interpretation of time-consuming expensive experiments. Some of this has been a result of sick, malnourished and obese test animals. The purpose of animal bioassays has seemingly been often ignored, and the results perceived as ends unto themselves, rather than to be extrapolated for use in preventing human disease.

The results of any animal bioassay are only as good as the animals used in the study and they, in turn, are dependent to a significant degree on the diets they are fed. The fact that we have been able to gather reliable information from improperly fed experimental animals is a tribute to the great resilience of the rat and mouse maintained under less than optimum conditions.

The following text and tables will delineate some of the important aspects of diets, their individual nutrients and contaminants, and how these can influence the results of bioassays.

Types of diets available

Table 1 lists the two categories of diets commonly used in animal experimentation and some of their advantages and disadvantages. Clearly,

---

†Present address: Mallory Institute of Pathology, Department of Pathology, Boston University School of Medicine, 784 Massachusetts Avenue, Boston, MA 02118

Table 1. Diets for experimental animal studies.

---

1. *Natural unrefined ingredient diets*
   Advantages:
     readily available
     relatively inexpensive
     consumed by all species
   Disadvantages
     quality control less than optimum
     cannot be used in some studies (i.e., effect of nutrients)
     excess of some nutrients (protein)
     may contain contaminants
2. *Semi-purified, defined diets*
   Advantages
     excellent quality control
     little chance of contaminants
     useful for studies of nutrient effects
   Disadvantages
     relatively expensive
     requires equipment/expertise to make them
     shelf-life may be short

---

both types of diets have their place in bioassay programmes, but the needs of a particular study dictate the type most appropriate. With the availability of diets such as those developed at the National Institutes of Health (i.e., NIH-007), the unrefined diets are much more satisfactory compared to the older 'chow-type' diets with closed formulas. These types of 'open-formula' diets, that is, formulae which tell you the ingredients and their amounts, are to be preferred to the 'closed-formula' types which list ingredients but without any indication as to the amounts present in the finished product. However, the natural ingredients in these crude diets can affect the results of bioassays. They usually contain an excess of protein and some of the other nutrients which can contribute to such unwanted anomalies as renal disease or obesity. They may also contain contaminants which can also result in aberrant results. Table 2 lists a few of the contaminants found in natural product crude diets (Conybeare, 1980; Newberne & Fox, 1980; Newberne & McConnell, 1980). The heavy metals are usually present, particularly lead and cadmium.

Nitrates are present in many plant products at relatively high levels but are not known to create problems for animal diets. Since nitrates are converted to nitrites in mammalian systems (Tannenbaum *et al.*, 1976; Lintas *et al.*, 1982; Newberne, 1982), studies related to nitrosamines, for example, might be affected if high levels of nitrates were present in the test animal diet. Obviously, preformed nitrosamines, often found in diets which contain fish meal, are to be avoided. Man-made antioxidants sometimes find their way into laboratory animal chow-type diets but levels observed so far are not considered significant.

Aflatoxin B_1 (AFB_1) is a potent hepatocarcinogen and its content in human staple foods and in animal products is closely monitored by regulatory agen-

Table 2. Some contaminants found in crude natural product diets.†

Contaminant‡	Level of contaminator in diet	
	Range	Mean ± s.d.
Mercury (p.p.m.)	0·1–1·2	0·2 ± 0·1
Cadmium (p.p.m.)	0·1–1·8	0·4 ± 0·2
Lead (p.p.m.)	0·8–4·8	1·2 ± 0·4
Arsenic (p.p.m)	0–1·3	0·1 ± 0·05
PCBs (p.p.m.)	0·5–30	1·8 ± 0·3
Nitrates (p.p.m.)	3–184	19 ± 2·4
BHA/BHT (p.p.m.)	0–4	0·04 ± 0·1
Nitrosamines (p.p.b.)		
N-Dimethylnitrosamine	1–42	± 9·1
N-Nitrosopyrrolidine	0–24	± 2·3
Aflatoxin B_1 (p.p.b.)	0–48	± 3·4

†From random sampling of at least three different samples from the same manufacturer.
‡Data from Newberne (1975) and P. M. Newberne (unpublished results).

cies. Since AFB_1 is permitted in human foods at only very low levels, staples such as corn and peanut meal, contaminated with AFB_1, may not be discarded but instead may be diverted from human foods to animal diets for economic reasons. This requires monitoring by manufacturers and by users of natural product diets on a continuing basis if they are to assure freedom from such unwanted toxic materials.

While some investigators complain about semi-purified diets because, they say, such diets do not support adequate growth, reproduction and maintenance, the evidence is in the other direction. In chronic studies with both rats and mice, extending through five generations, there were no differences in either sex with respect to growth and reproduction, between those eating semi-purified diets and those on diets composed of crude unrefined ingredients (Newberne *et al.*, 1972, 1973a,b).

A note of caution is in order for the American Institute of Nutrition (AIN) diet (ILAR News, 1978), offered by some diet manufacturers. This diet was developed primarily for short-term studies and has not been satisfactory in chronic (up to two years) studies. While improvements have been made, experience indicates that it still falls short of adequate nutrient support for chronic safety evaluations.

Influence of calories and their sources

Irrespective of the type of diet used in chronic safety evaluation, most rodents are overfed, and tend to become obese with the unwanted consequences (See

Table 3. Liver tumour incidence in rats on various diets, with and without AFB_1.

| Treatment | Liver tumour incidence (no./%) | | | | | |
| | 12 months | | 24 months | | Total | |
	Male	Female	Male	Female	Male	Female
Control, *ad libitum*	0/80	0/77	0/48	0/54	0/80	0/77
Control, *ad libitum* + AFB_1	3/79	1/78	41/53*	28/60	44/79*	29/78*
			(77·3)	(46·6)	(55·7)	(37·2)
75% Restricted	0/80	0/80	0/64	0/72	0/80	0/80
75% Restricted + AFB_1	0/80	0/79	19/60*	12/67*	30/80*	20/79*
			(31·7)	(17·9)	(37·5)	(25·3)

*Statistically significant ($P < 0·01$).

Part 1, pp. 38–42). Our laboratory has demonstrated the effect of nutrition and overweight on tumour induction by chemicals and on the incidence of 'spontaneous' tumours, particularly those associated with the endocrine system (pituitary, thyroid, adrenal, gonads). In a recent study, we have shown that simply restricting the amount of food fed to some groups of rats, to 75% of that consumed by *ad libitum* groups, reduced the incidence of aflatoxin-induced liver tumours to less than one half in both sexes (Table 3). Furthermore, and equally significant, other types of tumours were sharply reduced in incidence (Table 4). In addition, longevity was improved and renal disease diminished (Table 5).

Therefore we have the means at hand to improve the performance of rodents used for chronic studies by preventing obesity. This can be accomplished in at least three ways:

1. Pair feeding to a group fed *ad libitum* where the food consumption is measured and the test animals fed a percentage of this (we suggest 75%).
2. By permitting access to feed about six hours per day.
3. By feeding the test group to a predetermined maximum body weight in each sex.

In addition to an overall reduction in food intake and in total body weight with its accompanying benefits, the source of calories is also important. Table 6 lists the incidence of liver tumours in rats exposed to aflatoxin B_1 after 24 months' study with protein levels varying from 6% to 20%. One group was allowed to eat a 20% protein diet *ad libitum* and other groups were pair-fed to the 6% group in order to avoid effects of varying total food intake. The exact mechanism for this effect is not clear but at least a part of it is associated with modified metabolism of the carcinogen. Table 7 shows the effects of dietary protein concentration on microsomal characteristics and on formation of aflatoxin covalent adducts, which are believed to be the means by which liver tumours are induced by aflatoxin.

Table 4. Incidence of proliferative lesions other than hepatocellular in rats on various diets with and without AFB_1.

Proliferation site/type of lesion	Control *ad libitum*		*Ad Libitum* + AFB_1		75% of *ad libitum*		75% of *ad libitum* + AFB_1	
	Male[1]	Female[2]	Male[3]	Female[4]	Male[5]	Female[6]	Male[7]	Female[8]
Pituitary								
Hyperplasia	8	15	10	19	7	3	6	2
Adenoma	19*	37*	15	32	3*	8*	2*	3*
Thyroid								
Follicular								
Hyperplasia	2	3	1	2	2	1	0	1
Adenoma	3	2	3	2	0	1	0	0
Interstitial								
Hyperplasia	2	1	1	0	0	2	0	1
Adenoma	1	2	0	1	0	1	0	0
Adrenal								
Cortical								
Hyperplasia	2	1	2	2	1	2	2	0
Adenoma	0	2	2	1	0	1	0	0
Medullary								
Hyperplasia	2	2	1	2	2	1	1	2
Adenoma	1	0	1	1	0	1	0	0
Mammary								
Adenoma	2	11	1	10	1	2	0	1
Carcinoma	1	8	0	12	0*	1*	0*	2*

* Statistically significant ($P < 0.01$).
[1]$n = 80$, [2]$n = 77$, [3]$n = 79$, [4]$n = 78$, [5]$n = 80$, [6]$n = 80$, [7]$n = 80$, [8]$n = 79$.

Table 5. Renal lesions in rats, on various diets, with and without AFB_1.

Treatment	Incidence of lesion (no.)					
	Pelvic nephrocalcinosis		Tubule cell			
			Hyperplasia		Adenoma	
	Male	Female	Male	Female	Male	Female
Control, *ad libitum*	45/80*	18/77*	4/80	7/77	1/80	2/77
Control, *ad libitum* + AFB_1	39/79**	9/78	3/79	6/78	1/79	2/78
75% Restricted	7/80*	9/80*	0/80	1/80	0/80	0/80
75% Restricted + AFB_1	8/80**	10/79	2/80	1/79	0/80	1/79

*Statistically significant ($P < 0.01$).
**Statistically significant ($P < 0.01$).

Table 6. Influence of dietary protein concentration on response to AFB_1 in rats†.

Group no.	Dietary treatment (%) protein	Tumour incidence at 24 months	
		No.	%
1	20	21/26	80·7
2	20‡	17/28	60·7
3	15‡	10/29	34·4
4	10‡	4/30	13·3
5	6	2/27	7·4

† All animals exposed to aflatoxin B, received intragastrically 25 μg per day for 15 daily doses.
‡ Pair-fed to the 6% protein group.

In a series of trials using an indirect carcinogen (dimethylhydrazine, DMH) and a direct-acting carcinogen (*N*-methylnitrosourea, NMU) we have failed to observe an effect of dietary fat on tumour incidence or frequency (Nauss *et al.*, 1983; Locniskar *et al.*, 1985 a, b). In view of these negative results we developed an hypothesis that an enhancing effect of dietary fat might be restricted to special aspects of experimental conditions including the strain of rat. This was explored by using two different strains of rats, the Fischer-344

Table 7. Influence of dietary protein on liver microsomal characteristics and AFB_1-adduct formation in rats.

	Dietary protein		
	6%	20% pair-fed	20% *ad libitum*
Microsomal protein (mg/g liver)	6·8 (±0·49)	10·9 (±0·3)	12·2 (±0·10)
Cytochrome P-450 (nmol/mg protein)	0·11 (±0·02)	0·43 (±0·08)	0·40 (±0·03)
P-450 reductase, (nmol P-450 reduced mg protein^{-1} h^{-1})	6·7 (±0·09)	16·8 (±0·09)	17·1 (±1·1)
Covalent AFB_1 adducts (ng/mg/DNA)	6·7 (±0·09)	16·8 (±0·09)	17·1 (±1·1)

Six to ten rats per group, assayed in duplicate; for AFB_1 adduct studies, ^{3}H-AFB_1 and cold AFB_1 to specific activity 7 Ci/mol at dose of 1 mg/kg, killed six hours later for assay.
Results are expressed as mean ±s.d.

Table 8. Effect of caloric intake on colon tumour incidence and frequency†
in rats.

	Food intake interval		
	Lower third	Middle third	Upper third
Sprague–Dawley			
Tumour incidence (%)	23	30	58
Total no. of colon tumours	12	15	33
Mean caloric intake (kcal/d)	45 ± 3	53 ± 2	64 ± 5
Mean body wt. (g)	401 ± 40	420 ± 30	461 ± 63
Fischer-344			
Tumour incidence (%)	33	20	38
Total no. of colon tumours	17	12	17
Mean caloric intake (kcal/d)	30 ± 3	36 ± 1	42 ± 3
Mean body wt. (g)	253 ± 30	252 ± 34	283 ± 42

† Induced by DMH and measured after three months on the experimental
diets. Animals were divided into three intervals according to food consumption ($n = 40$ rats/interval).
Results are expressed as mean ± s.d.

(F-344) and the Sprague–Dawley (SD). We have demonstrated that rats of the
Sprague–Dawley strain that consumed more calories had more colon tumours,
induced by DMH; Table 8 illustrates typical results. Although this important
effect was observed in the Sprague–Dawley strain, the Fischer strain of rat did
not exhibit such an effect from increased calorie intake. Diets of different
nutrient composition were also used but the differences in fat were 5% or 20%
beef fat with or without added corn oil or 5% or 20% corn oil. Variations in
micronutrients did not appear to influence any parameters measured so the
results of these are not given here.

The salient features of this study shown in Table 8 clearly indicate that a
complex interaction exists between animal strain, nutrient availability and the
toxic response to a carcinogen. Even though the dose of DMH was adjusted
on a body-weight basis, SD rats tolerated the treatment better than F-344
animals. There was a significant effect of both dietary composition and fat
content on body weight gain (Table 9). Rats fed the beef-fat diet at either the
5% or 20% fat level grew faster than those fed corn oil diets. When the growth
rate of SD rats in the experiment was compared with an earlier study (Nauss
et al., 1983), where a lower dose of DMH was administered for five weeks,
it was obvious that prolonged carcinogen treatment had a deleterious effect on
weight gain. F-344 rats were more sensitive than the SD strain to the toxic
effects of DMH. Although initial growth rates were identical in animals fed
the two diets, after seven doses of carcinogen, rats fed the beef fat diet ceased
gaining weight.

The effect of dietary fat on colon tumour development was analysed
separately for each strain. In the F-344 animals, there were no significant

Table 9. Effect of strain and body weight differences on DMH†
colon tumour induction in rats on diets of different levels of fat.

| Dietary fat (%) | Mean final wt. | Tumour incidence | |
		No.	%
*Sprague–Dawley**			
Beef fat			
5%	495 ± 38	8/30	27
20%	580 ± 27	17/30	57
Corn oil			
5%	412 ± 30	9/30	30
20%	467 ± 35	10/30	33
*Fischer-344***			
Beef fat			
5%	342 ± 20	8/30	27
20%	373 ± 23	11/30	37
Corn oil			
5%	221 ± 12	8/30	27
20%	236 ± 14	10/30	33

† Subcutaneous DMH, 200 mg/kg, then 10 mg/wk for 20 doses;
10 more weeks then rats killed.
*$P = 0·07$; **$P = 0·06$.

differences in intestinal tumourigenesis between animals fed beef fat or corn
oil at either the 5% or 20% fat level (Table 9). In the Sprague–Dawley group
the percentage of animals bearing colon tumours was 57% in rats fed beef fat
at 20% compared to 27–33% in the other three groups ($P = 0·07$ when the
four groups were compared by a χ^2 test). When the 5% beef fat diet group
in F-344 animals was compared to the 20% beef fat group, the increase was
marginally significant ($P = 0·02$). High levels of dietary fat had no effect on
tumour frequency, tumour size, degree of differentiation, invasion, or the
number of metastatic lesions in the Sprague–Dawley strain (data not shown
in table).

Rodents are considered by some investigators to adjust to a diet of increased
caloric density by reducing their food intake so that the number of calories
consumed remains constant. This has not been the case in many of our studies
nor was it in this study. Sprague–Dawley strain rats fed the 20% fat diets
consumed more energy per day than animals fed the 5% fat diets, regardless
of whether intake was expressed as kcal/d or kcal day^{-1} 100 g body weight^{-1}
($P < 0·01$). Fischer strain rats fed 20% beef fat consumed more total calories
per day than those fed 5% beef fat but there were no differences when intakes
were expressed as a function of total body weight.

The important observation in this study was the wide variation within a
group in individual caloric intake. If animals within each strain were divided
into three equal groups according to caloric intake, SD animals in the upper
third had a two-fold increase in tumour incidence and frequency compared to

those in the lower third (Table 8). In this study, where caloric intake was examined, those rats of the SD strain, consuming more calories per day were at greater risk for colon tumours than those consuming calories at the lower third of food consumption. No such association between caloric intake and intestinal tumourigenesis was seen in Fischer animals.

These results indicate that diet composition has a major influence on the response of experimental animals to colon carcinogens and point to a significant effect of weight gain, particularly in the early three or four months of the rat's life, and final body weight. Furthermore, rat strain and the method used to evaluate the data are important in the interpretation of results.

Influence of retinoids on response to toxins and carcinogens

We have pointed out that both beta carotene (precursor for vitamin A) and preformed vitamin A are variable in concentration in crude-product commercial diets (Newberne & McConnell, 1980). Moreover, vitamin A or beta carotene can have profound effects on the response of experimental animals to toxins and carcinogens (Newberne & Schrager, 1983). Tables 10 and 11 illustrate the effects of vitamin A and the synthetic retinoid 13-*cis*-retinoic acid on the induction of lung cancer by benz[a]pyrene, and the acute response of rats of two age-groups to the toxic effects of aflatoxin B_1. In Table 10, the data clearly illustrate the protective effect of normal levels of vitamin A, but not elevated concentration, on lung cancer induction. Moreover, there was a remarkable response when the hamsters were given the synthetic retinoid as well as a normal dietary level of vitamin A (retinyl acetate).

Table 10. Effects of vitamin A and 13-*cis*-retinoic acid on lung cancer induction in the Syrian golden hamster.

Treatment (diet)	Malignant tumours of respiratory tract	
	No.	%
Control (2 μg/g retinyl acetate, BP)	46/89	51·7
Low vitamin A (0·3 μg/g retinyl acetate, BP)	102/127	80·3
High vitamin A (30 μg/g retinyl acetate, BP)	40/88	45·4
Control (2 μg/g retinyl acetate + 13-*cis*-retinoic acid during dosing BP)	38/83	45·8
Control (2 μg/g retinyl acetate + 13-*cis*-retinoic acid during and after dosing BP)	4/91	4·4
Control (2 μg/g retinyl acetate + 13-*cis*-retinoic acid after dosing BP)	11/84	13·1

From Newberne & McConnell (1980); abridged with permission.
Retinyl acetate = vitamin A.
BP = benzo[a]pyrene.

Table 11. Vitamin A deficiency and response to AFB_1 in two different age-groups of male rats.

Treatment or parameter	12 weeks old†	52 weeks old†
Liver vitamin A ($\mu g/g$)		
Control	$54 \cdot 8 \pm 4 \cdot 8$	$47 \cdot 2 \pm 7 \cdot 3$
A-Deficient	$6 \cdot 9 \pm 0 \cdot 9$	$2 \cdot 8 \pm 0 \cdot 2$
LD_{50}, AFB_1(mg/kg)^2		
Control	$7 \cdot 1(4 \cdot 8 - 9 \cdot 2)$	$15 \cdot 3(10 \cdot 1 - 19 \cdot 8)$
A-Deficient	$3 \cdot 8(3 \cdot 0 - 6 \cdot 1)$	$9 \cdot 2(6 \cdot 9 - 13 \cdot 1)$
GSH ($\mu g/g$ liver)		
Control	1541 ± 121	962 ± 83
A-Deficient	730 ± 60	448 ± 36
Microsomal protein ($\mu g/g$ liver)		
Control	$15 \cdot 9 \pm 0 \cdot 91$	$13 \cdot 6 \pm 0 \cdot 82$
A-Deficient	$14 \cdot 8 \pm 1 \cdot 13$	$11 \cdot 2 \pm 0 \cdot 94$
AFB_1–GSH conjugate§ (nmol/g liver/h)		
Control	$0 \cdot 08(0 \cdot 06 - 0 \cdot 09)$	$0 \cdot 12(0 \cdot 05 - 0 \cdot 10)$
A-Deficient	$0 \cdot 25(0 \cdot 06 - 0 \cdot 10)$	$0 \cdot 22(0 \cdot 06 - 0 \cdot 09)$

† Eight to twelve rats per group, on diet 7–8 weeks or 52 weeks before evaluation.
‡ LD_{50} with 95% confidence interval.
§ ^{3}H-AFB_1 (150 μCi; specific activity of 40 Ci/mmol, 24 h before killing.

Table 11 illustrates further the protective effect of vitamin A on AFB_1 toxicity and the enhanced conjugation of AFB_1 by glutathione (GSH), a major pathway for detoxification of this dietary contaminant.

Lipotropes and carcinogenesis

In a series of studies, we have established that lipotropic factors (methionine, choline, folate, B_{12}) have a profound effect on sensitivity to a number of chemical carcinogens (Rogers & Newberne, 1980), and that a deficiency of lipotropes alone results in a significant incidence of hepatocellular carcinoma (HCC) in mice and rats, without superimposing carcinogens (Newberne *et al.*, 1982, 1983). These observations, reported from other laboratories (Ghoshal & Farber, 1983; Mikol *et al.*, 1983) as well as ours, have generated considerable interest in the scientific community concerned with cancer research. Taking something out of the diet, rather than putting something into it, to induce cancer is a new concept. The following data illustrate some new and fascinating aspects of hepatocarcinogenesis.

Rodents can be depleted of lipotropes and become profoundly susceptible to carcinogens. Table 12 illustrates the remarkably enhanced sensitivity to chemical carcinogens of a broad variety of structure and reactivity.

Table 12. Chemical carcinogenesis in lipotrope deficiency.

Carcinogen	Tumour site	Tumour incidence (%)	
		Control	Deprived
AFB$_1$	Liver	15	87
DEN	Liver	70	80
DMN	Liver	28	27
DMN	Kidney	16	3
AAF	Liver	19	41
AAF	Mammary	80	79

From Rogers & Newberne (1980).
DEN, *N*-nitrosodiethylamine; DMN,
nitrosodimethylamine; AAF,
N-2-fluorenylacetamine.

In the lipotrope-deficient rat as liver fat increases the number of cells labelled by [^{3}H] thymidine also increases (Newberne *et al.*, 1982). In addition, we found that lipotrope deficiency alone causes a sharp increase in cell death, as others have reported (Ghoshal *et al.*, 1983). There is increased DNA synthesis and increased cell turnover, both of which are essential components of hyperplasia of the liver parenchyma.

The dietary effect is similar to that produced by a partial hepatectomy; however a key difference is that cell death and compensatory hyperplasia of the parenchyma continue as long as the choline-deficient diet is fed. Partial hepatectomy causes only a temporary wave of hyperplasia and this returns to normal when the pre-hepatectomy liver volume is approximated. Lipoperoxidation has been considered by some to be related to the initiation of transformation of hepatocytes and promotion of hepatocarcinogenesis (Ghoshal *et al.*, 1984). It is interesting that our laboratory published such a relationship more than 15 years ago (Newberne *et al.*, 1969) and confirmed the observations with more sophisticated techniques a few years later (Wilson *et al.*, 1973). The synthetic antioxidants BHA and BHT protected the kidney and liver from choline deficiency and returned serum and tissue lipids to near control values. Furthermore, our later observations confirmed the probable relationship between lipid peroxidation and choline-deficiency injury. Table 13 indicates TBA values and the free radical index (FRI) of the lipotrope-deficient liver.

Poirier's laboratory (Table 14) and our own investigations (Table 15) point towards hypomethylation as an important event in choline-deficiency carcinogenesis. Wilson *et al.* (1984) observed a 10–15% decrease in the 5-methyldeoxycytidine in the deficient liver, but only after about six months on diet. Our studies (P. Punyarit & P. M. Newberne, unpublished data) essentially confirm the data of Wilson *et al.* (1984) (Table 15), although our methods were slightly different. We maintained rats on diet for up to six months, performed a partial hepatectomy to enhance the synthesis of new DNA (and

Table 13. Lipotrope deficiency and liver lipids

Parameter	Treatment		
	Chow diet	Choline-deficient diet	Choline-supplemented diet
Hepatic lipid (% dry wt.)	$22 \cdot 2 \pm 0 \cdot 5$	$44 \cdot 6 \pm 2 \cdot 1$	$24 \cdot 0 \pm 1 \cdot 8$
Free radical index	464 ± 71	553 ± 85	303 ± 22
Liver TBA	$129 \pm 4 \cdot 2$	$21 \pm 9 \cdot 6$	$6 \cdot 2 \pm 2 \cdot 3$

Abridged from Wilson *et al.* (1973).
Values shown are mean ± s.e. of nine liver samples.

Table 14. Lipotrope deficiency and 5-methyldeoxycytidine content or hepatic DNA.

Treatment	% Deoxycytidine residues as 5-Me deoxycytidine	
	8 Weeks	22 Weeks
Control	$3 \cdot 33 \pm 0 \cdot 03$	$3 \cdot 27 \pm 0 \cdot 04$
Deficient	$3 \cdot 13 \pm 0 \cdot 05$	$2 \cdot 81 \pm 0 \cdot 04$

Abridged from Wilson *et al.* (1984).

Table 15. Lipotropes and 5'-methylcytosine in liver DNA.

Time on diet	5-Methylcytosine as % of cytosine	
	Control	Deficient
3 Weeks	$4 \cdot 8 \pm 0 \cdot 09$	$4 \cdot 5 \pm 0 \cdot 11$
3 Months	$4 \cdot 4 \pm 0 \cdot 13$	$4 \cdot 7 \pm 0 \cdot 20$
6 Months	$4 \cdot 5 \pm 0 \cdot 10$	$3 \cdot 3 \pm 0 \cdot 06$

From P. Punyarit & P. M. Newberne (unpublished results).
Two weeks before sacrifice a two thirds partial hepatectomy was performed.

accompanying methylation) and two weeks later killed the animals for DNA analyses. In agreement with Wilson *et al.* (1984), it was only after six months of continuous exposure to the lipotrope-deficient diet that we found a modest hypomethylation of cytosine. This indicates that it is a slow process and, if, involved with carcinogenesis, hypomethylation very likely requires chronic derangement of liver genetic material over long periods of time.

Gene activity frequently correlates with hypomethylation (Doerfler, 1983).

In addition to the data reported above it should be noted that Wainfan *et al.* (1986) have found that liver tRNA, isolated from rats fed a lipotrope-deficient diet, is hypomethylated and that there is an increase in the activity of N^2-guanine tRNA methyltransferase (NMG2), mimicking the effects of the liver carcinogen ethionine. Thus, not only is DNA hypomethylated but tRNA critical to normal cell proliferation is also hypomethylated in the choline-deficient liver.

Conclusions

There are several points which should be made with respect to the influence of diet and nutrition on the results of safety evaluations conducted using rodents. These are:

1. Commercial natural-product diets (chow-type) vary considerably in their nutrient content.
2. Chow-type diets may contain a variety of contaminants that can have a profound effect on the results of studies in animals fed such diets.
3. Calories do count in rodents, as in humans. Rodents, particularly rats, held on chronic studies (two years or for a lifetime) often become obese. This appears to affect the incidence of 'spontaneous' tumours, especially those associated with the endocrine system (pituitary, thyroid, adrenal, mammary gland), and also induced tumours. Renal lesions (nephrocalcinosis, etc.) also are increased in overweight rats.
4. Excessive protein can have an influence on a number of tumour types, apparently acting via the effect of protein on the enzyme systems responsible for the activation or deactivation of chemicals.
5. Many of the nutrients which vary in rodent diets can have profound effects on the response of rodents to toxins and carcinogens.

The problems associated with the care and feeding of experimental animals used for safety evaluations of drugs and other chemicals cannot be ignored. It behoves the investigators charged with proper testing and interpretation of results to accord these factors more attention than has been the case in the past.

Acknowledgements

We are indebted to Dr. Ronald Shank, University of California, Irvine for some of the DNA analyses listed in Table 15.

References

Conybeare, G., 1980, Effect of quality and quantity of diet on survival and tumour incidence in outbred Swiss mice. *Fd. Cosmet. Tox.*, **18**, 65–75.

Doerfler, W., 1983, DNA methylation and gene activity. *Ann. Rev. Biochem.*, **52**, 93–124.

Ghoshal, A. K. and Farber, E., 1983, Induction of liver cancer by a diet deficient in choline and methionine. *Proc. Am. Assoc. Cancer Res.*, **24**, 98.

Ghoshal A. K., Ahlrualia, M. and Farber, E., 1983, The rapid induction of liver cell death in rats fed a choline-deficient, methionine-low diet. *Am. J. Path.*, **113**, 309–314.

Ghoshal, A. K., Rushmore, T., Lim, Y. and Farber, E., 1984, Early detection of lipid peroxidation in the hepatic nuclei of rats fed a diet deficient in choline and methionine. *Cancer Res.*, **25**, 94–98.

ILAR News, 1978, *Control of Diets in Laboratory Animal Experimentation* (Washington, DC: National Academy of Sciences).

Lintas, C., Clark, A., Tannenbaum, S. R. and Newberne, P. M., 1982, *In vivo* stability of nitrite and nitrosamine formation in the dog stomach: effect of nitrite and amine concentration and of ascorbic acid. *Carcinogenesis*, **3**, 161–165.

Locniskar, M., Nauss, K. M., Kauffmann, P. and Newberne, P. M., 1985 a, Comparison of immune status and 1,2-dimethylhydrazine-induced tumorigenesis in Brown Norway and Fischer rats. *Cancer Lett.*, **25**, 311–323.

Locniskar, M., Nauss, K. M., Kauffmann, P. and Newberne, P. M., 1985 b, Interaction of dietary fat and route of carcinogen administration on 1,2-dimethylhydrazine-induced colon tumorigenesis in rats. *Carcinogenesis*, **6**, 349–354.

Mikol, Y. B., Hoover, K. L., Creasia, D. and Poirier, L. A., 1983, Hepatocarcinogenesis in rats fed methyl-deficient amino-acid defined diets. *Carcinogenesis*, **4**, 1619–1629.

Nauss, K. M., Locniskar, M. and Newberne, P. M., 1983, Effect of alterations in the quality and quantity of dietary fat on 1,2-dimethylhydrazine-induced colon tumorigenesis in rats. *Cancer Res.*, **43**, 4083–4090.

Newberne, P. M., 1975, Influence on pharmacological experiments of chemicals and other factors in diets of laboratory animals. *Fedn Proc. Fedn Am. Socs. exp. Biol.*, **34**, 209–218.

Newberne, P. M., 1982, Nitrates and nitrites in foods and in biological systems. In *Trace Substances and Health: A Handbook, Part II*, edited by P. M. Newberne (New York: Marcel Dekker), chap. 1, pp. 1–45.

Newberne, P. M. and Fox, J. G., 1980, Nutritional adequacy and quality control of rodent diets. *Lab. Anim. Sci.*, **30**, 352–365.

Newberne, P. M. and McConnell, R. G., 1980, Dietary nutrients and contaminants in laboratory animal experimentation. *J. envir. Path. Tox.*, **4**, 105–122.

Newberne, P. M. and Schrager, T., 1983, Promotion of gastrointestinal tract tumors in animals: dietary factors. *Envir. Hlth Perspect.*, **50**, 71–83.

Newberne, P. M., Bresnahan, M. R. and Kula, N., 1969, Effects of two synthetic antioxidants, vitamin E and ascorbic acid on the choline deficient rat. *J. Nutr.*, **97**, 219–231.

Newberne, P. M., Glaser, O., Friedman, L. F. and Stillings, B., 1972, Chronic exposure of rats to methyl mercury in fish protein. *Nature*, **237**, 40–41.

Newberne, P. M., Glaser, O., Friedman, L. F. and Stillings, B., 1973 a, Safety evaluation of fish protein concentrate over five generations of rats. *Toxic. appl. Pharmac.*, **24**, 357–368.

Newberne, P. M., Glaser, O. and Friedman, L. F., 1973 b, Biologic adequacy of fish protein concentrate in five generations of mice. *Nutr. Rep. Int.*, **7**, 181–189.

Newberne, P. M., deCamargo, J. L. V. and Clark, A., 1982, Choline deficiency, partial hepatectomy and liver tumors in rats and mice. *Toxic. Path.*, **2**, 95–109.

Newberne, P. M., Rogers, A. E. and Nauss, K. M., 1983, Choline, methionine and related factors in oncogenesis. In *Nutrition Factors in the Induction and Maintenance of Malignancy*, edited by C. Butterworth and M. Hutchinson (New York: Academic Press), pp. 247–271.

Rogers, A. E. and Newberne, P. M., 1980, Lipotrope deficiency in experimental carcinogenesis. *Nutr. Cancer*, **2**, 104–114.

Tannenbaum, S. R., Weisman, M. and Fett, D., 1976, The effect of nitrate intake on nitrite formation in human saliva. *Fd Cosmet. Tox.*, **14**, 549–552.

Wainfan, E., Drznik, M., Hlubaky M. and Balis, M. E., Alteration of tRNA methylation in rats fed lipotrope-deficient diets. *Carcinogenesis*, **7**, 473–476.

Wilson, R. B., Kula, N., Newberne, P. M. and Conner, M. W., 1973, Vascular damage and lipid peroxidation in choline deficient rats. *Exp. molec. Path.*, **18**, 357–368.

Wilson, M. J., Shivapurkar, N. and Poirier, L. A., 1984, Hypomethylation of hepatic nuclear DNA in rats fed with a carcinogenic methyl-deficient diet. *Biochem. J.*, **218**, 987–994.

The role of clinical pathology in the selection of animal species

Walter F. Loeb

Metpath, 5516 Nicholson Lane, Kensington, MD 20895, USA

The use of laboratory animals in biomedical research, as we currently know it, is being challenged today by groups ranging from the lunatic fringe to highly respected scientists. While research utilizing animals appears essential to the continued progress of modern medicine, its justification requires that the objectives of studies be clearly formulated and that the studies be designed so as to meet these objectives. Clinical laboratory studies may provide the data to resolve many of these objectives, however, the unique characteristics of each species must be considered to determine whether the numerical values generated truly answer the biological questions and whether they do in a manner representative of man. An understanding of clinical pathology and its relationship to the animal species does not often play a role in the selection of the optimal species and strain, but it may be a major consideration in determining whether a particular experiment, and especially a particular measurement, will resolve a particular objective. Exceptionally, when an extraordinary biochemical pathway, such as bilirubin metabolism in the Gunn Rat, specifically fulfils the research objective, clinical pathology may be the determinant of the optimal species and strain.

The applicability of the measurement of chemical analytes varies by species in several ways. The appropriate analyte to determine may vary with the species. While in man, the dog, and the guinea-pig the principal adrenal glucocorticoid is cortisol, in the rat and mouse it is corticosterone. There are species differences in the organ sites of synthesis. In man and in the rat, amylase is secreted in the saliva, therefore sialadenitis may result in increased serum amylase. Since the saliva of the dog does not contain amylase, sialadenitis is not a consideration in the evaluation of hyperamylasaemia in the canine species. Analytes vary in turnover time as a function of both species and disease. In the dog, the three principle serum isoenzymes of alkaline phosphatase, osteoblastic, biliary, and steroid-induced, have a mean half-life of 72 h, whereas in the cat, the mean half-life of the two principal isoenzymes of alkaline phosphatase, bone and biliary, is 6 h, or one twelfth that of the dog (Hoffman and Dorner, 1977). The effect of this is that elevations of alkaline phosphatase are more marked and diagnostically sensitive in the dog than in the cat. The marked elevation of lactic dehydrogenase, isocitric dehydrogenase, malic dehydrogenase, phosphohexose isomerase and aspartate aminotransferase in mice infected with Riley's agent is due to impaired reticuloendothelial clearance rather than to increased release. The biochemical clearance of a substance may vary by species. In man, hyperamylasuria follows hyperamylasaemia. If a patient is suspected of having had acute pancreatitis but now has normal serum amylase, urine amylase may be measured to determine whether he has recently been hyperamylasaemic. In the dog this is not true. Although renal impairment or urinary obstruction in the dog leads to hyperamylasaemia, suggesting that excretion is through the kidney, the enzyme is not found in the urine. It is speculated that the enzyme is inactivated by the kidney. Finally, the structure of an analyte may differ from one species to another. This is especially important in the immunoassay of protein or peptide substances. The insulin molecule in the dog is sufficiently similar to that of man that the radioimmunoassay for human insulin may be applied validly to dog serum. By contrast, the rat has two separate and distinct insulin molecules which require a different antibody, competitive antigen, and standards for accurate quantification. These are a few examples of the types and mechanisms of differences among species with respect to clinical pathology, and we will expand on them later in this chapter.

Some important considerations are more pragmatic and mundane than these. Can an adequate volume of specimen, such as serum, be collected from the experimental animal to make all the necessary measurements? Recently our laboratory was asked to perform several hormone measurements on sera from mice. The investigator was to provide a minimum of 500 μl of serum for the prescribed measurements, which would only permit each of the measurements to be analysed once, not in duplicate. The specimens received were each between 100 and 200 μl. A larger species of animal would have allowed the objectives to be fulfilled. Generally, it is experimentally disadvantageous to pool specimens from several animals. If at all possible, each measurement should be performed on a specimen from a single animal in order to develop appropriate statistics for the distribution of values of the analyte, range and variance as well as mean. If clinical pathology determinations are to be performed several times during the study, the volume of specimen required may compromise the animals, or alter subsequent values. One millilitre of whole blood can be drawn from a 250 g rat every two weeks without producing any detectable effect. Most specimens for coagulation studies are best drawn from an endothelial-lined space by atraumatic puncture. Blood can be collected from rats by jugular venipuncture, but blood collected from rats, mice or hamsters by orbital sinus puncture is contaminated with tissue thromboplastin and the trauma of blood collection results in the activation of procoagulants and potentially erroneous data.

A recent experience in our laboratory demonstrated the effect that blood collection may have on analytical values. In collecting terminal blood samples from mice for both haematology and clinical chemistry, one of the animal technicians devised a scheme to obtain greater volume yield. The mice were bled from the orbital sinus for the specimen for haematology and then for a clotted blood sample for serum until the physical effect of weakening or hyperpnoea occurred. The mice were then allowed to rest for about half an hour, after which they were bled a second time and exsanguinated. The two clotted samples from each mouse were pooled. The analytical results obtained in this manner were in the historical reference range except for lactate dehydrogenase, aspartate aminotransferase and alanine aminotransferase, all of which were markedly elevated. In a series of experiments, it was demonstrated that from 1 min to 24 h after an initial bleeding, a second blood sample had markedly elevated enzyme values without respect to the site or method of collection. The underlying mechanism has not been experimentally ascertained, but it is speculated that the initial bleeding produced hypovolaemic shock with resulting hepatocellular injury and release of enzymes. Since no other analytes were affected, enzymes in the initial blood sample and any remaining analytes were subsequently determined. A recent publication on the effect of blood collection site on results in rats revealed a similar phenomenon (Suber & Kodell, 1985).

The need for fasting or non-absorptive blood samples may be a determinant of appropriate species. Although dogs are in a basal or non-absorptive state after a 12 h fast, and rhesus and cynomolgus monkeys after a 14 h fast, food must be withheld from rats for 72 h to render them non-absorptive, obviously not a generally appropriate technique. For this reason, clinical chemical measurements are generally performed on rats in an absorptive state.

Excitement markedly affects several laboratory parameters, including erythrocyte count, leukocyte count, cortisol and glucose. In a recently published study (Fulmer *et al.*, 1984), it was demonstrated that intravenous glucose tolerance tests could be validly performed on rhesus and African green monkeys anaesthetized with either ketamine or pentobarbital. When African green monkeys or male rhesus monkeys were physically restrained, the glucose tolerance results were invalid, but female rhesus monkeys, which are more docile than males or African greens, could be validly tested while physically restrained. Street & Jonas (1982) reported that anaesthetic agents significantly alter oral glucose tolerance testing in monkeys, apparently by impairing the absorption of glucose.

Bar-Ilan & Marder (1980) demonstrated that light anaesthesia of guinea-pigs with thiopentane caused respiratory depression, leading to respiratory acidosis and mild metabolic acidosis, when compared to values obtained in unanaesthetized unrestrained animals implanted with chronic cannulas. Each of these observations demonstrates the difficulty of obtaining clinical pathology measurements in the absence of extraneous effects.

Certain analytes, in particular hormones, undergo rhythmic variation. Those occurring on a daily basis are termed circadian and are the result of light-dark cycles, or in some instances sleep–wake cycles. Other cycles of more or less than a day's duration may control secretion independently or are superimposed on a circadian rhythm. In the dog, cortisol has a circadian rhythm with its maximum at 10 a.m. and its minimum at 10 p.m. In the rat and mouse, corticosterone has a circadian rhythm, having its maximum at 5–8 p.m. and its minimum at 4–6 a.m. In the adult female rat, variation of corticosterone levels with the oestrus cycle is superimposed on the circadian rhythm, with highest levels in pro-oestrus (D'Agostino *et al.*, 1982; Ottenweller *et al.*, 1979). Newborn rat pups do not show circadian rhythm for corticosterone; the rhythm develops at 21–30 days of age as a result of contact with the mother or a foster mother. A study by Takahashi *et al.* (1982) demonstrated that this occurs even in rat pups blinded neonatally. If analytes having cyclic periodicity are measured, and especially if they are measured repeatedly in a study, it is essential to measure them in the appropriate phase of the cycle, and to measure them each time in the same phase.

One may now turn to some of the differences in clinical chemical analytes among species. Whereas uric acid is not generally an analyte of great importance, it is a good example of the effect under consideration. In man it is the end-product of purine metabolism and an insensitive indicator of renal function. In submammalian vertebrates, it is the principal end-product of nitrogen metabolism. Christen *et al.* (1970) studied serum uric acid and hepatic uricase (urate oxidase), the enzyme which converts uric acid to the more readily soluble allantoin, in various species of primates. In man and the great apes, no hepatic uricase was found and serum uric acid levels were 3–7 mg/dl. In Old World primates they found stable hepatic uricase associated with low serum levels of uric acid: levels of about $0 \cdot 5$ mg/dl, comparable to those seen in subprimate mammals. In the New World primates *Cebus* and *Lagothrix* and in the marmoset, *Saguinus*, low hepatic activity of an unstable uricase was associated with serum uric acid levels of 2–3 mg/dl. Finally, prosimians, like the Old World primates, had high hepatic activity of stable uricase associated with a low serum uric acid concentration.

Alanine aminotransferase, the enzyme formerly designated SGPT, has been very extensively utilized as a sensitive indicator of hepatocellular injury. In the dog, its high activity in the cytosol of hepatocytes and very low activity in other tissues justify this application. There are two isoenzymes of alanine aminotransferase, one found in the cytosol and the other in the mitochondria. In contrast to the cytosol isoenzyme, which is released from cells as a result of mild increases in cell membrane permeability, the mitochondrial isoenzyme is only released following cell necrosis. In the guinea-pig, the total concentration of hepatic alanine aminotransferase is low and the predominant isoenzyme is that of the mitochondria. Therefore, in the guinea-pig, alanine aminotransferase is neither sensitive nor hepatospecific.

The uniqueness of each animal species is, of course, coded in its sequence of DNA bases and expressed in the sequence of amino acids. Therefore, protein and peptide hormones vary in structure among species. Whether the antibody in an immunoassay recognizes the hormone in one species that it was intended to measure in another, and whether it binds to it with the same affinity, depends on the structural similarity between hormones of the two species. There is no general rule to determine whether a particular hormone from one species will cross-react validly with the same hormone in another species. This must be determined empirically and by the structure of the hormone. The ACTH molecule is a sequence of 39 amino acids. All mammals which have been studied, more than 40 species in all, including all common laboratory and domestic animals, share the same sequence in the first 24 amino acids to which the antibody is raised. Therefore, the radioimmunoassay for human ACTH accurately measures the ACTH of other mammals.

Canine insulin is structurally quite similar to human insulin, and it has been shown that the radioimmunoassay for human insulin measures canine insulin validly. By contrast, the rat, mouse and Syrian hamster have two different non-allelic insulin molecules that are present in all members of the species (Markussen, 1971). Neither of these is proinsulin or C peptide. Mouse insulin II is identical to rat insulin II, and mouse insulin I differs from rat insulin I by a single amino acid. Rat insulin I and rat insulin II are present in approximately equal concentrations. The assay used to measure rat or mouse insulin must recognize both molecules equally. The rat insulin assay measures mouse insulin validly, but when used for the mouse it should be calibrated with mouse insulin standards. Insulin from the pancreatic islets of the guinea-pig is structurally quite dissimilar to insulin of either the dog or the rat and cannot be validly measured with either assay. However, the guinea-pig also produces another insulin from non-pancreatic sources. This insulin, which does not play a major role in glucoregulation, is structurally quite similar to canine or human insulin. Therefore, using the human assay to measure guinea-pig insulin not only fails to measure the principal glucoregulatory insulin, but measures a different molecule potentially leading to fallacious conclusions (Rosenzweig *et al.*, 1980).

In summary, a number of mechanisms have been reviewed and some examples of species differences in clinical laboratory parameters have been presented. In the design of any study, the unique characteristics of the proposed test species should be considered to determine whether the experimental protocol with respect to clinical pathology can be accurately and validly carried out. Collection of specimens must not introduce artefact into the study. The numbers generated must truly yield the information required to fulfil the objectives in a fashion representative of the species for which the study is designed, most often man. If the proposed test species is inappropriate in this respect, an appropriate species must be utilized to meet these objectives.

References

Bar-Ilan, A. and Marder, J., 1980, Acid-base status in unanesthetized unrestrained guinea-pigs. *Pflügers Arch.* **384**, 93–97.

Christen, P., Peacock, W. C., Christen, A. E. and Wacker, W., 1970, Urate oxidase in primate phylogenesis. *Eur. J. Biochem.,* **12**, 3–5.

D'Agostino, J. B., Vaeth, G. F. and Henning, S. J., 1982, Diurnal rhythm of total and free concentrations of serum corticosterone in the rat. *Acta Endocrinol.,* **100**, 85–90.

Fulmer, R., Loeb, W. F., Martin, D. P. and Gard, E. A., 1984, Effects of three methods of restraint on intravenous glucose tolerance testing in Rhesus and African Green monkeys. *Vet. clin. Path.,* **13**, 19–25.

Hoffman, W. E. and Dorner, J. B., 1977, Disappearance rate of intravenously injected canine alkaline phosphatase isoenzymes. *Am. J. vet. Res.,* **38**, 1553–1555.

Markussen, J., 1971, Mouse insulins. Separation and structure. *J. Protein Res.,* **3**, 149–155.

Ottenweller, J. E., Meier, A. H., Russo, A. C. and Frenzke, M. E., 1979, Circadian rhythms of plasma corticosterone binding activity in the rat and the mouse. *Acta Endocrinol.,* **91**, 150–157.

Rosenzweig, J., Lesniak, M., Samuels, B., Yip, C., Zimmerman, A. and Roth, J. 1980, Insulin in the extrapancreatic tissues of guinea pigs differs markedly from the insulin in their pancreas and plasma. *Trans. Assoc. Am. Phys.,* **93**, 263–278.

Street, I. W. and Jonas, A. M., 1982, Differential effects of chemical and physical restraint on carbohydrate tolerance testing in non-human primates. *Lab. Anim. Sci.,* **32**, 263–266.

Suber, R. L. and Kodell, R. L., 1985, The effect of three phlebotomy techniques on haematological and clinical chemical evaluation in Sprague–Dawley rats. *Vet. clin. Path.,* **14**, 23–30.

Takahashi, K., Hayafuji, C. and Murakami, N., 1982, Foster mother entrains circadian adrenocortical rhythm in blinded pups. *Am. J. Physiol.,* **243**, E443–E449.

Species differences in toxic lesions

G. H. Hottendorf†

Pharmaceutical Research and Development Division, Bristol-Myers Company,
P. O. Box 4755, Syracuse, NY 13221-4755 USA

Introduction

Differences in toxic lesions between animal species and man are a persistent problem for the extrapolation of toxicological data developed in animals to human safety (Newberne *et al.*, 1967; Alden, 1985). Species differences in toxicity must not only be considered in the extrapolation from laboratory animals to man, but toxic lesions are often not consistent between the different species of animals used in the toxicological studies. When the toxic lesions induced by 50 chemical compounds were compared between rodents and non-rodents, 40% of the compounds produced lesions in different target organs in different species (Heywood, 1981). Tumours are a particularly ominous toxic lesion, but rats cannot predict tumours in mice and vice versa (Di Carlo, 1984; Hottendorf, 1985). This review will attempt to summarize some reported species differences in toxic lesions produced in animals and examine the implications of such a recapitulation when the human experience is added.

Reports surveyed

Seventeen reports of species differences in toxic lesions were found in the literature and are outlined in Table 1. Three additional examples of species differences were obtained from in-house studies performed at Bristol-Myers Company Pharmaceutical Research and Development Division. Searching for reports of species differences in toxic lesions is difficult if such differences are not identified in the title. Therefore the depth of this search of the literature is unknown but is undoubtedly incomplete.

The majority of the comparisons listed involve pharmaceutical agents; this provided the opportunity to add toxicity data in man to the comparisons. The human safety data represented in Table 1 come either from the specific

†Present address: Medical University of South Carolina, 171 Ashley Avenue, Charleston, S.C. 29425-2216

Table 1. Comparisons of species differences in toxic lesions.

References	Chemicals	Toxicity compared	Rat	Dog	Mouse	Rabbit	Monkey	Guinea-pig	Hamster	Man
1	Acetaminophen	Nephrotoxicity	(+)	(−)	(−)					(+)
2	BL-4162	Thrombocytopenia	(−)	(−)	(−)	(−)	(+)	(−)		(+)
3	BL-5111	Cardiomyopathy	(+)	(−)	(−)					(−)
4	Benzylpenicillin	Delayed enterotoxaemia	(−)	(−)	(−)			(+)	(+)	(−)
5	Bromocriptine	Uterine tumours	(+)							(−)
6	Capreomycin	Nephrotoxicity	(+)	(−)	(−)	(−)	(−)	(−)		(+)
7	Ceforanide	Nephrotoxicity	(+)	(+)	(+)	(+)				(−)
8	Chloroform	Nephrotoxicity	(+)	(+)		(+)			(−)	(+)
9	Cinoxacin	Retinal atrophy	(−)	(−)						(−)
10	Cyclacillin	Nephrotoxicity	(+)	(−)						(−)
11	Decalin	Nephrotoxicity	(+)	(−)	(−)		(−)	(−)		(−)
12	Dimethylhydrazine	Colonic tumours	(+)	(+)	(+)		(−)	(−)	(+)	
13	Imipramine	Testicular atrophy	(−)	(+)						(+)
14	Indomethacin	Ulcerogenesis	(+)	(+)	(+)	(−)	(−)	(−)	(−)	(−)
15	Lysinoalanine	Nephrocytomegaly	(+)	(−)	(−)	(+)	(−)	(+)		(−)
16	Mepirizole	Ulcerogenesis	(+)	(+)	(−)	(−)	(−)	(−)		
17	Minoxidil	Cardiomyopathy	(−)	(+)	(−)		(−)			(−)
18	Probucol	Cardiomyopathy	(−)	(+)	(−)		(−)			(−)
19	Salbutamol	Mesoviral leiomyomas	(+)							
20	SCH 19927	Tapetopathy	(−)	(+)			(−)	(−)	(−)	(−)
		No. of comparisons	20	17	16	10	8	8	5	14

1, Cobden et al. (1982), Newton et al. (1983), Newton et al. (1985).
2, B-M data (unpublished data).
3, B-M data (unpublished data).
4, Boyd & Fulford (1961),
5, Richardson et al. (1984)
6, Muraoka et al. (1968), Physicians Desk Reference (1985)
7, B-M data (unpublished data), Smyth and Hottendorf (1980).
8, Klaassen and Plaa (1967), Deutsch & Van Dam (1971), Heywood et al. (1979), Smith et al. (1985).
9, Physicians Desk Reference (1985)
10, Tucker et al. (1974).

11, Alden (1985).
12, International Agency for Research on Cancer (1974), Wilson (1976).
13, Physicians Desk Reference (1985).
14, Wilhelmi (1974), Mariani & Bonanomi (1978).
15, DeGroot et al. (1976).
16, Ishihara et al. (1983).
17, Carlson & Feenstra (1977), Sobota et al. (1980).
18, Molello et al. (1973).
19, Jack et al. (1983).
20, Schiavo et al. (1984).

literature reports and/or from adverse reactions, mentioned in the package inserts as represented in the *Physician's Desk Reference* (1985).

The toxicities compared (Table 1) are the primary toxicities of most of these chemicals. Nephrotoxicity is well represented since it was involved in 7 out of 20 comparisons. Three of the comparisons involved tumours as the toxicity. These tumours have been included because data were available which involved more species than mice and rats, the two most common species used in carcinogenicity bioassays. The remaining toxicities are varied but do not represent the entire spectrum of potential toxic lesions.

Eight species are included in Table 1; all these species were not however tested with every chemical. Excluding man, the number of animal species per comparison ranged from three to seven with an average of four species per comparison. Although the duration of dosing in the toxicological studies may vary from acute single-dose studies to two year carcinogenicity studies, the length of dosing among the species tested with an individual chemical were usually similar.

Results

The rat is one of the most popular species utilized in toxicological studies and was present in all 20 comparisons cited in Table 1. As summarized in Table 2, the rat exhibited the toxic lesion in 12 of the 20 comparisons (60%). The dog is the second most popular toxicological species and was represented in 17 of the 20 comparisons; the dog was positive for the indicated toxicity in 6 of these 17 comparisons (35%). Toxicological data were obtained in the mouse in 16 of the 20 comparisons and the mouse was positive in only 3 of 16 comparisons (19%). Ten of the 20 comparisons included the rabbit which was positive in 3 (30%). Monkeys and guinea-pigs were represented in 8 of the comparisons and were positive once and twice, respectively (13 and 25%). The hamster was represented in the fewest number of comparisons but was positive

Table 2. Toxic lesions: Percentage positive by species.

Species	Positive/no. of comparisons	%
Rat	12/20	60
Dog	6/17	35
Mouse	3/16	19
Rabbit	3/10	30
Monkey	1/8	13
Guinea-pig	2/8	25
Hamster	2/5	40
Man	5/14	36

Table 3. Toxic lesions: comparisons with only a single animal species positive.†.

Species	Only species positive/no. of comparisons	%
Rat	8/15	53
Dog	5/12	42
Monkey	1/8	13
Rabbit	1/10	10
Mouse	0/15	—
Guinea-pig	0/4	—
Hamster	0/3	—

† Five comparisons involving toxicity in more than one animal species excluded.

in two of five (40%). The human experience could be added to 14 comparisons; man revealed the toxic lesion in 5 of 14 (36%) comparisons.

Of the 20 comparisons, 15 indicated a toxicity that was confined to one of the various animal species (Table 3). The rat had the highest incidence as the only animal to express the species-specific toxic lesion (53%). The dog was the only animal species positive in 42% of such comparisons in which it was included. Although the mouse was included in all 15 of these comparisons, it never exhibited the species-specific toxic lesion.

"Surprisingly little effort has been made to correlate toxicity in animals and adverse effects in man" (Heywood, 1981). Despite the bias inherent in selecting comparisons that demonstrate species differences in toxic lesions and the small numbers of comparisons (five) which include human toxicity, a correlation of the toxicity displayed in animals with human toxicity should therefore be of interest (Tables 4 and 5). The rat predicted for man (either positive or negative) in 71% of the comparisons. The rat falsely predicted human toxicity in 3 of 14 comparisons (21%), but failed to predict a toxic lesion that subsequently developed in man in only 1 of 14 comparisons (7%). The mouse correctly

Table 4. Toxic lesions: correlation of toxicity with man.

	Rat	Mouse	Dog	Rabbit	Monkey	Guinea-pig	Hamster
Comparisons with man	14	11	11	8	6	5	3
Like man (+ or −)	10 (71%)	8 (73%)	5 (45%)	4 (50%)	5 (83%)	1 (20%)	1 (33%)
False-positive	3 (21%)	0 —	4 (36%)	1 (13%)	0 —	1 (20%)	1 (33%)
False-negative	1 (7%)	3 (27%)	2 (18%)	3 (37%)	1 (17%)	3 (60%)	1 (33%)

Table 5. Toxic lesions: prediction of toxicity in man.

Species	Predicted/no. of comparisons	%
Rat	4/5	80
Mouse	2/5	40
Dog	1/3	33
Rabbit	1/4	25
Monkey	1/2	50
Guinea-pig	0/3	—
Hamster	0/1	—

predicted the human toxic potential (either positive or negative) of 73% of 11 chemicals. Reflecting its low rate of positive reactions, there were no false-positives noted in the mouse but 3 (27%) false-negatives are indicated. The dog was included in 11 of the comparisons which involved man, but the dog was like man (either positive or negative) in only 5 (45%) comparisons. The dog also had a 36% false-positive indication of human toxicity and an 18% false-negative prediction. Several comparisons of the toxicity of anti-cancer agents between animals and man have been reported (Schein *et al.*, 1970; Schein, 1977; Rozencweig *et al.*, 1981). The dog also had a high false-positive prediction rate in these anti-cancer data, particularly those involving the liver and kidney. The rabbit was like man in 50% of the 8 comparisons in which both species were represented. The rabbit gave a false-positive in one of these 8 (13%) comparisons and a false-negative in 3 (37%). Monkeys were included in 6 comparisons with man and were like man in 5 (83%). Monkeys predicted the human toxicity in only one comparison, however. Guinea-pigs and hamsters were similar to man in their expression of toxicity in only 1 of 5 and 1 of 3 comparisons, respectively.

Discussion

The data base presented in Table 1 is limited to only 20 comparisons biased by selection for the demonstration of species differences in toxicity. The actual incidence of species differences in toxic lesions, particularly in the common toxicology species, remains unknown.

There are a wide range of factors that contribute to species susceptibility to xenobiotics (Caldwell, 1981; Calabrese, 1984). Although the main difference between the biotransformation of xenobiotics in man and animals is more quantitative than qualitative (Williams, 1963; Hottendorf, 1975), species differences in conjugation, acetylation, hydroxylation and biliary excretion have been established (Caldwell, 1981; Calabrese, 1984). Species differences in biotransformation led to the production of a toxic metabolite in the affected species given cyclacillin (Jansen *et al.*, 1974; Tucker *et al.*, 1974) and BL-5111

(Bristol-Myers, unpublished data). However, with BL-5111 the main determinant was the amount of the metabolite produced rather than a true species difference in the qualitative metabolic pattern. The differences in the ulcerogenic potential of indomethacin in various species is also more quantitative than qualitative, with the rat and man being more sensitive than the mouse or guinea-pig (Wilhelmi, 1974; Mariani & Bonanomi, 1978). The dog is listed as negative for the nephrotoxicity induced by chloroform. However, at acute doses approaching lethality chloroform administration to the dog may result in nephrotoxicity (Klaassen & Plaa, 1967). In 13 of the 20 comparisons in Table 1 the effect of different doses was not a quantitative concern because the negative species were given doses at least equivalent to the dose producing the effect in the sensitive species.

The majority of the species differences in toxicity as described in Table 1 are unexplained. Six of the 20 examples of toxic differences between species listed in Table 1 may be explained. The tapetopathy which developed in dogs with SCH-19927 involved the tapetum lucidum of the canine eye (Schiavo *et al.*, 1984). This structure is not present in rats, rabbits, most monkeys and man. A species difference in renal physiology is involved in the nephrotoxicity of decalin. The species-specific nephrotoxicity observed in rats but not in the mouse, dog and guinea-pig is believed to be a consequence of the proteinuria which develops spontaneously in aged rats (Alden, 1985). The uterine tumours that appeared after administration of bromocriptine in the rat, but not in the mouse, dog or man, are believed to involve species-specific differences in various sex hormones (Richardson *et al.*, 1984). As qualified above, species-specific differences in metabolism may account for the toxicity distribution between various species after administration of cyclacillin (Tucker *et al.*, 1974), chloroform (Klaassen and Plaa, 1967) and BL-5111 (Bristol-Myers unpublished data).

Some species involvements may be somewhat misleading, as represented in Table 1. Stump-tailed monkeys exhibited the thrombocytopenia produced in man with BL-4162, but the rhesus, cynomolgus and squirrel monkeys, as well as chimpanzees, did not indicate this unusual toxicity (Bristol-Myers, unpublished data). In addition to species differences, several strain and sex differences are included in Table 1. Fischer 344 but not Sprague–Dawley male rats displayed the nephrotoxicity of acetaminophen (Newton *et al.*, 1983, 1985). The nephrotoxicity of cyclacillin showed a sex as well as a species preference, being confined to male rats (Tucker *et al.*, 1974).

These comparisons of species differences in toxicity are limited in number (20) and are biased by selection towards a lack of species correlation. Nevertheless, the paucity of such toxicity data, coupled with the inclusion of the human experience in 14 of 20 comparisons and an average of four animal species per comparison, are believed to have made an analysis of the correlations worthwhile. When both positive and negative reactions are considered, the mouse and rat predicted 73% and 71% for man. A more disappointing level of agreement was observed between the dog and man (45%). Monkeys predicted for man 83% in a smaller number of comparisons (six) in which they were included. The ability to predict the five toxicities produced in man was good with the rat (80%), but poor with the other species (40% or less). The monkey and man were both included in only two comparisons, and the monkey predicted human toxicity in one of them (Table 5).

The only valid conclusion that can be drawn from these limited data is that additional comparisons of the toxicities produced by chemicals in various species including man are surely indicated. These limited data suggest that the rat and mouse predict toxicity better for man than the dog. The predictive value of toxicological studies performed in animal species and the incidence of species differences in toxicity could and should be placed in sharper perspective with an expanded data base.

References

Alden, C. L., 1985, Species, sex, and tissue specificity in toxicologic and proliferative responses. *Toxic. Path.*, **13**, 135–140.

Boyd, E. M. and Fulford, R. A., 1961, The acute oral toxicity of benzylpenicillin potassium in guinea-pigs. *Antibiot. Chemother.*, **11**, 276–283.

Calabrese, E. J., 1984, Suitability of animal models for predictive toxicology. Theoretical and practical considerations. *Drug. Metab. Rev.*, **15**, 505–523.

Caldwell, J., 1981, The current status of attempts to predict species differences in drug metabolism. *Drug. Metab. Rev.*, **12**, 221–237.

Carlson, R. G. and Feenstra, E. S., 1977, Toxicologic studies with the hypotensive agent minoxidil. *Toxic. appl. Pharmac.*, **39**, 1–11.

Cobden, I., Record, C. O., Ward, M. K. and Kerr, D. N. S., 1982, Paracetamol-induced acute renal failure in the absence of fulminant liver damage. *Br. Med. J.*, **284**, 21–22.

DeGroot, N. P., Slump, P., Feron, V. J. and Van Beek, L., 1976, Effects of alkali-treated proteins: feeding studies with free and protein-bound lysinoalanine in rats and other animals. *J. Nutr.*, **106**, 1527–1538.

Deutsch, S. and Van Dam, L. D., 1971, General anesthesia 1: volatile agents. In *Drill's Pharmacology in Medicine*, edited by J. R. Di Palma (New York: McGraw-Hill), pp. 162–163.

Di Carlo, F. J., 1984, Carcinogenesis bioassay data: correlation by species and sex. *Drug Metab. Rev.,* **15**, 409–413.

Heywood, R., Sortwell, R. J., Noel, P. R. B., Street, A. E., Prentice, D. E., Roe, F. J. C., Wadsworth, P. F. and Worden A. N., 1979, Safety evaluation of tooth paste containing chloroform, III. Long-term study in beagle dogs. *J. envir. Path. Tox.*, **2**, 835–851.

Heywood, R., 1981, Target organ toxicity. *Toxic. Lett.*, **8**, 349–358.

Hottendorf, G. H., 1975, Pharmacokinetic considerations in toxicology. *Proc. Eur. Soc. Toxic.*, **17**, 255–261.

Hottendorf, G. H., 1985, Carcinogenicity testing of antitumor agents. *Toxic. Path.*, **13**, 192–199.

International Agency for Research on Cancer (IARC), 1974, *Evaluation of Carcinogenic Risk of Chemicals to Humans. IARC Monograph*, Vol. 4, (Lyon: International Agency for Research on Cancer), pp. 145–152.

Ishihara, Y., Yoshiharu, Y., Hata, Y. and Susumu, O., 1983, Species and strain differences in mepirizole-induced duodenal and gastric lesions. *Dig. Dis. Sci.*, **28**, 552–558.

Jack, D., Poynter, D. and Spurling, N. W., 1983, Beta-adrenoceptor stimulants and mesovarian leiomyomas in rat. *Toxicology*, **27**, 315–320.

Jansen, F. W., Young, E. M., Kirkman, S. K., Agersborg Jr, H. P. K., Tucker Jr, W. E. and Ruelius, H. W., 1974, Metabolic and pathologic investigation of 1-aminocyclohexanecarboxylic acid (ACHC), a metabolite of 6-(1-aminocyclo-hexanecarboxamido)-penicillanic acid (cyclacillin). *Toxic. appl. Pharmac.*, **29**, 19–34.

Klaassen, C. D. and Plaa, G. L., 1967, Relative effects of various chlorinated hydrocarbons on liver and kidney functions in dogs. *Toxic. appl. Pharmac.*, **10**, 119–131.

Mariani, L. and Bonanomi, L., 1978, Resistance of the guinea pig to indomethacin ulcerogenesis. *Toxicol. appl. Pharmac.*, **45**, 637–639.

Molello, J. A., Gerbig, C. G. and Robinson, V. B., 1973, Toxicity of [4,4-(isopropylidenedithio) bis (2,6-di-*t*-butylphenol)], probucol, in mice, rats, dogs and monkeys: demonstration of a species-species phenomenon. *Toxic. appl. Pharmac.*, **24**, 590–593.

Muraoka, Y., Hayashi, Y. and Minesita, T., 1968, Studies on capreomycin nephrotoxicity. *Toxic. appl. Pharmac.*, **12**, 250–259.

Newberne, J. W., Gibson, J. P. and Newberne, P. M., 1967, Variation in the toxicologic response of species to an analgesic. *Toxic. appl. Pharmac.*, **10**, 233–243.

Newton, J. F., Yoshimoto, M., Bernstein, J., Rush, G. F. and Hook, J. B., 1983, Acetaminophen nephrotoxicity in the rat. 1. Strain differences in nephrotoxicity and metabolism. *Toxic. appl. Pharmac.*, **69**, 291–306.

Newton, J. F., Pasino, D. A. and Hook, J. B., 1985, Acetaminophen nephrotoxicity in the rat: quantitation of renal metabolic activation *in vivo*. *Toxic. appl. Pharmac.*, **78**, 39–46.

Physicians Desk Reference (PDR), 1985, 39th edn (Oradell, NJ: Medical Economics Co.).

Richardson, B. P., Turkalj, I. and Flückiger, E., 1984, Bromocriptine. In *Safety Testing of New Drugs*, edited by D. R. Laurence, A. E. M. McLean and M. Weatherall (London: Academic Press), pp. 19–63.

Rozencweig, M., Von Hoff, D. D., Staquet, M. J., Schein, P. S., Penta, J. S., Goldin, A., Muggia, F. M., Freirech, E. J. and DeVita Jr, V. T., 1981, Animal toxicology for early clinical trials with anticancer agents. *Cancer Clin. Trials*, **4**, 21–28.

Schein, P. S., 1977, Preclinical toxicology of anticancer agents. *Cancer Res.*, **37**, 1934–1937.

Schein, P. S., Davis, R. D., Carter, S., Newman, J., Schein, D. R. and Rall, D. P., 1970, The evaluation of anticancer drugs in dogs and monkeys for the prediction of qualitative toxicities in man. *Clin. Pharmac. Ther.*, **11**, 3–40.

Schiavo, D. M., Sinha, D. P., Black, H. E., Arthaud, L., Massa, T., Murphy, B. F., Szot, R. J. and Schwartz, E., 1984, Tapetal changes in beagle dogs. 1. Ocular changes after oral administration of a beta-adrenergic blocking agent— SCH-19927. *Toxic. appl. Pharmac.*, **72**, 187–194.

Smith, J. H., Hewitt, W. R. and Hook, J. B., 1985, Role of intrarenal biotransformation in chloroform-induced nephrotoxicity in rats. *Toxic. appl. Pharmac.*, **79**, 166–174.

Smyth, R. D. and Hottendorf, G. H., 1980, Application of pharmacokinetics and biopharmaceutics in the design of toxicological studies. *Toxic. appl. Pharmac.*, **53**, 179–195.

Sobota, J. T., Martin, W. B., Carlson, R. G. and Feenstra, E. S., 1980, Minoxidil: right atrial cardiac pathology in animals and man. *Circulation*, **62**, 376–387.

Tucker, Jr, W. E., Janssen, F. W., Agersborg Jr, H. P. K., Young, E. M. and Ruelius, H. W., 1974, Sex and species-related nephropathy of 6-(1-aminocyclohexane-carboxamido) penicillanic acid (cyclacillin) and its relationship to the metabolic disposition of the drug. *Toxic. appl. Pharmac.*, **29**, 1–18.

Wilhelmi, G., 1974, Species differences in susceptibility to the gastro-ulcerogenic action of anti-inflammatory agents. *Pharmacology*, **11**, 220–230.

Williams, R. T., 1963, Detoxification mechanisms in man. *Clin. Pharmac. Ther.*, **4**, 234–254.

Wilson, R. B., 1976, Species variation in response to dimethylhydrazine. *Toxic. appl. Pharmac.*, **38**, 647–650.

PART 3

Metabolic and pharmacokinetic considerations in species selection

Section editor:
A. G. E. Wilson

Retrospective evaluation of appropriate animal models based on metabolism studies in man

Mitchell N. Cayen

Department of Biochemistry, Ayerst Laboratories Research, Inc., CN 8000, Princeton, NJ 08540, USA

Introduction

A major goal of modern toxicology and therapeutics is to assess the causes of inter-species differences in susceptibility to xenobiotics, with the hope of trying to improve upon present capability of predicting human responses based on animal studies. There are, of course, no generally appropriate animal models which are usually predictive of human exposure and responses to foreign compounds. Retrospective evaluation of animal data following metabolism and pharmacokinetic studies in man can uncover similarities between a given species and man in the disposition of a specific xenobiotic or class of xenobiotics. Since the source of species similarities and differences is often due to the metabolic disposition of the compound, such evaluations expand our knowledge on the range of factors that contribute to differential species susceptibility to xenobiotics. The goal of this brief overview is to discuss some of the disposition factors to be considered in species comparisons. This aspect of safety assessment, which can be defined as the science which predicts from animal experiments the safety of a chemical in man under the likely condition of exposure, can help increase our chances of valid extrapolations of animal data to those in man. The disposition factors discussed are those which may be considered in the rational design of toxicity studies and clinical trials, and are by no means comprehensive.

Sources of species differences in the metabolic disposition of xenobiotics

The major causes of species variation in the pharmacology and/or toxicology of xenobiotics are shown in Figure 1. The exposure phase comprises factors which regulate the amount of foreign compound available for absorption by the applied route of administration (e.g., digestion, inhalation, skin contact),

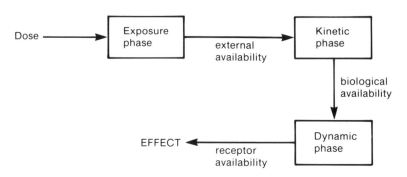

Figure 1. Sources of species variation in the action of xenobiotics.

and involves dose frequency, dose magnitude and dosage form, that is, factors which determine whether the xenobiotic acts as a pharmacological or therapeutic agent, or as a toxicant. The kinetic (pharmacokinetic or toxicokinetic) phase involves the processes of absorption, distribution, biotransformation and excretion. The pharmaco- (or toxico-) dynamic phase consists of processes involved in the interaction of the active agent and the target molecule(s) (i.e., receptors) – frequently bipolymers, such as functional proteins. This discussion will be restricted to some of the variables within the kinetic phase.

Biotransformation

Probably the most important cause of species differences in susceptibility or exposure to foreign compounds is differential biotransformation, and this topic has been reviewed elsewhere (Williams, 1967; Walker, 1978; Caldwell, 1980). Species variations in biotransformation can occur in one of three forms (Caldwell, 1981), detailed below.

Species-specific deficiency in a particular metabolic reaction

Although most species have the capacity to carry out the common reactions of xenobiotic metabolism, there exist various combinations of species and substrate from which one of these reactions is absent. Such species can be termed deficient in this particular reaction. For example, the rat is deficient in the *N*-hydroxylation of aliphatic amines, the dog in acetylations, the cat in glucuronidation reactions and the pig in most sulphation reactions. Awareness of such deficiencies is important in predicting species differences in xenobiotic metabolism.

Species-specific limitation in a particular metabolic reaction

There are several types of metabolic reactions which occur only in certain species or class of species. Most interest has centered on those reactions which are predominant in man and other primates, but are absent in other mammals. For example, reactions limited to man and certain other primates (Caldwell, 1981) are N^1-glucuronidation of sulphadimethoxine and other methoxy-sulphonamides, the aromatization of quinic acid to yield benzoic acid which is then excreted as hippuric acid, conjugation of arylacetic acids with glutamine, glucuronic acid conjugation of cyproheptadine to yield its quarternary glucuronide, and O-methylation of 3,5-di-iodo-4-hydroxybenzoic acid.

Variations in activities of competing metabolic reactions

Most xenobiotics possess within their chemical structure a number of possible sites for metabolic attack. Although most species are capable of carrying out these metabolic reactions, it is common to encounter species variation in the relative extents of potential biotransformation processes. For example, the multifunctional benzodiazepine skeleton can undergo hydroxylation or cleavage at six different sites on the molecule, and the relative-contributions of these processes vary between rat, dog and man (Caldwell, 1981).

An ultimate goal in predicative toxicology is to assess whether species patterns exist in the metabolism of xenobiotics. It has been known for some time that, in general, lower animals metabolize drugs more rapidly than man (Quinn *et al.*, 1958). This is due in part to the fact that the main organ in which drug metabolism takes place is the liver, and the relative liver size is generally greater in lower animals (e.g., 4% of body weight in rats compared to 2% in man). Also, the activities of most mammalian hepatic drug metabolizing enzymes tend to decrease (expressed as units of activity per kilogram body weight) as body weight increases (Krasovskii, 1976). For example, rat liver contains five times the concentrations of cytochrome P-450 than does human liver (Walker, 1978). However, in spite of these observations, it does not appear valid to make generalizations about rates of unknown metabolic reactions. Many exceptions can be found to the apparent tendency of the rate of biotransformation processes to decrease with body size (or surface area). Different qualitative pathways may dominate in different species and toxicity may sometimes be associated with the concentration of an active intermediate that represents only a minor metabolic pathway. However, once species patterns are recognized for a particular chemical series, it may then be possible to predict the metabolic profile of a novel compound in that series. For example, excellent data are available on the biotransformation of amphetamines in various species (Caldwell, 1976, 1981). The general structure of amphetamines and their sites of biotransformation are shown in Figure 2. The

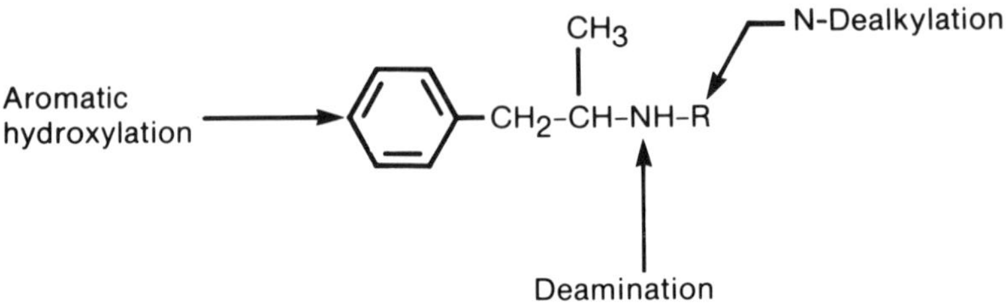

Figure 2. Amphetamines and their sites of biotransformation.

Table 1. Species variations in the metabolism of amphetamines.

| Species | No. of compounds | Relative extent of metabolism† | | | |
		Aromatic hydroxylation	*N*-Dealkylation	Deamination	Excreted unchanged
Rat	11	+ + + +	+ + +	+	+ +
Guinea-pig	6	0	+ +	+ + + +	+ +
Rabbit	8	+	+ +	+ + + +	+
Marmoset	4	+	n.a.	+	+ + + +
Rhesus monkey	4	+ + +	n.a.	+ + +	+ +
Man	13	+ +	+	+ + +	+ + +

† 0 (absent) to + + + + (extensive): adapted from Caldwell, 1981.
n.a., Data not available.

major metabolic routes of up to 13 amphetamines in six species are shown in Table 1. The major finding from these data is that although major species differences exist in the metabolism of amphetamines, even between primate species, the metabolic profile *within* a species is very similar, and it would therefore be expected that the metabolic fate of novel amphetamine analogues can be predicted in these six species.

Plasma protein binding

Most analytical techniques to measure plasma or serum drug concentrations determine total (free plus bound) drug. Free-circulating concentrations are inherently more reliable indices of the intensity of drug action than are total concentrations (Greenblatt *et al.*, 1982), and thus species differences in protein binding are major factors to consider when assessing drug exposure, especially for those drugs which are very highly protein bound. Table 2 presents comparisons of data obtained in our laboratories on the protein binding of clofibric acid (CPIB), the circulating active form of the anti-hyperlipidaemic drug clofibrate (Cayen, 1983), the non-steroidal anti-inflammatory drug

Table 2. Binding of drugs to plasma proteins.

Compound	Unbound drug (%)					
	Rat	Mouse	Dog	Rabbit	Rhesus monkey	Man
CPIB	25	65	15	n.a.	5·0	3·0
Etodolac	0·7	5·2	1·7	0·5	1·2	0·8
Tolrestat	1·7	4·0	2·0	1·0	1·4	0·7
Pelrinone	28	78	20	26	21	11
Benoxaprofen	0·7	1·1	0·8	0·4	0·4	0·2

n.a., Data not available.

etodolac (Cayen *et al.*, 1981; Ferdinandi *et al.*, 1986), the aldose reductase inhibitor tolrestat (Cayen *et al.*, 1985), the basic cardiotonic drug pelrinone, and in other laboratories with benoxaprofen (Chatfield & Green, 1978) (structures are shown in Figure 3). The generalities which emerge are that protein binding is highest in human serum, weakest in mouse serum, and somewhat variable with other species. The implication is that for any given serum or plasma concentration of total drug, the potential exposure to free or unbound drug is often greater in laboratory animals than in man. The higher the binding

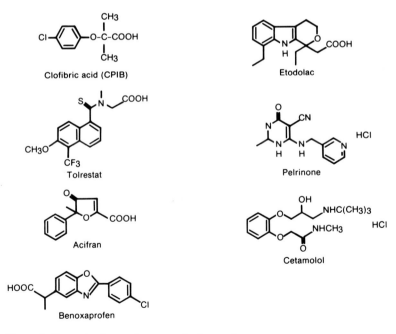

Figure 3. Some structures of compounds discussed.

to plasma proteins, the greater the extent to which species variation in binding can potentially affect the therapeutic and toxic properties of a foreign compound.

Biliary excretion

The rat and dog are very efficient in biliary excretion; guinea-pigs, monkeys and man are relatively inefficient; the mouse is somewhere in between. Such species differences have pronounced toxicological implications, especially when biliary excretion is followed by reabsorption and return to the liver by the portal system, i.e., enterohepatic circulation takes place. The degree of enterohepatic circulation and/or renal excretion can markedly affect the pharmacokinetics and metabolism, and therefore the therapeutic and toxic properties of xenobiotics (Levine, 1978). For example, the intestinal toxicity of indomethacin in five species of laboratory animals is inversely proportional to the exposure of the intestinal mucosa to the drug as a consequence of enterohepatic circulation. Therefore, the extent of cumulative exposure expressed as a percentage of dose was found to be in the order dog > rat > monkey > guinea-pig > rabbit > man, with the minimum toxic dose

Table 3. Radioactivity excretion following oral administration of ^{14}C-labelled drugs.

Drug	Class or drug	References	Percentage of dose excreted within 7–14 d[†]							
			Rat		Mouse		Dog		Man	
			Ur	Fe	Ur	Fe	Ur	Fe	Ur	Fe
CPIB	Hypo-lipidaemic	Cayen (1983)	90§	3	n.a.	n.a.	60	36	96	2
Acifran	Hypo-lipidaemic	Cayen et al. (1986)	62‖	29	95	1	90	2	69	6
Etodolac	NSAID	Cayen et al. (1981) Ferdinandi et al. (1986)	21§	81	53	44	11	84	73	14
Tolrestat	AR-inhibitor‡	Cayen et al. (1985) Hicks et al. (1984)	16§	86	55	39	30	57	69	27
Cetamolol	β-Blocker	Unpublished	23§	74	n.a.	n.a.	43	44	74	18
Pelrinone	Cardiotonic	Scatina et al. unpublished results	58§	39	88	12	80	8	91	5

Ur, Urine; Fe, Faeces;
NSAID, Non-steroidal anti-inflammatory drug.
n.a., Data not available.
† Some of these data are unpublished.
‡ Aldose reductase inhibitor (for complications of diabetes).
§ Drug undergoes enterohepatic circulation.
‖ Drug does not undergo enterophepatic circulation.

ranging from 0·5 mg/kg/d in dogs to 20 mg/kg/d in rabbits (Duggan & Kwan, 1979). Examples from our laboratories of some species differences in the route of drug excretion are shown in Table 3. All the compounds are well absorbed (at least 70% of the dose) in all species, therefore high faecal excretion is not due to poor absorption, but to biliary excretion of absorbed drug. The molecular weight or organic anions will often determine the extent of urinary and biliary exretion in some species of lower animals (Hirom *et al.*, 1972). In rats and dogs, well absorbed drugs can be excreted in both urine and faeces, independent of whether enterohepatic circulation takes place. For example, CPIB (Cayen, 1980) and tolrestat (Cayen *et al.*, 1985) undergo enterohepatic circulation in rats, a process which contributes to the plasma profile of the drugs, but 90% of the dose of CPIB and 16% of tolrestat is excreted in the urine.

Pharmacokinetics

The application of pharmacokinetic principles to safety assessment forms an integral part of extrapolating data from animals to man. Extensive literature is available on this topic, which has been recently reviewed (Clarke & Smith, 1984). The use of comparative pharmacokinetics is based on the principle that the intrinsic sensitivity of different species to a given xenobiotic is similar, that is, a characteristic effect is observed when a particular tissue concentration is attained. Thus, the goal of pharmacokinetics is to correlate the profile of the circulating xenobiotic with dose (i.e., dose magnitude, dose frequency, dosage form, route of administration, etc.). The following endpoints must be considered in rational selection for toxicity or clinical studies:

1. The range of dose-independent kinetics.
2. Single-dose and steady-state circulating drug levels.

These endpoints can vary due to species variation in the parameters discussed previously as well as variations in clearance (Boxenbaum & Fertig, 1984) and volume of distribution, processes which are regulated by such factors as first-pass effect (pre-systemic drug elimination) and plasma protein binding. Both these parameters independently influence the elimination half-life ($t_{½}$). Clearance can be viewed as the efficiency of the eliminating organs to remove the drug, and volume of distribution as the ability of tissues to take up the drug from the circulation. Knowledge of the range of dose-independent kinetics − the range in which the circulating drug levels increase linearly with dose − assists the rational dose selection in toxicity studies. The steady-state concentrations are the average maximum and minimum drug levels achieved daily, and imply a constant exposure of the test species and its organs to the drug throughout the toxicity test (or clinical trial).

Active metabolites

Consideration of the pharmacokinetics of a metabolite is of importance when the activity of this metabolite can contribute to toxicity or to therapeutic action; in such instances, the determination of the parent drug alone may cause misleading toxicological, pharmacological or clinical interpretations (Drayer, 1982; Clark & Smith, 1984; Garattini, 1985). As a general rule, metabolites with slower elimination rates than the parent compound are likely to be of more significance in safety evaluation, particularly when their rate of formation is high. Similarly, the metabolites with more rapid elimination will be of less significance since their behaviour is predictable from the kinetics of the parent compound. However, it should be noted that low levels of some chemically and highly reactive (mainly oxidized) metabolites can mediate such toxic manifestations as carcinogenesis, mutagenesis and cellular necrosis.

Isomers and enantiomers

Some drugs are given in the form of two or more isomers, with only one having the desired pharmacological activity. The other isomer(s) may be inactive, partially active or contribute to side-effects or toxicity. Some compounds may form rotamers in the body. Most analytical procedures used to monitor plasma drug levels measure both isomers together. Several drugs given as racemates undergo stereoselective bioavailability, distribution, clearance and metabolism (Ariens, 1984). For example, following oral administration of racemic propranolol, the pharmacologically active enantiomer S-propranolol attains higher concentrations than the inactive R-enantiomer in man (S/R ratio = 1·4), but less than the R-enantiomer in the dog (S/R ratio = 0·5); these differences were associated with species-specific stereoselectivity in plasma protein binding, extra-vascular distribution and hepatic metabolism (Walle *et al.*, 1982; Walle, 1985). Also, the N-dealkylation pathway of the quinidine-like anti-arrhythmic agent disopyramide in dogs and the aryl hydroxylation pathway of the drug in rats are stereoselective, illustrating species differences in stereoselective metabolism (Cook *et al.*, 1982). Although the pharmacological and toxicological properties of a racemate are composites of those of the component isomers and their specific metabolites, pharmacokinetic data derived for the active form can be misleading if all isomers or enantiomers are analysed and reported as a single entity. A pragmatic approach is to be aware of the limitations when deriving kinetic data, and to take into account potential species differences in stereoselective metabolism and disposition when extrapolating data from animals to man.

Other sources of species differences

The purpose of this overview is not to provide an exhaustive review of the sources of species differences in the disposition of xenobiotics, but to illustrate with a few examples the strengths and weaknesses in the usefulness of animal models for predictive toxicology to man. Differences based on administration only by the oral route have been discussed. Other routes of administration, such as percutaneous absorption (Wester & Noonan, 1980), provide species differences in the rate and extent of delivery of xenobiotics to the systemic circulation.

Appropriate animal models

Hopefully, I have conveyed the message that extrapolation of animal data to man is a science which involves dissecting and evaluating the basis for species differences and similarities. However, the rat is not 'a little man', and the best model for man is man. It is well known that, in general, the best animal model for man is the non-human primate, specifically Old World Monkeys such as the rhesus monkey, for reasons such as their same limited metabolic reactions, no species defects in xenobiotic biotransformations, similar plasma protein binding and similar susceptibility to teratogenic agents. It should be noted, however, that although the rhesus monkey is more similar to man regarding xenobiotic biotransformation, it appears to be no better or no worse than other species when considering xenobiotic pharmacokinetics. For example, the data in Table 4 illustrate that the elimination half-life of CPIB and of several non-steroidal anti-inflammatory drugs in the rhesus monkey show differences to man, as do other animal species. One reason for the lack of similarity in the pharmacokinetics of drugs between man and rhesus monkey is that although the patterns of metabolism are generally similar in man and Old World Monkeys, the rate processes are often different.

Because of their high cost and limited availability, the rhesus monkey is used less often than more available less expensive lower animals to evaluate the

Table 4. Elimination half-life of some drugs in laboratory animals and man.

Drug	Reference(s)	Elimination half-life ($t_{1/2}$; h)				
		Rat	Dog	Mouse	Rhesus monkey	Man
CPIB	Cayen (1980) Walmsley (1984)	6	40	2	2	21
Benoxaprofen	Chatfield & Green (1978)	28	11	24	12	23
Naproxen	Runkel *et al.* (1972)	5	35	n.a.	2	14
Phenylbutazone	Bertelli & Casali (1977)	6	6	n.a.	8	72
Tolmetin	Grindel (1981)	0·7	n.a.	1·4	3·5	2·8
Isoxicam	Borondy & Michniewicz (1984)	31	41	n.a.	29	31
Suprofen	Mori *et al.* (1985)	3·7	1·9	1·8	1·9	0·7

n.a., Data not available.

pharmacological and toxicological properties of foreign compounds. The rat, which has become the superspecies of the laboratory animal colony, can be effectively used to predict human risk and exposure only if the differences between rat and man are effectively evaluated. Calabrese (1984) compared some biochemical and physiological differences between rat and man; some of these are presented in Table 5. He concluded that, even though profound differences exist between the two species that can result in differential susceptibilities to foreign compounds, valid predictions to man based on rat data can be made using appropriate extrapolations.

The purpose of retrospective evaluation of animal data following metabolic studies in man is to identify animal species which are similar to man. A fascinating example where toxicity testing in various animal species, including non-human primates, is not predictive of toxicity in man is with chenodeoxycholate (CDCA) and ursodeoxycholate (UDCA), which are naturally occurring bile acids used for the dissolution of cholesterol gallstones in the gall bladder. The first species in which CDCA was administered as a therapeutic agent was man in 1972, when Danzinger *et al.* (1972) found that the bile acid was effective in dissolving gallstones. These studies were borne out in long-term trials, and expanded with the finding that the 7β-epimer of CDCA, UDCA, was more potent but equally as safe as CDCA (Bachrach & Hoffmann, 1982). Using a backwards approach to toxicity testing, these bile acids were subsequently tested in animals, and found to be hepatotoxic in the rat,

Table 5. Some metabolic differences of potential pharmacological and toxicological significance between rat and man.†

	Relative amount/activity	
Parameter	Rat	Man
Flora in stomach, proximal small intestine‡	Numerous	Little or none
Intestinal β-glucuronidase	Very high	Low
Skin stratum corneum/vasculature	Thin	Thick
Plasma protein binding	Lower	Higher
Biliary excretion	High	Low
Conjugations		
Glucuronidation	High	Low
Sulphation	Low	High
Acetylation	Effective	Effective or slow§
Amino acid with phenylacetic acid	Glycine	Glutamine
Urine concentration	Higher	Lower
Urinary excretion of xenobiotics	Lower	Higher

† Adapted from Calabrese (1984).
‡ Sites of absorption from gastro-intestinal tract.
§ Genetically determined.

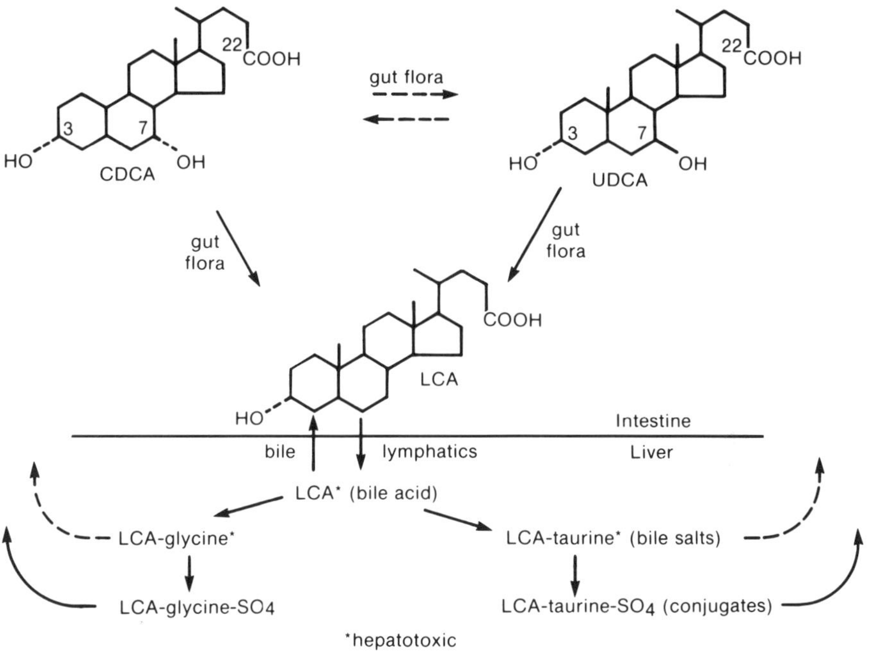

Figure 4. Biotransformation of chenodeoxycholate (CDCA) and ursodeoxycholate (UDCA).

hamster, rabbit, dog, rhesus monkey and baboon; the only species without hepatotoxicity were the squirrel monkey, chimpanzee and man (Bazzoli *et al.*, 1982, Suzuki *et al.*, 1985). The toxicity of UDCA and CDCA was found to be due to species-specific metabolism (Figure 4) (Bazzoli *et al.*, 1982; Suzuki *et al.*, 1985). Lithocholic acid (LCA), formed in the gastro-intestinal tract by dehydroxylation, and salts of LCA formed in the liver were responsible for the hepatotoxicity of CDCA and UDCA. Man, the squirrel monkey and the chimpanzee were the only species in which LCA and its salts were very efficiently sulphated in the liver, and this species-specific detoxification mechanism was the reason for the safety of CDCA and UDCA in these species. The toxicity in the other species is an example where the pathogenesis involves absorption of a toxic bacterial metabolite which is not readily detoxified in the liver. As far as this author is aware, CDCA and UDCA are the only drugs which exhibit such strikingly different toxicities in man and the commonly tested non-human primates. They are probably the only such known drugs because during the normal course of drug development, any drug which manifests this degree of toxicity in rats, dogs and the commonly tested non-human primates is unlikely to be administered to man.

Conclusions

The use of animal models for quantitative assessment of the potential exposure by man to xenobiotics is a slowly growing science. We are under constant pressure, especially in the area of potential carcinogens, to become more precise and quantitative in our predictions. As the science of predictive toxicology continues to expand, we should not only attempt to determine which animal species most closely resembles man, but to identify species differences to explain findings in a given species, and to assess whether similar events are likely to occur in man. The ultimate goal of predictive toxicology is to protect society from chemically-induced tragedies. Research investigators in drug metabolism are continually searching for patterns of species similarities and differences to assist colleagues in toxicology and clinical research in the rational design of drug testing programmes.

References

Ariens, E. J., 1984, Stereochemistry, a basis for sophisticated nonsense in pharmaco-kinetics and clinical pharmacology. *Eur. J. clin. Pharmac.*, **26**, 663–668.
Bachrach, W. H. and Hofmann, A. F., 1982, Ursodeoxycholic acid in the treatment of cholesterol cholelithiasis. *Dig. Dis. Sci.*, **27**, 737–761; 833–856.
Bazzoli, F., Fromm, H., Sarve, R. P., Sembrat, R. F. and Ceryak, S., 1982, Comparative formation of lithocholic acid from chenodeoxycholic and ursodeoxycholic acids in the colon. *Gastroenterology*, **83**, 753–760.
Bertelli, A. and Casali, I., 1977, Extrapolation of data on metabolism of drugs from the animal to man: problems and difficulties. *Adv. clin. Pharmac.*, **13**, 169–181.
Borondy, P. E. and Michniewicz, B. M., 1984, Metabolic disposition of isoxicam in man, monkey, dog, and rat. *Drug. Metab. Disp.*, **12**, 444–451.
Boxenbaum, H. and Fertig, J. B., 1984, Scaling of antipyrine intrinsic clearance of unbound drug in 15 mammalian species. *Eur. J. Drug Metab. Pharmacokin.*, **9**, 177–183.
Calabrese, E. J., 1984, Suitability of animal models for predictive toxicology: theoretical and practical considerations. *Drug Metab. Rev.*, **15**, 505–523.
Caldwell, J., 1976, The metabolism of amphetamines in mammals. *Drug Metab. Rev.*, **5**, 219–280.
Caldwell, J., 1980, Comparative aspects of detoxication in mammals. In *Enzymatic Basis of Detoxication*, Vol. 1, edited by W. B. Jacoby (New York: Academic Press), chap. 5.
Caldwell, J., 1981, The current status of attempts to predict species differences in drug metabolism. *Drug. Metab. Rev.*, **12**, 221–237.
Cayen, M. N., 1980, Metabolic disposition of antihyperlipidemic agents in man and laboratory animals. *Drug. Metab. Rev.*, **11**, 291–323.
Cayen, M. N., 1983, Metabolism and pharmacokinetics of antihyperlipidemic agents. In *Progress in Drug Metabolism*, Vol. 7, edited by J. W. Bridges and L. F. Chasseaud (London: John Wiley), pp. 173–227.
Cayen, M. N., Kraml, M., Ferdinandi, E. S., Greselin, E. and Dvornik, D., 1981, The metabolic disposition of etodolac in rats, dogs, and man. *Drug Metab. Rev.*, **12**, 339–362.
Cayen, M. N., Hicks, D. R., Ferdinandi, E. S., Kraml, M., Greselin,E. and Dvornik,

D., 1985, Metabolic disposition and pharmacokinetics of the aldose reductase inhibitor tolrestat in rats, dogs, and monkeys. *Drug Metab. Disp.*, **13**, 412–419.

Cayen, M. N., Gonzalez, R., Ferdinandi, E. S., Greselin, E., Hicks, D. R., Kraml, M. and Dvornik, D., 1986, The metabolic disposition of acifran, a new antihyper-lipidemic agent, in rats and dogs. *Xenobiotica*, **16**, 251–263.

Chatfield, D. H. and Green, J. N., 1978, Disposition and metabolism of benoxaprofen in laboratory animals and man. *Xenobiotica*, **8**, 133–144.

Clark, B. and Smith, D. A., 1984, Pharmacokinetics and toxicity testing. *CRC Crit. Rev. Tox.*, **12**, 343–385.

Cook, C. S., Karim, A. and Sollman, P., 1982, Stereoselectivity in the metabolism of disopyramide enantiomters in rat and dog. *Drug Metab. Disp.*, **10**, 116–121.

Danzinger, R. G., Hofmann, A. F., Schoenfield, L. J. and Thistle, J. L., 1972, Dissolution of cholesterol gallstones by chodeoxycholic acid. *New Engl. J. Med.*, **286**, 1–8.

Drayer, D. E., 1982, Pharmacologically active metabolites of drugs and other foreign compounds. Clinical, pharmacological, therapeutic and toxicological considerations. *Drugs*, **24**, 519–542.

Duggan, D. E. and Kwan, K. C., 1979, Enterohepatic recirculation of drugs as a deter-minant of therapeutic ratio. *Drug Metab. Rev.*, **9**, 21–41.

Ferdinandi, E. S., Sehgal, S. N., Demerson, C. A., Dubuc, J., Zilber, J., Dvornik, D. and Cayen, M. N., 1986, Disposition and biotransformation of ^{14}C-etodolac in man. *Xenobiotica*, **16**, 153–166.

Garattini, S., 1985, Active drug metabolites. An overview of their relevance in clinical pharmacokinetics. *Clin. Pharmacokin.*, **10**, 216–227.

Greenblatt, D. J., Sellers, E. M. and Koch-Weser, J., 1982, Importance of protein binding for the interpretation of serum or plasma drug concentrations. *J. clin. Pharmac.*, **22**, 259–263.

Grindel, J. M., 1981, The pharmacokinetic and metabolic profile of the antiinflam-matory agent tolmetin in laboratory animals and man. *Drug Metab. Rev.*, **12**, 363–377.

Hicks, D. R., Kraml, M., Cayen, M. N., Dubuc, J., Ryder, S. and Dvornik, D., 1984, Tolrestat kinetics. *Clin. Pharmac. Ther.*, **36**, 493–499.

Hirom, P. C., Millburn, P., Smith, R. L. and Williams, R. T., 1972, Species variation in the threshold molecular weight factor for the biliary excretion of organic anions. *Biochem. J.*, **129**, 1071–1077.

Krasovskii, G. N., 1976, Extrapolation of experimental data from animals to man. *Envir. Hlth Perspect.*, **13**, 51–58.

Levine, W. G., 1978, Biliary excretion of drugs and other xenobiotics. *Ann. Rev. Pharmac. Tox.*, **18**, 81–96.

Mori, Y., Kuroda, N., Sakai, Y., Yokoya, F., Toyoshi, K. and Baba, S., 1985, Species differences in the metabolism of suprofen in laboratory animals and man. *Drug Metab. Disp.*, **13**, 239–245.

Quinn, G. P., Axelrod, J. and Brodie, B. B., 1958, Species, strain and sex differences in metabolism of hexobarbitone, aminopyrine, antipyrine and aniline. *Biochem. Pharmac.*, **1**, 152–159.

Runkel, R., Chaplin, M., Boost, G., Segre, E. and Forchielli, E., 1972, Absorption, distribution, metabolism, and excretion of naproxen in various laboratory animals and human subjects. *J. Pharm. Sci.*, **61**, 703–708.

Suzuki, H., Hamada, M. and Kato, F., 1985, Metabolism of lithocholic and chenodeoxycholic acids in the squirrel monkey. *Gastroenterology*, **89**, 631–636.

Walker, C. H., 1978, Species differences in microsomal monooxygenase activity and their relationships to biological half-lives. *Drug. Metab. Rev.*, **7**, 295–323.

Walle, T., 1985, Stereochemistry of the *in vivo* disposition and metabolism of propranolol in dog and man using deuterium-labeled pseudoracemates. *Drug Metab. Disp.*, **13**, 279–282.

Walle, T., Oatis Jr, J. E., Walle, U. K. and Knapp, D. R., 1982, New ring-hydroxylated metabolites of propranolol. Species differences and stereospecific 7-hydroxylation. *Drug. Metab. Disp.*, **10**, 122–127.

Walmsley, L. M., 1984, Dose-dependent pharmacokinetics of clofibric acid in the non-human primate. *Archs. Tox.*, (Suppl.) **7**, 272–277.

Wester, R. C. and Noonan, P. K., 1980, Relevance of animal models for percutaneous absorption. *Int. J. Pharm*, **7**, 99–110.

Williams, R. T., 1967, Comparative patterns of drug metabolism. *Fedn Proc. Fedn Am. Socs exp. Biol.*, **26**, 1029–1039.

The role of studies of absorption, metabolism, distribution and elimination in animal selection and extrapolation

Michael J. McKenna

Department of Pathology and Experimental Toxicology,
Warner-Lambert/Parke-Davis, Ann Arbor, Michigan, USA

Introduction

A primary goal of the efforts of toxicologists is to predict safety for man. A pivotal step in achieving that goal is the clear understanding of the test systems used in the laboratory assessment of toxicity. This chapter aims to provide some examples of how the study of pharmacokinetics and metabolism provides a tool which furthers our understanding of chemical biology in laboratory animals and the ability to extrapolate our results to man. This general overview of the utility of pharmacokinetic and metabolic data in toxicity evaluation is from the perspective of a toxicologist who uses the tool of pharmacokinetics. Further, the review intends to draw upon my own experiences in the laboratory, which are related to problems associated with chemical exposure via the inhalation route of administration. However, it must be pointed out that the observations that follow are equally applicable to any other route.

Although the modelling of pharmacokinetic data has played an important role in toxicity evaluation and extrapolation of animal data between species, this aspect of pharmacokinetics will not be dealt with to any great extent. Most toxicologists do relatively little modelling, but gain most benefit in studying relatively simple data sets in the context of the toxicity observed in laboratory animals.

Broadly defined, pharmacokinetics is the study of chemical fate. This definition includes the processes of absorption, distribution, metabolism and excretion (ADME). As toxicologists, we often find that we deal with the additional categories of metabolism as it relates to detoxification or intoxication, as well as the interaction of chemicals with critical macromolecules, its relationship to toxicity, and the repair of such events. Thus in toxicity evaluation, as in all research, one thing usually leads to another.

In general, one can divide the applications of ADME data into three categories relative to toxicity evaluations: study design, interpretation and extrapolation. In the first two categories, ADME data aid in the understanding of the animal model and often provide explanations or clues to unusual or unexpected results. As an aid to extrapolation, such investigations not only provide a means of comparison between animals and man, but often allow extension of the dose–response curve beyond the boundaries of observable toxicity as assessed by conventional laboratory methods. Each of these areas of application of ADME data in toxicology will be dealt with, and some examples of such applications provided.

Study design

Although the collection of vast amounts of ADME data in various test species might be of use in the selection of the species that is most like man for toxicity evaluation, it is hardly a practice that would be either efficient or cost effective. Species selection in toxicity assessment is often for reasons other than being representative of man. Primary considerations of the study objectives and the criteria of response are usually the determinant of the animal species and strain employed. Factors such as availability, economy of care and housing, uniformity, hardiness, regulatory guidelines, statistical power and historical experience, all have an impact on animal selection. Particularly important in laboratories where large numbers of test compounds are evaluated in 'routine' toxicity testing, is the need for reliable and predictable animal models that are well studied.

Often toxicologists and others express concern over the adequacy of currently used animal models and study designs. However, many mistakenly equate this dissatisfaction with a particular animal model with a lack of utility or suitability for providing useful data. In fact, substantial progress has been made in improving models of toxicity over recent years. Healthy reliable uniform animal strains and species are now used, which have been selectively bred for laboratory research, to employ in experiments where uniformity and reliability are paramount. Therefore, any shortcomings in models should be worked on so they are more thoroughly understood, and their utility in extrapolating to man is maximized.

Just as confidence in experimental models of toxicity is enhanced by the experience gained by the consistent use of a particular laboratory animal model, so, too, is it strengthened by a knowledge of chemical disposition and metabolism in that model. Often attempts are made to interpret findings in terms of what is known about the metabolism and elimination of a chemical in the laboratory species under study. Target-organ toxicity is often correlated with the tissue distribution of a test chemical or its metabolites. Conversely, the ability to detoxify the administered chemical may be a determining factor also in the expression of toxicity, particularly when that ability is compromised or overwhelmed.

Perhaps the most significant contribution of pharmacokinetics in the design and/or interpretation of toxicity studies is the concept of dose-dependent or non-linear kinetics. Many of the physiological and biochemical processes which affect the disposition of chemicals in the body are capacity limited or saturable. When any of the rate-limiting processes of absorption, distribution, metabolism or excretion become saturated, the internal concentration of either the parent chemical or its metabolites may not be directly proportional to the administered dose. Disproportionate increases or decreases in internal concentrations may occur, with concurrent effects upon toxicity. Some of the criteria which suggest that saturation may be occurring include the following (Levy, 1968):

1. The decline of levels of chemicals in the body does not follow an exponential time-curve.

2. The biological half-life increases with increasing dose.

3. The area under the plasma concentration versus time curve is not proportional to increasing doses.

4. The composition of excretory products may be changed both quantitatively and qualitatively with increasing dose.

5. Competitive inhibition by other chemicals metabolized by the same enzymatic systems is likely.

6. Dose–response curves show unusually large increases in response with increasing dose, starting with the dose level where saturation effects first become evident.

The utility of pharmacokinetic and metabolic data in study design, as well as the impact of non-linear pharmacokinetics on study design, can be illustrated by studies on pharmacokinetics of inhaled methylene chloride in rats (McKenna *et al.*, 1982). These experiments also serve to point out a common pitfall in inhalation toxicology – that exposure concentration is not always representative of the 'dose' achieved by the experimental animal model.

Initial experiments were designed to evaluate the effect of increasing exposure concentrations on methylene chloride plasma levels. Male Sprague–Dawley rats were exposed to methylene chloride concentrations of 50, 500 and 1500 p.p.m. for six hours, and plasma samples were obtained frequently for analysis by gas chromatography in order to determine the uptake and post-exposure elimination of the solvent (Figure 1). An apparent steady-state plasma concentration of methylene chloride was attained after approximately two hours of inhalation exposure. When compared to that attained during the 50 p.p.m. exposure, the steady-state exposure concentrations attained by rats exposed to 500 and 1500 p.p.m. were disproportionately greater than expected from the relative increase in exposure concentration. Similarly, measurement of the area under the plasma methylene chloride curves (*AUC*) revealed a non-linear response with increasing exposure concentrations (Table 1). After

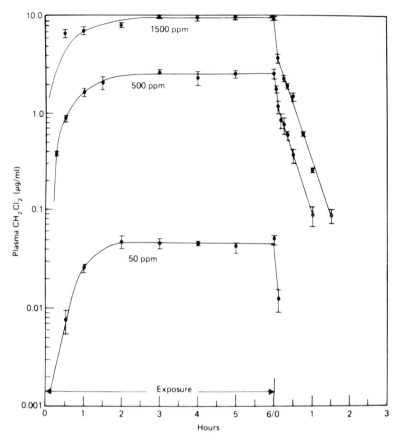

Figure 1. Plasma concentrations of methylene chloride in rats during and after a six hour inhalation exposure. Each point represents the mean and s.d. for two to four rats. (Reprinted from McKenna *et al.*, 1982, with permission.)

exposure, plasma concentrations of methylene chloride declined in a biexponential manner, with apparent half-lives of 2 and 15 min for the rapid and slow components of elimination, respectively. There were no differences in the rates of elimination of methylene chloride from plasma following either the 500 or 1500 p.p.m. exposures.

Material balance experiments with [14C]-labelled methylene chloride provided further insight into the non-linear pharmacokinetics observed in the previous experiment, and suggested that the kinetic non-linearity may be due to saturable metabolism. In these experiments we exposed rats by inhalation to [14C]-methylene chloride for six hours and thereafter followed the excretion of the radiolabel for 48 h after exposure. [14C]-Methylene chloride *per se* was excreted only in expired air following inhalation exposure (Table 2). The major metabolites of the solvent, [14C]-carbon monoxide and [14C]-carbon

Table 1. Apparent steady-state plasma concentrations and area under the curve (*AUC*) values for rats exposed to methylene chloride.

Exposure conc. (p.p.m.)	Plasma CH_2Cl_2 (μg/ml)†	*AUC* (μg/h/ml)‡	Normalized *AUC* (50 p.p.m.)‡
50	$0 \cdot 05 \pm 0 \cdot 01$	$0 \cdot 23$	$1 \cdot 0$
500	$2 \cdot 38 \pm 0 \cdot 42$	$12 \cdot 65$	$55 \cdot 8$
1500	$8 \cdot 94 \pm 0 \cdot 39$	$49 \cdot 90$	$220 \cdot 1$

† Values represent the mean and s.d. for three rats.
‡ *AUC* values obtained from the data in Figure 1.

dioxide, were also excreted in expired air. The percentage of the body burden excreted as unchanged methylene chloride in the expired air increased with increasing exposure concentration, much the same as previously observed for the plasma methylene chloride data. This increase in unchanged methylene chloride excretion at higher exposure concentrations was accompanied by a decrease in the percentage of the body burden metabolized to carbon monoxide and carbon dioxide. The percentage of radioactivity remaining in the body at 48 h following the inhalation exposure also decreased with increasing exposure concentrations.

Of particular importance to considerations of study design was the relationship between the exposure concentration, the body burden, and the body burden of metabolized methylene chloride observed in these experiments. The body burden of ^{14}C activity resulting from a six-hour inhalation exposure to [14C]-methylene chloride was calculated from the total radioactivity recovered during the first 48 h after exposure (Table 3). Values for metabolite burden were obtained by subtracting the recovery of exhaled [14C]-methylene

Table 2. Disposition of [14C]-methylene chloride in rats following inhalation exposure for six hours.

	(%) Body burden after exposure to [14C]CH_2Cl_2 at various concentrations.		
	50 p.p.m.	500 p.p.m.	1500 p.p.m.
Expired air			
Methylene chloride	$5 \cdot 42$	$30 \cdot 40$	$55 \cdot 00$
Carbon dioxide	$26 \cdot 20$	$22 \cdot 54$	$13 \cdot 61$
Carbon monoxide	$26 \cdot 67$	$18 \cdot 09$	$10 \cdot 23$
Urine	$8 \cdot 90$	$8 \cdot 41$	$7 \cdot 20$
Faeces	$1 \cdot 94$	$1 \cdot 85$	$2 \cdot 33$
Carcass	$23 \cdot 26$	$11 \cdot 56$	$7 \cdot 24$
Skin	$6 \cdot 85$	$6 \cdot 72$	$3 \cdot 97$
Cage wash	$0 \cdot 75$	$0 \cdot 42$	$0 \cdot 43$

Values represent the mean of three rats per exposure group.

Table 3. Net body burden and metabolized [^{14}C]-methylene chloride in rats after inhalation exposure for six hours.

Exposure conc. (p.p.m.)	Body burden (mg-Equiv./kg)†	Metabolized	
		(mg-Equiv./kg)†	%
50	5·53 ± 0·33	5·23 ± 0·32	94·6
500	48·41 ± 4·33	33·49 ± 0·33	69·2
1500	109·14 ± 3·15	49·08 ± 1·37	45·0

† Values represent recovery of radioactivity following inhalation exposure and are the mean ± s.d. for three rats.

chloride from the body burden values. Thus, the values shown in Table 3 represent net uptake and metabolism resulting from the six hour exposures and do not account for excretion of volatile metabolites during the actual exposure period. The influence of metabolism on the dose-dependent accumulation of ^{14}C activity is clearly evidenced by the data for net uptake and metabolism of [^{14}C]-methylene chloride.

Figure 2 is a graphic representation of the relationship between exposure concentration and metabolite burden following a single six hour inhalation exposure. Increasing the methylene chloride exposure concentration results in diminishingly smaller increments in the metabolism of the solvent. If the expression of an observed biological response due to methylene chloride were dependent upon metabolism, one might expect that the dose–response relationship at higher concentrations would more nearly approximate relative rates of metabolism rather than the relationship between exposure concentrations. This was in fact the case, when the data from a chronic inhalation toxicity study of methylene chloride in rats was analysed for dose–response relationships (Burek *et al.*, 1984).

In this study rats were exposed to 0, 500, 1500 or 3500 p.p.m. methylene chloride for six hours daily, five days a week, for 24 months. The observed incidence and severity of treatment-related effects noted in the study (e.g. hepatocellular alterations, altered spontaneous tumour incidences, and blood carboxyhaemoglobin levels) were markedly different than that predicted by a relative exposure concentration relationship of 1:3:7, but were closely approximated by the relative rates of metabolism at the three concentrations − 1:1·6:2·0. That the animals' capacity to metabolize the solvent was exceeded at all three exposure concentrations was suggested by the observation that the post-exposure blood carboxyhaemoglobin levels were about 10–12% for all exposed rats, irrespective of the exposure concentration. Unfortunately, due to the proximity of the 'effective doses' in this experiment, a no-observed-effect level was not achieved, and a subsequent chronic toxicity study was initiated at exposure concentrations of 500 p.p.m. and lower, which would be expected to result in a more linear pharmacokinetic response as indicated by Figure 2.

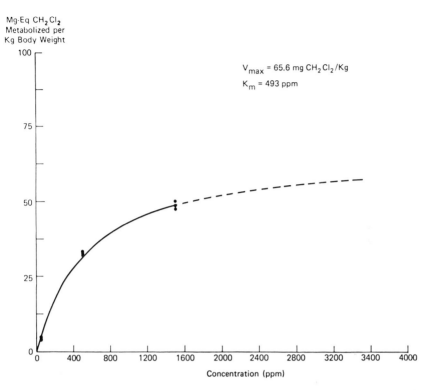

Figure 2. Methylene chloride exposure concentration versus metabolite burden in rats after a single six hour inhalation exposure. Each point represents an individual animal. The dotted line is a computer-generated extrapolation of the curve, based on the Michaelis–Menten equation.

In retrospect, this example serves to show both the importance of pharmacokinetic and metabolism data in dose selection and the importance of obtaining such information in a timely manner. Had these data been available at the time when the dose-selection criteria were prepared for the chronic inhalation study, we might well have spread the exposure concentrations or added additional exposure groups to the experiment and thereby more appropriately covered the range of both linear and non-linear kinetic responses. However, it is also important to recognize that the use of pharmacokinetic data is not a ready substitute for other experimental parameters of toxicity which traditionally are used to determine the so-called maximum tolerated dose (MTD), that is the highest intended dose for studies such as the chronic rodent bioassay. The primary use of kinetic and metabolic data is as an aid in establishing an adequate 'spread' of doses for the experiment, once the 'MTD' has been established by clinical, biochemical and pathological endpoints. A recent report from the National Toxicology Program provides an excellent discussion of the utility of pharmacokinetic data in study design, along with several theoretical examples of the use of such data in a combination with the MTD concept in establishing doses for chronic rodent bioassays (National Toxicology Program, 1984).

Study interpretation

Quite often the assessment of drug or chemical toxicity in one or more laboratory species results in markedly different results. Inter-species differences in the response to test material administration may be qualitative, in terms of the target organ affected, or quantitative , with respect to the dose or exposure concentration resulting in injury, the threshold or no-observed-effect level (NOEL) for a particular effect, and recovery or repair of chemically induced injury. In such instances the ability to interpret such inter-species differences is often enhanced by a knowledge of chemical disposition and metabolism as it relates to the observed toxicity. Once again it it useful to understand the relationship between the 'effective dose' and that which was administered to the test animals. The effective dose may be defined in terms of absorption, metabolism or the concentration of parent compound or metabolite at the target organ. The influence of the route of administration of the test chemical, as well as the influence of metabolism on the expression of toxicity, are of significance to the interpretation of inter-species differences in toxicity. Studies to compare the pharmacokinetics and metabolism of vinylidene chloride (1,1-dichloroethylene) in laboratory rats and mice are a useful example of the utility of such data in the interpretation of inter-species differences in response (McKenna *et al.*, 1977, 1978; Reitz *et al.*, 1980).

Inhalation exposure of rats to vinylidene chloride results in a decrease of hepatic glutathione concentrations (Jaeger *et al.*, 1974). Further depletion of glutathione stores and enhancement of vinylidene chloride-induced hepatotoxicity are achieved by fasting before exposure in order to deplete hepatic glutathione. Subsequent experiments with inhaled [^{14}C]-vinylidene chloride indicated a correlation between centrilobular hepatic necrosis and covalently bound ^{14}C activity in the livers of exposed rats (McKenna *et al.*, 1978). These experiments led to the hypothetical metabolic scheme for vinylidene chloride shown in Figure 3.

Several chronic oncogenicity studies in rats have failed to show evidence of carcinogenic potential for vinylidene chloride when administered by inhalation (25, 75 or 100 p.p.m.) or in the drinking water (up to 220 p.p.m.) (Maltoni *et al.*, 1977; Rampy *et al.*, 1977; Viola & Caputo, 1977). In contrast, two investigators have reported a tumourigenic response to vinylidene chloride in mice following chronic inhalation exposure to 25 or 55 p.p.m. (Maltoni *et al.*, 1977; Lee *et al.*, 1978). Maltoni *et al.* (1977) suggested that male mice were more sensitive to the effects of vinylidene chloride than female mice. The target organ in male mice was the kidney, and the tumourigenic response to

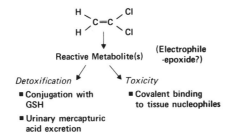

Figure 3. Hypothetical metabolic pathway for vinylidene chloride in the rat and its relationship to toxicity.

vinylidene chloride was accompanied by substantial non-tumour pathology in the same organ. These authors also reported that exposure of mice to 10 p.p.m. vinylidene chloride resulted in an absence of both tumours and non-tumour pathology in the kidneys. We undertook a series of studies to investigate the biochemical and metabolic possibilities that may explain the difference in target organs and tumourigenic response to vinylidene chloride in the rat and the mouse (McKenna *et al.*, 1978; Reitz *et al.*, 1980).

Initial experiments compared the disposition of [^{14}C]-vinylidene chloride in male Sprague–Dawley rats and male Ha(ICR) mice (Table 4). Inhalation exposure to [^{14}C]-vinylidene chloride at 10 p.p.m. for six hours resulted in no significant qualitative differences in the fate of the chemical in rats and mice. However, the net body burden of radioactivity in mice was nearly twice that acquired by the rat under identical exposure conditions. The inhaled

Table 4. Comparative disposition of [^{14}C]-vinylidene chloride in rats and mice following inhalation exposure to 10 p.p.m. for six hours.

	% Body burden	
	Rats	Mice
Expired vinylidene chloride	$1 \cdot 63 \pm 0 \cdot 14$	$0 \cdot 65 \pm 0 \cdot 07$
Carbon dioxide	$8 \cdot 74 \pm 3 \cdot 72$	$4 \cdot 64 \pm 0 \cdot 17$
Urine	$74 \cdot 72 \pm 2 \cdot 30$	$80 \cdot 83 \pm 1 \cdot 68$
Faeces	$9 \cdot 73 \pm 0 \cdot 10$	$6 \cdot 58 \pm 0 \cdot 81$
Carcass	$4 \cdot 75 \pm 0 \cdot 78$	$5 \cdot 46 \pm 0 \cdot 41$
Cage wash	$0 \cdot 44 \pm 0 \cdot 28$	$1 \cdot 83 \pm 0 \cdot 84$
	mg-Eq. [^{14}C]-vinylidene chloride/kg	
Body burden	$2 \cdot 89 \pm 0 \cdot 24$	$5 \cdot 30 \pm 0 \cdot 75$
Total metabolized	$2 \cdot 84 \pm 0 \cdot 26$	$5 \cdot 27 \pm 0 \cdot 74$

All values represent the mean ± s.d. for three animals.

[^{14}C]-vinylidene chloride was also more extensively metabolized by the mouse than the rat.

The greater body burden and more extensive metabolism of vinylidene chloride (A) by mice suggested that the production of reactive metabolites in mice might be greater than observed in rats, thus rendering them more susceptible to the adverse effects of vinylidene chloride exposure (McKenna *et al.*, 1977). Covalently bound ^{14}C-activity (B) in the liver and kidneys of the two species are compared in Table 5. A marked increase in covalently bound ^{14}C-labelled metabolites in the mouse liver and kidney was observed when compared to rats. The enhanced production of reactive metabolites in mouse tissue could not be attributed solely to the increased metabolism of vinylidene chloride over that of the rat, as indicated by the normalized binding data which accounts for differences in metabolism (B/A ratio). Not only was the metabolism of vinylidene chloride greater in the mouse than in the rat, but the production of reactive metabolites in target tissues for vinylidene chloride-induced toxicity was markedly greater.

Subsequently, Reitz *et al.* (1980) examined the effects of [^{14}C]-vinylidene chloride exposure on DNA damage and repair in the target tissues from both rats and mice. These experiments resulted in little if any significant effect of vinylidene chloride on alkylation or repair of DNA damage. In contrast, significant cytotoxic activity was observed in the form of increased DNA synthesis in the mouse kidney, the target organ for tumour development. Similar increases in DNA synthesis were not seen in organs of the mouse where tumours did not develop, nor in the rat, which did not develop vinylidene chloride-induced tumours in any target tissue.

Thus these investigations contributed substantially to the final interpretation of the tumourigenicity data obtained for vinylidene chloride in the rat and the mouse. The pharmacokinetic data revealed that the mouse metabolized the test chemical at a faster rate than the rat did, and therefore produced more reactive metabolites. This resulted in an enhanced binding to inner-cellular macromolecules in the organs susceptible to tumour formation in the mouse (i.e., the

Table 5. Vinylidene chloride metabolism and covalently bound ^{14}C activity in rats and mice after a 10 p.p.m. inhalation exposure.

A Metabolized vinylidene chloride (mg-Equiv./kg)	Species	Tissue	B Covalent binding (μg-Equiv./g protein)	B/A†
$2 \cdot 84 \pm 0 \cdot 26$	Rat	Liver	$5 \cdot 28 \pm 0 \cdot 14$	$1 \cdot 86$
		Kidney	$13 \cdot 14 \pm 1 \cdot 25$	$4 \cdot 63$
$5 \cdot 27 \pm 0 \cdot 74$	Mouse	Liver	$22 \cdot 29 \pm 3 \cdot 77$	$4 \cdot 23$
		Kidney	$79 \cdot 55 \pm 19 \cdot 11$	$15 \cdot 09$

All values represent the mean ± s.d. for three animals.
† Covalent binding data normalized to account for differences in vinylidene chloride metabolism.

kidney). Further, the increased DNA synthesis observed in the target tissue for tumour development in the mouse, but not in non-target tissues of the mouse or in the rat, correlated well with the observed chronic tissue damage which preceded tumour development in the mouse kidney. This latter observation had significant implications for the mechanisms of tumourigenicity in the mouse and the attendant risk assessment of vinylidene chloride (Watanabe *et al.*, 1980).

Extrapolation from animal data to man

In general, there are two approaches to the problem of extrapolation of animal toxicity data to man. In both instances, ADME data are helpful in facilitating the extrapolation process.

The first situation, which I will call 'qualitative extrapolation', is simply trying to determine the suitability of the animal model of toxicity as a reasonable representative for man. In this case, we are usually seeking assurance that a given effect observed in our animal testing can be expected to occur in man. In other words, we need to determine whether the animal model is comparable to man in terms of chemical disposition and metabolism. Such information is also useful in dealing with the absence of adverse effects as well.

In the second situation, 'quantitative extrapolation', we are usually faced with the problem of estimating exposure, or the potential for resultant injury in man, based upon limited knowledge of human chemical disposition and more substantial data for laboratory animals. This is almost always a more difficult task. However, recent advances in mathematical modelling techniques, most notably the use of physiological-based modelling as a tool for 'scale-up' from rat to man, have greatly improved our capability in this area. I believe that this type of modelling will see increasing use in the future in toxicology, and will eventually replace traditional compartmental analysis as a tool for pharmacokinetic analysis. This should be a distinct advantage to the toxicologist as an extrapolation tool, since, as its name implies, physiological-based modelling is more intuitively understood by most biologists.

The application of physiological-based modelling will be discussed in the next chapter. However, an example follows of a comparative chemical disposition study and how relatively simple data can be used to increase our confidence in the reliability of animal models as predictors for man.

Data on the pharmacokinetics and metabolism of methylene chloride in rats was explained above. Of particular interest at the time these data were obtained was the question of whether one could expect a similar profile of dose-dependent pharmacokinetics in man and, more specifically, whether saturation of the metabolic pathway leading to carbon monoxide might limit the formation of carboxyhaemoglobin in man as it did in rodents. In order to answer

Table 6. Steady-state measurement and calculated uptake rates obtained for six male volunteers during inhalation of methylene chloride.

Methylene chloride (p.p.m.)			Uptake rate (mg/min)
Inhaled air	Exhaled air	Blood	
100	44 ± 3	1·05 ± 0·10	1·02 ± 0·26
350	194 ± 8	5·86 ± 0·49	2·83 ± 0·72

All values represent the mean ± s.d. for six men. Uptake rates were calculated as described in the text.

these questions we conducted a study of the pharmacokinetics of inhaled methylene chloride in normal male volunteers (McKenna *et al.*, 1980).

In two well-separated experiments, six healthy male volunteers were exposed to 100 and 350 p.p.m. methylene chloride during each of two exposure periods lasting for six hours. Measurements of blood methylene chloride and carboxy-haemoglobin levels, and methylene chloride and carbon monoxide in expired air, were performed during exposure and for the 24 h period thereafter. Evidence for the dose-dependent pharmacokinetics of inhaled methylene chloride is evident from an analysis of the measurements of the solvent in whole blood and expired air at apparent steady-state during the inhalation exposure (Table 6). A 3·5-fold increase in the concentration of methylene chloride in the inspired air resulted in disproportionately greater increments in the concentration of the solvent found in both the expired air and blood. These data suggest that with increasing exposure concentration the net result is less metabolism (i.e., net uptake of the solvent is less, resulting in greater expired air concentrations) and therefore higher circulating blood levels of methylene chloride.

Table 6 also summarizes the calculated rates of uptake of the solvent at steady state during exposure to either 100 or 350 p.p.m. methylene chloride. Given the assumption that once steady-state is achieved and further uptake of the solvent is proportional to the rate of biotransformation, an uptake rate was calculated for each individual using the concentrations in inspired and exhaled air and respiratory minute volume. This technique has been applied previously to the uptake of anaesthetic gases (Fiserova-Bergerova & Holaday, 1979). Although the data might suggest dose dependency, the variability in respiratory minute volume measurements among individual participants in the study makes it difficult to fully appreciate.

A more consistent indicator, and one which allowed for reliable comparison with data from other investigators, was to simply remove the variable of respiratory minute volume from the calculation, and look at the difference in inspired versus expired air concentrations of the solvent at apparent steady state. Such an evaluation of the data from our experiment, as well as similar

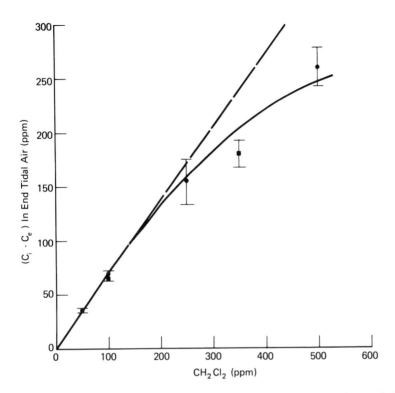

Figure 4. Dose-dependent uptake of methylene chloride at apparent steady state during inhalation exposure of normal male volunteers. The graph is a composite of results from experiments in two laboratories. (See text for details.) ●, Stewart *et al.* (1976), ■, McKenna *et al.* (1980).

data calculated from studies by Stewart and co-workers (1976) are shown in Figure 4. For this comparison, we used only the difference between inspired and expired air concentrations at apparent steady state during exposure. Combining the data from the two laboratories allowed a clear demonstration of the influence of dose-dependent metabolism of methylene chloride over a wide range of exposure concentrations, 50–500 p.p.m. The data indicate a deviation from linear or first-order metabolism at approximately 200–250 p.p.m.

The metabolic pathway for methylene chloride leading to carbon monoxide was of particular interest. Figure 5 shows the influence of methylene chloride exposure concentration of the formation of carboxyhaemoglobin; data from Dr Stewart's experiments are shown as well as our own. Despite the variability in end-exposure carboxyhaemoglobin measurements there is still good agreement between both experiments. These data indicate the dose-dependent character of carboxyhaemoglobin formation following methylene chloride exposure, and a maximum carboxyhaemoglobin concentration of 10–12% is suggested. The curve deviates from linearity at about 200–250 p.p.m.

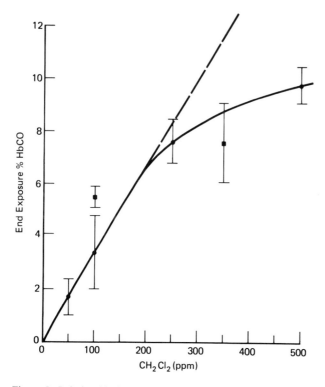

Figure 5. Relationship between end-exposure blood carboxyhaemoglobin values and methylene chloride exposure concentrations from studies of the pharmacokinetics of inhaled methylene chloride in normal male volunteers. The data are a composite of results from experiments in two laboratories. (See text for details.) ●, Stewart *et al.* (1976); ■, McKenna *et al.* (1980).

In summary, these experiments suggest that the dose-dependent phar-macokinetics of inhaled methylene chloride in man is similar to that observed in the rat. In both species, saturable metabolic pathways influen:e the uptake of the solvent and the ultimate body burden acquired during exposure. Devia-tion from linear pharmacokinetics occurs in both species at exposure concen-trations of approximately 200–250 p.p.m. methylene chloride. Also, the rela-tionship between solvent exposure and resultant blood carboxyhaemoglobin values is similar in both species. Thus it appears that, at least from a phar-macokinetic standpoint, the rat is a reasonable laboratory animal model for extrapolation to man. However, in making such comparisons it is important to emphasize that the relationship between the dose-dependent metabolism of methylene chloride and the toxicity of the solvent is not fully understood. Although pharmacokinetic data provide useful tools to the toxicologist, they are of limited value without a perspective on their relevance to toxicity. Therefore, we must recognize that although similarity in metabolic and kinetic behaviour of chemicals in laboratory animals and man lends credibility to the use of a particular animal model, the process of risk assessment must encompass all the data available from both laboratory studies and our daily experience in the use of such chemicals.

In concluding, I hope that this brief overview of the application of ADME data has provided some useful ideas to approaching the design and interpretation of laboratory assessments of toxicity as well as extrapolation to man. As with many of the tools which the toxicologist has at his disposal, the technology in this particular area has grown rapidly over recent years. The challenge for the future is to fully integrate these tools into the assessment of toxicity and safety for man.

References

Burek, J. D., Nitschke, K. D., Bell, T. J., Wackerle, D. L., Childs, R. C., Beyer, J. E., Dittenber, D. A., Rampy, L. W. and McKenna, M. J., 1984, Methylene chloride: a two-year inhalation toxicity and oncogenicity study in rats and hamsters. *Fund. appl. Tox.* **4**, (1), 30–47.

Fiserova-Bergerova, V. and Holaday, D. A., 1979, Uptake and clearance of inhalation anesthetics in man. *Drug. Metab. Rev.*, **9**, 43–60.

Jaeger, R. J., Connally, R. and Murphy, S. D., 1974, Effect of 18-hour fast and glutathione depletion on 1,1-dichloroethylene-induced hepatotoxicity and lethality in rats. *Exp. Molec. Path.*, **20**, 187–198.

Lee, C. C., Bhandari, J. C., Winston, J. M., Dixon, R. L. and Woods, J. S., 1978, Carcinogenicity of vinyl chloride and vinylidene chloride. *J. Tox. Envir. Hlth.*, **4**, 15–30.

Levy, G., 1968, Dose-dependent effects in pharmacokinetics. In *Importance of Fundamental Principles in Drug Evaluation*, edited by D. H. Tedeschi and R. E. Tedeschi (New York: Raven Press), pp. 141–172.

Maltoni, C., Cotti, G., Morisi, L. and Chieco, P., 1977, Carcinogenicity bioassays of vinylidene chloride: research plan and early results. *Medicina del Lavoro*, **68**, 241–262.

McKenna, M. J., Watanabe, P. G. and Gehring, P. J., 1977, Pharmacokinetics of vinylidene chloride. *Envir. Hlth. Perspect.*, **21**, 99–105,

McKenna, M. J., Zempel, J. A., Madrid, E. O. and Gehring, P. J., 1978, The pharmacokinetics of ^{14}C-vinylidene chloride in rats following inhalation exposure. *Toxic. appl. Pharmac.*, **45**, 599–610.

McKenna, M. J., Saunders, J. H., Boeckler, W. H., Karbowski, R. J., Nitschke, K. D. and Chenoweth, M. B., 1980, The pharmacokinetics of inhaled methylene chloride in human volunteers. *Society of Toxicology Abstracts of Papers*, March 1980. (Washington, DC: Academic Press), Abstract No. 176.

McKenna, M. J., Zempel, J. A. and Braun, W. H., 1982, The pharmacokinetics of inhaled methylene chloride in rats. *Toxic. appl. Pharmac.*, **65**, 1–10.

National Toxicology Program, 1984, *Report of the NTP ad hoc Panel on Chemical Carcinogenesis Testing and Evaluation* (Research Triangle Park, NC: US Dept of Health and Human Services (PHS)), pp. 125–140.

Rampy, L. W., Quast, J. F., Humiston, C. G., Balmer, M.F. and Schwetz, B. A., 1977, Interim results of two year toxicological studies in rats of vinylidene chloride incorporated in the drinking water or administered by repeated inhalation. *Envir. Hlth. Perspect.*, **21**, 33–43.

Reitz, R. R., Watanabe, P. G., McKenna, M. J., Quast, J. F. and Gehring, P. J., 1980, Effects of vinylidene chloride on DNA synthesis and DNA repair in the rat and mouse: a comparative study with dimethylnitrosamine. *Toxic. appl. Pharmac.*, **53**, 357–370.

Stewart, R. D., Hake, C. L. and Wu, A., 1976, Use of breath analysis to monitor methylene chloride exposure. *Scand. J. Work, Environ. Hlth.*, **2**, 57–70.

Viola, P. L. and Caputo, A., 1977, Carcinogenicity studies on vinylidene chloride. *Envir. Hlth. Perspect.*, **21**, 45–47.

Watanabe, P. G., Reitz, R. H., Schumann, A. M., McKenna, M. J., Quast, J. F. and Gehring, P. J., 1980, Implications of the mechanisms of tumorigenicity for risk assessment. In *The Scientific Basis of Toxicity Assessment*, edited by H. Witschi, (New York: Elsevier/North-Holland Biomedical Press), pp. 69–89.

Physiologically based pharmacokinetics and methylene chloride cancer risk assessment considerations[†]

Melvin E. Andersen, Harvey J. Clewell III and Richard H. Reitz[‡]

Biochemical Toxicology Branch, Toxic Hazards Division, Armstrong Aerospace Medical Research Laboratory, Wright-Patterson AFB, OH 45433–6573, USA and ‡Toxicology Research Laboratory, Dow Chemical USA, 1803 Building, Midland, MI, 48674, USA

Introduction

Inhalation bioassays of methylene chloride (CH_2Cl_2; dichloromethane; DCM) have been conducted with Golden Syrian hamsters, Fischer 344 rats and B6C3F1 mice (Burek *et al.*, 1984; National Toxicology Program, 1985). The studies in hamsters at exposure concentrations up to 3500 p.p.m., six hours/day, five days/week for two years, were essentially negative. Results with rats were equivocal but showed an increase in benign mammary tumours at exposure concentrations of 2000 or 4000 p.p.m. In contrast, the recent bioassay in mice showed very significant dose-related increases in the incidence of tumours in both liver and lung at exposure concentrations of 2000 and 4000 p.p.m. (Table 1). These observations have prompted the US Environmental Protection Agency (EPA) to review their DCM risk assessment with an eye towards its control as a suspect human carcinogen (EPA, 1985). This review has included a traditional risk assessment involving linear extrapolation of external dose in exposed mice, combined with an inter-species correction factor based on body surface area.

There has been increasing interest among regulatory agencies in incorporating pharmacokinetic principles into the cancer risk assessment process. DCM is a good candidate for a pharmacokinetic risk assessment because its metabolism, distribution and kinetic profiles have been thoroughly examined in several animal species. A physiologically-based pharmacokinetic (PB-PK) model has been developed for dihalomethanes (Gargas *et al.*, 1986) and is especially well suited for its use in risk calculations because it easily supports

---

† This work is a condensation of a paper, "Physiologically-Based pharmacokinetics and the Risk Assessment Process for Methylene Chloride" (Andersen *et al.*, 1987), which has been published in *Toxicology and Applied Pharmacology*.

Table 1. Incidence of lung and liver tumours in B6C3F1 mice with lifetime exposure to dichloromethane (six hours/day, five days/week).

	Incidence of tumours after exposure to CH_2Cl_2 at various conc.					
	Liver tumours			Lung tumours		
	0 p.p.m.	2000 p.p.m.	4000 p.p.m.	0 p.p.m.	2000 p.p.m.	4000 p.p.m.
Males						
Adenoma	20[a]	29	29	6	38	48
Carcinoma	26	31	53	4	20	56
Combined	44	49	67	10	54	80
Females						
Adenoma	4	13	46	4	48	58
Carcinoma	2	23	67	2	27	60
Combined	6	33	83	6	63	85

[a] Results are percentage of exposed group with a particular tumour type. In all cases initial group sizes were 50. For purposes of this report note the clear-cut dose response as exposure concentration is increased from 2000 to 4000 p.p.m. (National Toxicology Program, 1985).

both dose-route and inter-species extrapolations of kinetic behaviour. This PB-PK model permits calculation of internal doses by integrating information on administered dose, physiological properties of the mammalian species, and biochemical and physiochemical properties of methylene chloride. Predicted measures of internal dose can be correlated with toxicity or tumour incidence to yield hypotheses for the mechanisms of toxicity. In this chapter, we develop a PB-PK model for DCM, use the model to support a proposed mechanism of DCM carcinogenicity, and compare cancer risk calculated by this model with risk estimated by the more conventional regulatory approaches to the cancer risk assessment.

Methods

The PB-PK model

The model developed for DCM considered metabolism in both target tissues, the lung and liver, and accounted for metabolism by both mixed-function oxidation (MFO) and by conjugation (Figure 1) with glutathione (GSH). The model itself was very similar to that described by Ramsey & Andersen (1984) for styrene, except for the explicit inclusion of a lung tissue (Figure 2) with specified volume, DCM solubility and DCM-metabolizing activities. With any PB-PK model, three kinds of data are required: tissue partition coefficients, physiological parameters for the test species, and biochemical constants for binding/metabolism of the chemical in biological tissues.

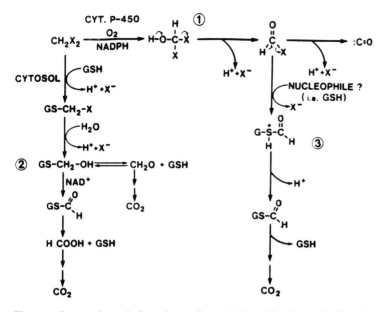

Figure 1. Proposed metabolic pathways for methylene chloride metabolism (based on Ahmed & Anders (1978) and Kubic *et al.* (1974)). Potentially reactive intermediates are formed in each pathway: formyl chloride in the CYT P-450 (MFO) pathway and chloromethyl glutathione in the cytosolic (GST) pathway. Either metabolic pathway can produce carbon dioxide in this scheme, but only the MFO pathway yields carbon monoxide and elevated carboxyhaemoglobin concentrations.

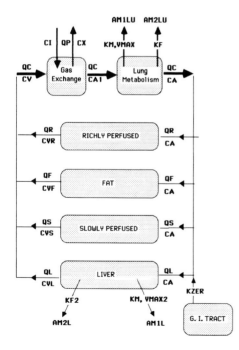

Figure 2. Diagram of the physiologically-based pharmacokinetic (PB-PK) model utilized for dichloromethane (DCM). This model is an adaptation of the one used previously by Ramsey & Andersen (1984) to describe the metabolism of styrene. Body tissues are grouped into five compartments: lung, fat, liver, richly perfused and slowly perfused. Metabolism occurs in the lung and liver compartments. DCM enters the body through inhalation with absorption into pulmonary blood in the gas exchange compartment or by ingestion with absorption directly into the liver compartment.

Partition coefficients

Partition coefficients were estimated by a vial-equilibration method (Sato & Nakajima, 1979). Blood/air partition coefficients were determined in mouse (B6C3F1), rat (Fischer 344), hamster (Golden Syrian) and human blood. Tissue partitions were determined for rat and hamster samples. The tissue partitions for human and mouse tissues were not determined directly but were set equal to those of the rat (Table 2).

Table 2. Kinetic constants and model parameters used in the physiologically-based pharmacokinetic model for dichloromethane.

Constants/parameters	B6C3F1 Mice[†]	Human
Weights (kg)		
Body weight	0·0345	70·0
Lung ($\times 10^3$)	0·410	772·0
% body weight		
Liver	4·0	3·14
Rapidly perfused tissues	5·0	3·71
Slowly perfused tissues	78·0	62·1
Fat	4·0	23·1
Flows (l/h)		
Alveolar ventilation	2·32	348·0
Cardiac output	2·32	348·0
% Cardiac output		
Liver	0·24	0·24
Rapidly perfused tissues	0·52	0·52
Slowly perfused tissues	0·19	0·19
Fat	0·05	0·05
Partition coefficients		
Blood/air	8·29	9·7
Liver/blood	1·71	1·46
Lung/blood	1·71	1·46
Rapidly perfused/blood	1·71	1·46
Slowly perfused/blood	0·960	0·82
Fat/blood	14·5	12·4
Metabolic constants		
Oxidation: $V_{max \text{ (mg/h)}}$	1·054	118·9
K_m(mg/l)	0·396	0·580
Conjugation clearance (ml/h)	4·67	1174
A1[‡]	0·416	0·00143
A2[§]	0·137	0·0473

[†] Parameters correspond to the average body weight of B6C3F1 mice in the NTP Bioassay (National Toxicology Program, 1985).
[‡] Ratio of lung mixed-function oxidase and liver mixed-function oxidase activity (from Lorenz *et al.*, 1984).
[§] Ratio of lung glutathione-*S*-transferase and liver glutathione-*S*-transferase activity (from Lorenz *et al.*, 1984).

Physiological constants

Values chosen for physiological constants were similar to those used in other physiological models (Ramsey & Andersen, 1984; Gargas *et al.*, 1986). Lung weight was estimated from Leith (1976) and ventilation rates were based on the results of gas-uptake studies with soluble, well-metabolized vapours at concentrations where metabolism was not saturated. The ventilation rates in mice were observed to be larger than expected from the allometric constant determined by Guyton (1947). The allometric constant for mice was twice as large as that used for rats.

Biochemical constants

DCM is metabolized by mixed-function oxidation and by conjugation with GSH. In small experimental animals, whole-body rates of metabolism by these two pathways can be determined by gas-uptake techniques (Gargas *et al.*, 1986). For the present study, whole-body metabolism for these two pathways was apportioned between lung and liver by assuming the distribution of enzymes metabolizing DCM was the same as the distribution of enzymes acting upon the model substrates, 7-ethoxycoumarin for oxidation and 2,4-dinitrochlorobenzene for GSH conjugation (Lorenz *et al.*, 1984). With humans, there is ample evidence to establish *in vivo* kinetic constants for DCM oxidation (Andersen *et al.*, 1987), but the activity of the GSH pathway must be estimated indirectly. For this model, the human GSH activity was set equal to the highest activity found in experimental animals. Thus in rats and mice, the weight-adjusted clearance was 60 ml/h with a body weight exponent of 0·7. This same value was used with the human, giving a GSH pathway clearance of 1174 ml/h (Table 2).

The mass-balance equations for lung and liver contained terms accounting for the rate of loss of DCM by metabolism in these tissues (dAM_{ti}/dt; mg/h):

$$\frac{dAM_{ti}}{dt} = \frac{V_{max,ti} \times C_{v,ti}}{K_m + C_{v,ti}} + kf \times V_{ti} \times C_{v,ti}$$

In this equation the first term accounts for loss of DCM by microsomal oxidation, which is described as a saturable metabolic process. The second term accounts for metabolism by GSH conjugation, described as a first-order process at all accessible DCM concentrations. Clearance by the GSH pathway is equivalent to the ($kf \times V_{ti}$) term. $V_{max,ti}$ is the maximum velocity of oxidation in a particular tissue (mg/h); K_m is the Michaelis constant for the binding of DCM to the enzyme (mg/l); $C_{v,ti}$ is the DCM concentration in venous blood from the tissue (mg/l); V_{ti} is the tissue volume (l); and kf is the first-order rate constant for the GSH pathway (h^{-1}). A more complete development of this model is provided by Gargas *et al.* (1986).

Results

Kinetic results

Kinetic results for DCM metabolism in mice were estimated from a series of closed-chamber exposures (Figure 3). Similar studies have been conducted with hamsters and rats (not shown) and provide the kinetic constants for metabolism (Table 2). Human oxidative kinetic constants were set from studies conducted by R. J. Nolan & M. J. McKenna (unpublished data) at Dow Chemical Company. The complete PB-PK model accounted for the behaviour of DCM inhalation in humans and of intravascular injection in mice (Figure 4).

Analysis of dose surrogates

The PB-PK model for DCM in mice was used to analyse two bioassays conducted in this species. One bioassay, conducted for the National Coffee Association by ingestion of DCM in drinking water at 250 mg/l was essentially negative (Serota *et al.*, 1984). The inhalation bioassay was positive, with a clear-cut dose dependence between 2000 and 4000 p.p.m. (Table 1). The DCM model was used to estimate lung and liver exposure to parent chemical and to

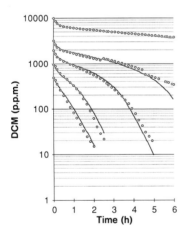

Figure 3. Gas uptake results with male B6C3F1 mice. Groups of about 15 mice are placed in a 9 l desiccator jar chamber. A small amount of DCM is injected and the loss of chamber DCM from the chamber is followed for a period of three to six hours. Semi-logarithmic plots are chamber concentration versus time after injection for a variety of initial concentrations. The complex curves can be analysed by computer simulation utilizing a physiological model. This analysis provides estimates of the kinetic constants for both oxidative metabolism and metabolism of DCM by conjugation with GSH (Table 1). The smooth curves are from the physiological model developed in this paper and in Andersen *et al.* (1987).

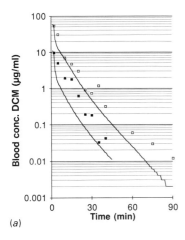
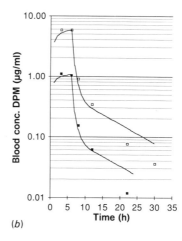

(a)

(b)

Figure 4. Validation of the PB-PK Model with experimental data. (a) Shows blood concentration/time data obtained in B6C3F1 mice following intravenous administration of 10 or 50 mg DCM/kg (Angelo *et al.*, 1984). (b) Presents data obtained in humans during and following inhalation exposure for six hours to 100 or 350 p.p.m. with a 24 h post-exposure observation (R. J. Nolan & M. J. McKenna, Dow Chemical USA, unpublished data, 1984). In each case, the simulated data is presented as a solid line, while the experimental data is shown with closed or open symbols. The model faithfully reproduces behaviour in both species.

the metabolites produced by each of two pathways of DCM metabolism. Exposure to parent is expressed as the area under the time-course curve for parent chemical in the target tissue. This measure of tissue exposure has units of (mg × h)/l. For short-lived reactive metabolites, the actual time-course of reactive intermediate in tissue cannot be determined and a surrogate measure of exposure must be developed. In this case, the surrogate should be proportional to the area under the tissue concentration versus time-course curve for the metabolite. The surrogate used for both pathways was total amount metabolized/tissue volume (Andersen *et al.*, 1987). When these dose surrogates are calculated for the mouse bioassays, tumour incidence is seen to correlate with parent chemical or glutathione pathway conjugates, but not with metabolites produced by oxidation (Table 3). Because of its low reactivity, DCM is unlikely to be directly involved in tumour initiation, and the most likely hypothesis is that metabolites of the GSH pathway are involved in cancer initiation.

Predicting human tissue doses

The human PB-PK DCM model can be exercised to predict tissue exposure as a function of the particular environmental exposure concentration. For instance, the predicted target tissue doses resulting from inhalation of various concentrations of DCM for six hours were calculated for the two species of

Table 3. Calculated target tissue dose surrogates for the two mouse bioassays conducted with dichloromethane.

	Target tissue dose	
	Inhalation study†	Drinking water study‡
Microsomal oxidation§		
Liver	5420	5650
Lung	2640	1580
Glutathione conjugation§		
Liver	1480	8·3
Lung	207	0·6
Methylene chloride‖		
Liver	1100	6·2
Lung	1120	3·1

† The inhalation bioassay conducted at 2000 and 4000 p.p.m. The calculations are for the 400 p.p.m. exposures.

‡ The National Coffee Association drinking water study. Calculations are for the highest concentration used, 250 mg/l, and were done assuming zero-order absorption during the day (Andersen *et al.*, 1987).

§ Units are mg metabolized by the pathway/volume of target tissue for a 24 h period in the study.

‖ Units are mg DCM/h/l for any 24 h period in the study. For this study note that there are large differences in the two studies when GSH conjugate or DCM area under the curve are calculated but not for the microsomal oxidation pathway.

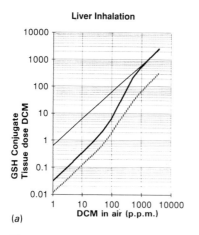
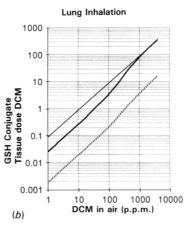

(a)   (b)

Figure 5. Relationship of tissue dose and external exposure concentration for both humans and mice: glutathione pathway. The PB-PK model was used to determine target tissue dose from the GSH pathway in both liver (*a*) and lung (*b*) at various exposure concentrations in humans and mice. Tissue dose is given as the total amount metabolized during a 24 h period divided by tissue volume, a surrogate proportional to the area under the toxic metabolite concentration versus time curve in the target tissues (Andersen *et al.*, 1987). Dose surrogates for mice are the solid lines; those for humans are the heavy dashed lines. A reference line depicting linear back extrapolation to 1 p.p.m. is shown as the lighter solid line to facilitate comparison of curvature in the other curves.

interest, mouse and human, and the two tissues of interest, liver and lung (Figure 5). These figures show a third line generated by linear back-extrapolation of the behaviour at the experimental concentrations of the bioassay. These curves show that target tissue dosage in humans is expected to be lower than that in mice at all concentrations and the tissue dose in mice at low concentrations is less than expected by a linear back-extrapolation of the high-concentration behaviour.

Discussion

PB-PK models and risk analysis

Model output of target tissue dose can be used as the basis for risk analysis in humans. On the simplest level, we can analyse the curves in Figure 5 to evaluate human tissue dose for six hours per day inhalation exposure dose. For the liver, the mouse tissue dose at 1 p.p.m. is 20·8-fold lower than predicted by linear back extrapolation. The non-linear behaviour in the mouse occurs because the oxidative pathway is favoured at low concentrations but is readily saturated at inhaled concentrations above several hundred parts per million. The human dose is some 2·74 times lower than that for the mouse. In total then, the human tissue dose at 1 p.p.m. is some 57 times lower than expected by linear back extrapolation of the results in mice. In contrast, the EPA approach is to increase the dose value obtained by linear back extrapolation by 2·95 to account for differences in surface area and breathing rates between mouse and humans. The net result is that tissue dose and risks estimated by the PB-PK model are lower by a factor of $57 \times 2·95$ or about 168, than those calculated by the approach currently used by the EPA (1985).

When a similar analysis is conducted for tissue dose to the lung, the PB-PK assessment predicts an internal tissue dose at 1 p.p.m. that is lower by a factor of 143 than that calculated in the more conventional approach to risk assessment (Andersen *et al.*, 1987 for details of these calculations). When appropriate data are available, PB-PK models can be useful in providing a better estimation of delivered dose in real-world human exposure situations. These PB-PK models have great promise for improving risk analysis because they are readily amenable to the low-dose, inter-species, and dose-route extrapolations necessary to convert validated animal models to be predictive of pharmacokinetic behaviour in humans.

Several additional experimental pieces of data would be useful to refine the DCM model for humans. They include: (1) the distribution of oxidizing and conjugating activities for DCM in human lung and liver and (2) the total glutathione transferase activity toward DCM in humans *in vivo*. For this model, the former was estimated from Lorenz *et al.* (1984) with non-DCM substrates while the latter was estimated by allometric scaling of DCM gas-uptake results in three rodent species (i.e., mouse, rat and hamster). Even lacking these data at the moment (studies are underway to determine these constants), this PB-PK model for DCM appears sufficiently well-validated to be used for risk assessment calculations and can be improved as newer data are obtained.

PB-PK models provide more complete understanding of target tissue dose in various species under various exposure situations. By applying these improved estimates of tissue dose, the risk-assessment process can be similarly refined. However, there is a fundamental underlying assumption in using animal toxicity results to estimate human risk − that all species are equally sensitive to chemical injury once the appropriate measure of tissue dose is defined. This fundamental assumption may not be valid with DCM. Excess tumours were not observed in inhalation bioassays with hamsters, even though tissue doses of DCM and its metabolites should be nearly as great as those achieved in the B6C3F1 mice. Perhaps the production of a particular tissue dose is a necessary but not sufficient stimulus to cause tumours. It may be that DCM or its GSH metabolite(s) act to promote rather than to initiate a carcinogenic response. In this case host factors such as intrinsic background cancer rates may be important in the ultimate response to DCM.

References

Ahmed, A. E. and Anders, M. W., 1978, Metabolism of dihalomethanes to formaldehyde and inorganic halide. I. *In vitro* studies. *Drug Metab. Disp.*, **4**, 357–361.

Andersen, M. E., Clewell III, H. J., Gargas, M. L., Smith, F. A. and Reitz, R. H., 1987, Physiologically-based pharmacokinetics and the risk assessment process for methylene chloride. *Toxic. appl. Pharmac.* **87**, 185–205.

Angelo, M. J., Bischoff, K. B., Pritchard, A. B. and Presser, M. A., 1984, A physiological model for the pharmacokinetics of methylene chloride in B6C3F1 mice following iv administration. *J. Pharmac. Biopharm.*, **12**, 413–436.

Burek, J. D., Nitschke, K. D., Bell, T. J., Waskerle, D. L., Childs, R. C., Beyer, J. D., Dittenber, D. A., Rampy, L. W. and McKenna, M. J., 1984, Methylene chloride: a two-year inhalation toxicity and oncogenicity study in rats and hamsters. *Fund. appl. Tox.*, **4**, 30–47.

EPA, 1985, Addendum to the health assessment document for dichloromethane (methylene chloride). Updated Carcinogen Assessment for Dichloromethane, EPA-600/8-82-004F (Washington, DC: Environmental Protection Agency).

Gargas, M. L., Clewell III, H. J., and Andersen, M. E., 1986, Metabolism of inhaled dihalomethanes *in vivo*: differentiation of kinetic constants for two independent pathways. *Toxic. appl. Pharmac.*, **2**, 211–223.

Guyton, A. C., 1947, Respiratory volumes of laboratory animals. *Am. J. Physiol.*, **150**, 70–77.

Kubic, V. L., Anders, M. W., Engel, R. R., Barlow, C. H. and Caughey, W. S., 1974, Metabolism of dihalomethanes to carbon monoxide. I. *In vivo* studies. *Drug Metab. Disp.*, **2**, 211–223.

Leith, D. E., 1976, Comparative mammalian respiratory mechanics. *Physiologist*, **19** 485–510.

Lorenz, J., Glatt, H. R., Fleischmann, R., Ferlinz, R. and Oesch, F., 1984, Drug metabolism in man and its relationship to that in three rodent species: monooxygenase, epoxide hydrolyase, and glutathione-*S*-transferase activities in subcellular fractions of lung and liver. *Biochem. Med.*, **32**, 43–56.

National Toxicology Program, 1985, NTP Technical Report on the Toxicology and Carcinogenesis Studies of Dichloromethane in F-344/N Rats and B6C3F1 Mice (Inhalation Studies), NTP-TR-306 (Board Draft), (Springfield, VA: Nat. Tech. Information Service).

Ramsey, J. R. and Andersen, M. E., 1984, A physiologically based description of the inhalation pharmacokinetics of styrene in rats and humans. *Toxic. appl. Pharmac.*, **73**, 159–175.

Sato, A. and Nakajima, T., 1979, Partition coefficients of some aromatic hydrocarbons and ketones in water, blood, and oil. *Br. J. ind. Med.*, **36**, 231–234.

Serota, D., Ulland, B. and Carlborg, F., 1984, Hazelton Chronic Oral Study in Mice. Food Solvents Workshop I: Methylene Chloride, 8–9 March, Bethesda, Maryland.

Route of exposure: an important consideration in animal selection and the design of toxicity studies

James S. Bus†

Department of Biochemical Toxicology and Pathobiology, Chemical Industry Institute of Toxicology, Research Triangle Park, NC 27709 USA

Introduction

Toxic responses associated with exposure to environmental agents are a reflection of a complex series of interactions within the organism. Environmental exposure to a chemical is not always indicative of the likelihood of a toxic response, as biological factors such as absorption, distribution, metabolism (including both toxication and detoxication reactions) and excretion all play important roles in modulating chemical toxicity (Bus & Gibson, 1985). Thus, the amount of chemical or metabolite that is delivered to the macromolecule(s) responsible for eliciting cell toxicity ultimately involves the interplay of numerous biological factors.

The first factor that serves as a critical modulator of chemical toxicity is the barrier to absorption, whether that be at the lung, skin, gastro-intestinal tract or other sites. Since the route of administration clearly affects the nature of the initial absorption barrier that a chemical encounters, and consequently the amount of chemical that is absorbed, it is an important factor to be considered when designing or interpreting toxicology studies. There are two questions that need consideration when determining the involvement of the route of administration in toxicology studies. First, what variations in toxicity might result when similar routes of administration are employed across species lines? This question is of obvious importance when the toxicologist is faced with the problem of extrapolating results obtained in animal models to what might potentially occur in man, even though the animal model may have been exposed by the route most relevant to man. The second question is what variations in toxicity may occur when different routes of administration are employed for a chemical within or across species lines? Thus depending on the chemical being studied, selection of an inappropriate route of administration may have major consequences on the interpretation of the toxicological study.

†Present address: Upjohn Company, Pathology/Toxicology Research, Kalamazoo, MI 49007.

The primary purpose of this chapter is to address the above questions through the use of several examples in which the route of administration has been shown to be a factor relevant to understanding the toxic potential associated with a chemical exposure. The examples are not meant to be comprehensive, but rather to provide a basis for perspective when issues relating to route of administration are encountered in toxicology studies.

Inhalation as a route of administration

Formaldehyde is an example of an inhaled toxicant with a widespread environmental distribution. It is of interest in that it is not only an irritant of the upper respiratory tract but, more importantly, has been identified in a recent animal bioassay to produce tumours of the upper respiratory tract (Swenberg *et al.*, 1983). Formaldehyde serves as an example of the situation described in the first question described above – the use of similar routes of administration resulting in dissimilar toxicological responses. Two species, rats and mice, were evaluated in the rodent bioassay of formaldehyde. Chronic exposure of rats to approximately 15 p.p.m. formaldehyde resulted in a 44% incidence of squamous cell carcinoma in the nasal cavity. Mice similarly exposed exhibited only a 1% incidence of this tumour. At an exposure of 6 p.p.m., the incidence of squamous cell carcinoma was reduced to 1% in rats and 0% in mice. The bioassay results obtained with formaldehyde, therefore, suggest a significant variation in species sensitivity although similar routes of administration were evaluated.

A series of investigations have provided insight into the mechanism of the marked difference in the response of rats and mice to formaldehyde. The upper respiratory tracts of mammals contain receptors which respond to the stimuli of irritant materials by initiating a reflex which results in a rapid decrease in respiratory rate (Alarie, 1973). Since the decrease in respiratory rate is not compensated for by an increase in tidal volume, the net result of the activation of the reflex is a reduction in minute volume. It is thought that the purpose of the reflex mechanism is to reduce exposure of the cells lining the upper respiratory tract to irritant compounds. In the case of formaldehyde exposure, however, it has been shown that the species used in the bioassay do not exhibit quantitatively similar reflex responses (Chang *et al.*, 1983). Rats responded to 15 p.p.m. formaldehyde with only a slight reduction in minute volume while mice showed a significantly greater reduction in minute volume (Figure 1(*a*)).

The fact that formaldehyde is a very water-soluble gas, and therefore is effectively scavenged by the upper respiratory tract (Egle, 1972), and that rodents are obligatory nose breathers, which results in passage of the entire inhaled dose through the upper respiratory tract, allows for a more direct calculation of the true 'delivered dose' in both species. Morphometric tech-

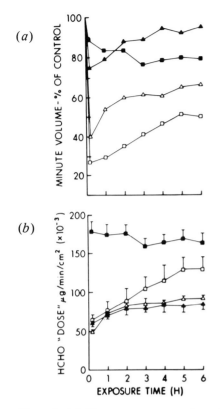

Figure 1. (*a*) Time–response curves for minute volume from rats and mice exposed to 6 or 15 p.p.m. formaldehyde for 6 hr. (*b*) Time-weighted averages of the theoretical formaldehyde dose available for deposition on cells of the nasal cavity of rats and mice during a six hour exposure to 6 or 15 p.p.m. formaldehyde. Reprinted with permission from Swenberg *et al.* (1983). ■, Rats (15 p.p.m.); □, mice (15 p.p.m.); ▲, rats (6 p.p.m.); △, mice (6 p.p.m.).

niques have led to the estimation of the surface area of the nasal cavities of both mice and rats (Gross *et al.*, 1982), from which the delivered dose of formaldehyde to the upper respiratory tract can be more realistically estimated by the following formula:

$$\text{Delivered dose} = \frac{\text{HCHO concentration } (\mu g/l) \times \text{minute volume } (l/min)}{\text{nasal cavity surface area } (cm^2)}$$

When the environmental exposure to formaldehyde is 'corrected' in this manner, it becomes apparent that the upper respiratory tract cells of mice receive a substantially lower dose of formaldehyde at equivalent external exposures (Figure 1(*b*)). In fact, because of the marked reduction in minute volume in

Table 1. Formaldehyde-induced tumour incidence in rats and mice: exposure concentration versus delivered dose.

Species	Exposure concentration (p.p.m.)	Delivered† dose	Tumour incidence (%)
Mice	15	57·1	0·83
Rats	6	76·0	0·93
Rats	15	124·5	44·40

† Delivered dose expressed as area under the curve (AUC). taken from HCHO delivered dose versus exposure time graph (Figure 1(*b*); data from Swenberg *et al.*, 1983)

mice exposed to 15 p.p.m. formaldehyde, the actual delivered dose to the nasal cavity at this concentration was comparable to that of rats exposed to 6 p.p.m. of the gas (Table 1). An important outcome from these calculations is that they indicate that equivalent delivered doses result in equivalent tumourigenic responses, suggesting that upper respiratory tract tissue may be intrinsically similar in its biological response to formaldehyde. In addition, the example of formaldehyde indicates that cross-species variations associated with inhalation exposure to upper respiratory tract irritants potentially may be better understood when examined in the context of delivered dose.

Skin as a route of administration

Absorption of chemicals through the skin represents a second major route of exposure to environmental chemicals. Consequently, a significant amount of research has been directed to the development of animal models which predict dermal absorption of chemicals in man (Bronaugh & Maibach, 1985; Wester & Maibach, 1985).

A number of chemicals have been comparatively evaluated for dermal absorption *in vivo* in man and various animal models (Bartek *et al.*, 1972; Bartek & LaBuddle, 1975; Table 2). In general, rabbit skin was the most permeable of the animal systems evaluated, while human skin was the least permeable. Of the non-primate animal models, the skin of the pig appeared to be the best predictor of percutaneous absorption in man, although monkeys most closely approximated dermal absorption *in vivo*. Wester & Maibach (1985), however, have recently commented that comparisons such as those made in Table 2 involve application of the chemical at different sites of the body in the different species tested (the back for rat, rabbit, pig and monkey, and forearm for man). Thus, the differences noted in dermal absorption may not be entirely attributable to true species differences, but also may include

Table 2. Percutaneous absorption of various chemicals *in vivo* by rat, rabbit, pig, monkey and man.

Chemical	% Dose absorbed				
	Rat	Rabbit	Pig	Monkey	Man
Haloprogin	95·8	113·0	19·7	—	11·0
Acetylcysteine	3·5	2·0	6·0	—	2·4
Cortisone	24·7	30·3	4·1	—	3·4
Caffeine	53·1	69·2	32·4	—	47·6
Butter Yellow	48·2	100·0	41·9	—	21·6
Testosterone	47·4	69·6	29·4	—	13·2
DDT	—	46·3	43·4	1·5	10·4
Lindane	—	51·2	37·6	16·0	9·3
Parathion	—	97·5	14·5	30·3	9·7
Malathion	—	64·6	15·5	19·3	8·2

Data from Bartek *et al.* (1972) and Bartek & LaBuddle (1975).

factors such as variations in the composition of skin at the sites examined, and age, sex or condition of the skin evaluated (Wester & Maibach, 1985).

Comparative studies of dermal absorption have been conducted also across species lines using model systems *in vitro* (Bronaugh & Maibach, 1985). The availability of human skin makes this technique somewhat attractive, and several comparative studies have indicated that general ranking of skin permeability across species lines approximates that seen in studies *in vivo* (Table 2; Wester & Maibach, 1985). However, Wester & Maibach (1985) have pointed out that there is little quantitative agreement between the models *in vivo* and *in vitro*, and that the primary value of the systems used *in vitro* may be to qualitatively differentiate between compounds of high permeability and those of low permeability. These authors concluded that the model systems *in vitro*, therefore, will require further validation before results obtained from different animal skins can be evaluated for their relevance to man.

Comparison of toxicity associated with use of different routes of administration within and across species

The interpretation of toxicity data obtained from animal models in which different routes of administration are used for a given chemical is complicated by additional factors beyond those encountered when similar routes of administration are employed. First, agents which are potent irritants may produce their primary toxic effect at the site of application, for example, the upper respiratory tract, skin, or gastro-intestinal tract. Thus, upper respiratory tract tumours resulting from formaldehyde inhalation exposure (Swenberg *et al.*,

1983) would not be expected to occur after oral administration of this agent. A second example is that of a 'first pass' effect, in which the majority of a compound absorbed from a specific site passes through an organ of high metabolic capacity (particularly the liver) for that compound (Klaassen, 1980). Thus, the compound may not escape that organ for systemic distribution to other sites, the result being a reduction in the delivered dose to organs beyond the initial site of absorption. Thirdly, the rate or completeness of absorption may vary with the route of administration. A chemical poorly absorbed from the gut, for example, would be expected to produce significantly less toxicity when administered orally compared to intravenous or other parenteral routes.

Summary

The route of administration is an important determinant in the expression of toxicity associated with environmental exposure to chemicals, as it is the first step which modulates the actual dose delivered to the responsive tissue. Therefore, an appreciation of the potential similarities and differences between species with respect to the role of the route of administration in expression of chemical toxicity is an important element in the extrapolation of animal toxicity data to man.

References

Alarie, Y., 1973, Sensory irritation by airborne chemicals. *CRC Crit. Rev. Tox.*, **2**, 299–363.

Bartek, M. J., LaBuddle, J. A and Maibach, H. I., 1972, Skin permeability *in vivo*: comparison in rat, rabbit, pig and man. *J. Invest. Derm.*, **48**, 114–123.

Bartek, M. J. and LaBuddle, J. A., 1975, Percutaneous absorption *in vitro*. In *Animal Models in Dermatology*, edited by H. I. Maibach (New York: Churchill Livingstone), pp. 103–120.

Bronaugh, R. L. and Maibach, H. I., 1985, *In vitro* models for human percutaneous absorption. In *Models in Dermatology*, Vol. 2, edited by H. I. Maibach and N. J. Lowe (Basel: Karger), pp. 178–188.

Bus, J. S. and Gibson, J. E., 1985, Body defence mechanisms to toxicant exposure. In *Patty's Industrial Hygiene and Toxicology*, Vol 3B: *Biological Responses*, edited by L. Cralley and L. Cralley (New York: John Wiley), pp. 143–174.

Chang, J. C. F., Gross, E. A., Swenberg, J. A. and Barrow, C. S., 1983, Nasal cavity deposition, histopathology, and cell proliferation after single or repeated formaldehyde exposures in B6C3F1 mice and F-344 rats. *Toxic. appl. Pharmac.*, **68**, 161–176.

Egle Jr, J. L., 1972, Retention of inhaled formaldehyde, propionaldehyde and acrolein in the dog. *Archs. envir. Hlth.* **25**, 119–124.

Gross, E. A., Swenberg, J. A., Fields, S. and Popp, J. A., 1982, Comparative morphometry of the nasal cavity in rats and mice. *J. Anat.*, **135**, 83–88.

Klaassen, C. D., 1980, Absorption, distribution, and excretion of toxicants. In *Toxicology: The Basic Science of Poisons.*, edited by J. Doull, C. D. Klaassen and M. O. Amdur (New York: MacMillan), pp. 28–55.

Swenberg, J. A., Barrow, C. S., Borieko, C. J., Heck, H.D'A., Levine, R. J., Morgan, K. T. and Starr, T. B., 1983, Non-linear biological responses to formaldehyde and their implications for carcinogenic risk assessment. *Carcinogenesis*, **4**, 945–952.

Wester, R. C. and Maibach, H. I., 1985, Animal models for percutaneous absorption. In *Models in Dermatology*, Vol. 2, edited by H. I. Maibach and N. J. Lowe (Basel: Karger), pp. 159–169.

PART 4

Animal selection considerations in carcinogenic and reproductive toxicity

Section editor:
W. P. Ridley

The short-term assays: the challenges and problems of adolescence

Andrew J. Sivak

Life Sciences Section, Arthur D. Little, Inc. Cambridge, MA 02140, USA

The bioassays, now known as the short-term tests, were introduced into the armamentarium of the toxicologist initially to identify those chemicals that interacted in some way with DNA, and thus had a presumption of potential carcinogenicity. These tests were escalated into high visibility almost single handedly by Ames, who provided a rapid and inexpensive test to detect agents that could induce gene mutations in a set of special strains originally derived from the bacterium *Salmonella* (Ames *et al.*, 1973, 1975).

In the 15 years that have elapsed since, the flush of initial enthusiasm, which led some to suggest rashly that regulatory decisions might be made on the basis of an Ames assay alone, give way to the sombre realities that the large database now available for many assay systems is thrust upon us. The tests have reached their adolescence with many of the uncertainties and confusions that accompany that age, along with the opportunity for analysis and reflection to determine how best to use this valuable resource.

A number of multiple-assay multiple laboratory investigations have been carried out with a wide range of chemical agents of different chemical classes. The results of these studies clearly indicate that inter-assay correlations among the genetic end-points themselves leave much to be desired (Ashby *et al.*, 1982; Purchase *et al.*, 1982; Ashby *et al.*, 1985); and that correlations of genetic end-points to *in vivo* carcinogenesis, in general, are not convincing in support of the short-term tests as rigorous predictive tools. What then is to be their fate in the future. It appears that these assays have significant uses in several areas, some related to their original purpose of identifying potentially harmful chemicals and others that could help us understand better how to interpret the animal bioassay. As will be shown later, their use as a species-selection tool is not so promising.

In considering the first of these uses as a predictive tool, the premise that a chemical agent that induces some sort of genetic lesion in several of the test systems deserves attention and further study is a useful starting point.

With now a considerable experience on short-term bioassays, it is recognized that the assays develop information at several levels of relevance. The consequence of this observation is that considerable care needs to be exercised in the interpretation of genetic toxicity bioassays with respect to whether the assays

151

Table 1. Characteristics of short-term assays.

Assay type	Information type
Gene mutation	Direct/surrogate
Chromosome aberrations	Surrogate
Sister chromatid exchange	Surrogate
Excision repair induction	Surrogate
Neoplastic transformation	Direct/surrogate

measure an effect that is directly related to a transmittable lesion or is a surrogate (Table 1).

As Table 1 indicates, only the direct gene mutation and neoplastic transformation assay measure the response that may directly be the cause of a health problem. Yet even with these assays, there is an element of indirectness, since the results of the short-term gene mutation assay are used to predict cancer-causing potential or germ-cell damage, even though the necessity for a specific somatic mutation in cancer induction is certainly not proven and the correlation between cellular somatic mutation tests and germ cell lesions *in vivo* awaits a larger database for verification.

Several attempts have been presented recently to deal with the issue of the qualitative and quantitative relationships among the short-term tests and their end-points *in vivo*. These efforts are encouraging and exciting, because they move us from the accuracy, precision, false-positive and false-negative calculations that have taken so much, often non-productive, energy and time to a higher level of analysis that, with additional study, may yield more effective ways to address the issue of the appropriate contemporary use of the short-term tests.

The four analyses to be considered are:

1. Brusick and co-workers' weight of evidence proposals presented at the recent International Conference on Environmental Mutagenesis (Brusick *et al.*, 1985).
2. Ashby's pair-wise comparisons (Ashby *et al.*, 1982).
3. Mendelsohn's analysis using the Kappa statistic (M. Mendelsohn, personal communication).
4. Tennant's analysis of National Toxicology Program data (Tennant *et al.*, 1986).

The first analysis to be examined is the weight of evidence scheme proposed by Brusick and co-workers at the International Conference on Environmental Mutagens in 1985 (Brusick *et al.*, 1985). The rationale for this approach is that no single test is adequate to detect lesions from the multiple possible mechanisms and that target cells of different phylogenetic levels are necessary to provide a net to catch activity across chemical classes. Figure 1 is a presenta-

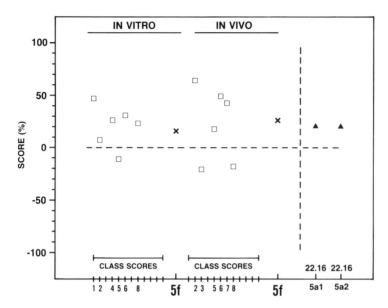

Figure 1. Weighted short-term test data for vinyl chloride (Brusick *et al.*, 1985).

tion of weighted data for vinyl chloride. The process merges individual test scores into class scores for each type of assay, combines family scores for assays *in vitro* or *in vivo*, and finally determines an agent score. This presentation then describes the intrinsic behaviour of a test battery with a single chemical. To anchor the system, one can take the class scores for any single assay and compare them to the carcinogenic response, for example. Although this relationship is not presently available, a separate expert committee is groping with this issue.

One can compare how results in any one class of assays compares with all other classes. For chromosome aberrations *in vitro*, the data are reasonably well behaved with only two false-positives and two false-negatives (Figure 2). For prokaryote gene mutation assays, the situation is considerably less correlated with a substantial number of bacterial negatives which score positively in other systems (Figure 3).

An alternative way to make similar comparisons is to compare pairs of assays for selected chemicals, as Ashby *et al.* have done (1985). Comparing chromosome aberrations to mammalian gene cell mutation, a rather good concordance is obtained among this limited set of chemicals (Figure 4). Comparing chromosome aberrations to *Salmonella* mutation results, the correspondence is less agreeable (Figure 5).

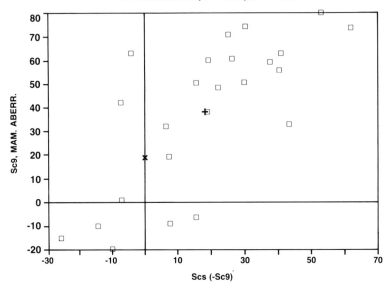

Figure 2. Correlation of *in vitro* chromosome aberration results with combined results of all other classes (Brusick *et al.*, 1985).

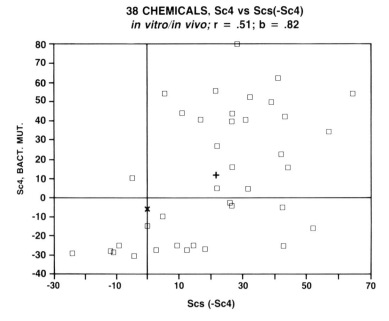

Figure 3. Correlation of prokaryotic gene mutation results with combined results of all other classes (Brusick *et al.*, 1985).

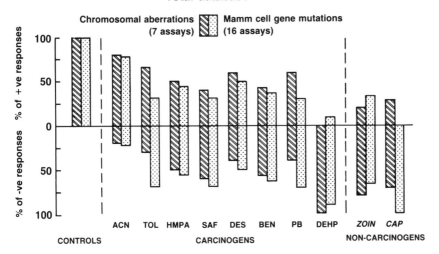

Figure 4. A comparison of the performances of the mammalian cell gene mutation assays and seven chromosomal aberration assays (Ashby *et al.*, 1982).

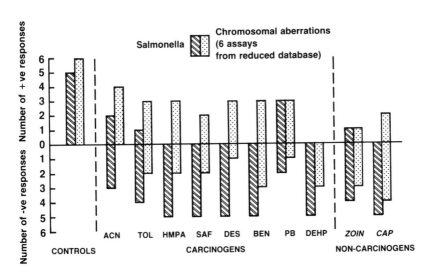

Figure 5. A comparison of the performance of the chromosomal aberration assays with that of the *Salmonella* assay (Ashby *et al.*, 1982).

The previous analyses have demonstrated how one could look at responses by assay, clusters of assays or by chemical. In each of these analyses, there was no direct correlation attempted with carcinogenicity.

The next two analyses will attempt comparisons to carcinogenicity. The first of these is a global approach described by M. Mendelsohn (personal communication, 1985). The basis for this analysis is a traditional sorting of carcinogenesis data based on the IARC scheme of sufficient, limited or insufficient data and genotoxicity data as positive, equivocal and negative. To reduce the matrix to be as manageable and unambiguous as possible in a two-by-two system, the genotoxicity equivocals were pooled with the negatives as were the carcinogenic limited data-sets, although this may not be completely justified because an inadequate evaluation by IARC could mean a negative carcinogenic response or insufficient data.

Table 2 shows the number of data-sets in each category. For example, positive genotoxicity sets for IARC carcinogens numbered 288. Positive carcinogens for negative or equivocal toxicity studies numbered 156.

The analysis of this data is carried out by a procedure that makes the two axes equivalent. Most calculations for these sorts of correlations take cancer data, human and animal, as the truth and take the genotoxicity data as the dependent variable. An alternative way of measuring the relationships of this sort of matrix is to use the Kappa statistic which was originally derived to test agreement among observers (Fleiss, 1981) Since it assumes no primacy of axis, the approach corrected for chance expectations is equivalent for both the carcinogenicity and the genotoxicity test data summaries. The original expression of the Kappa statistic was transformed to have the range of $+1$ to 0, where $+1$ is perfect agreement and 0 is disagreement. When one looks at the data set shown in Figure 6, one is struck by the consistency across the entire range of tests. The values are in the $0\cdot5-0\cdot7$ range. The exceptions are an insect chromosome set that had only four items and neoplastic transformation. Further analysis will need to be done to verify this finding, but it does suggest that

Table 2. Classification and distribution of IARC carcinogenicity data and short-term test data.

Test result	S	L,I	Total
+	288	128	416
? −	156	209	365
Total	444	337	781

From M. Mendelsohn (personal Communication).
S, Sufficient carcinogenicity data; L, limited carcinogenicity data; I, inadequate carcinogenicity data; +, significant positive in one or more assays; ?, contradictory or equivocal result; −, negative in one or more short-term assays.

KAPPA STATISTIC ANALYSIS

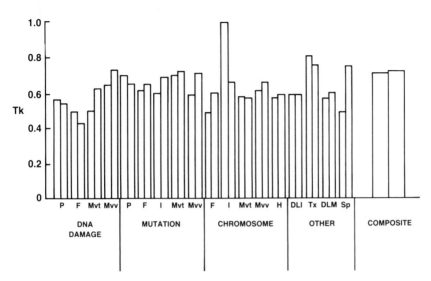

Figure 6. Kappa statistic analysis of the agreement between carcinogenicity data and short-term test data (M. Mendelsohn, personal communication).

transformation assays measure something rather different biologically than the usual genotoxicity assays.

Another analysis demonstrating how genotoxicity tests could be used after the fact to help understand mechanisms and be of some guidance in the risk-assessment process is based on the NTP set analysed by Tennant *et al.* (1986). The assays that can be compared in various ways to different types of experimental carcinogenicity data are shown in Table 3.

The evaluation shown in Table 4 compares genotoxicity test data to results with carcinogens that showed activity in both bioassay test species and both sexes.

Generally, the tumours were at more than one organ site, often at sites

Table 3. Genetic toxicity assays – NTP database.

Salmonella mutagenesis
Drosophila mutagenesis
Mouse lymphoma mutagenesis
Chromosome aberrations
Sister chromatid exchanges
Unscheduled DNA synthesis
Transformation

Table 4. Genetic toxicity versus trans-sex/species carcinogens.

Chemical	Positive	Equivocal	Negative
1, 2-Dibromo-3-chloropropane	6		5
Diglycidylresorcinol ether	10		5
4, 4'-Oxydianiline	16		5
Ethylene dibromide	9		3
Diethylhexylphthalate†	1		17
2,3,7,8-TCDD†			13
Polybrominated biphenyls†			15

Source: Tennant *et al.* (1986).
† Hepatic malignant tumours only.

where the spontaneous tumour rate is low. The information has some very important implications for understanding mechanism and for application to risk evaluations. Those carcinogens below the dotted line in Table 4, to which could be added butylated hydroxyanisole and dichloromethane, present a clear challenge for some innovative thinking in dealing with how one proceeds to carry out a risk evaluation with essentially non-genotoxic carcinogens. The carcinogenicity data could be forced into the various standard methods used for genotoxic carcinogens, and they have been for 2,3,7,8-tetrachloro-benzodioxin. The risk assessment that then becomes the basis for regulatory decisions is clearly faulty and has no mechanistic supportable basis. While there are solutions to how risk assessments can be done for these sorts of compounds, some candour in admitting ignorance of mechanism and exploring alternatives would undoubtedly be a healthy (less risky) endeavour.

Returning to a consideration of the analysis, as one moves to a lesser degree of animal carcinogenicity, the genotoxicity tests unsurprisingly perform less well (Table 5). For putative negative carcinogens, the bulk of tests are negative, although the inordinate contribution of chromosome aberrations'

Table 5. Genetic toxicity versus unisex/species carcinogens.

Chemical	Positive	Equivocal	Negative
Allyl isothiocyanate	4†		12
11-Aminoundecanoic acid	2		17
D&C Red 9	3	1	7
Melamine	0		14
α-Biphenylamine	3		8
Methyl chloroform	2‡	1	11

Source: Tennant *et al.* (1986).
†3/4 Cytogenetic positive.
‡2/2 Cytogenetic positive.

Table 6. Genetic toxicity versus non-carcinogens.

Chemical	Positive	Equivocal	Negative
Benzoin	4†		13
Bisphenol A	0		15
Caprolactam	1		14
2-(Chloromethyl)pyridine	6‡	1	6
Diallylphthalate	0		9

Source: Tennant *et al.* (1986).
†2/4 Cytogenetic positive.
‡4/6 Cytogenetic positive.

Table 7. DNA repair activity (erg/mm^2 U.V. light equiv.).

	DNA repair activity		
	Syrian Golden hamster	Sprague–Dawley rat	Hartley guinea-pig
IQ	11·9	21·0	9·4
MCIQ	9·0	7·3	1·7
2-AF	40·4	8·2	14·2
IQ/2-AF	1·3	2·9	5·5
MeIQ/2-AF	0·3	2·6	0·7

Source: Loury & Byard (1985).

false-positives is not unexpected (Table 6). The contribution of non-genetic cytotoxicity to these sorts of lesions is well documented (Galloway *et al.*, 1985)

Since one of the critical variables in a carcinogenicity bioassay is the selection of the test species (strain) for exposure, any guidance that can be obtained from short-term tests would be extremely valuable. The available data are not encouraging with respect to species selections based on genotoxicity data. The hepatocyte DNA repair system (Williams, 1977) is one of the few that is able to provide species comparisons by using the same cell type from each of the species to be studied.

The results of two studies are instructive examples of species variability in this type of assay that makes application of such data for species selection in studies *in vivo* difficult. Loury & Byard (1985) have examined the effects of mutagens isolated from fried foods and report a range of responses that exhibit no correlated pattern for either species or chemical (Table 7). In another study by Kornbrust & Barfknecht (1984), a similar pattern emerges with respect to variations that do not appear to be species or chemical specific (Table 8).

Table 8. DNA repair in rat and hamster hepatocytes.

	DNA repair			
	Sprague–Dawley rat		Syrian golden hamster	
Chemical	% Cells grains/cell	≥ 5 Grain	% Cells grains/cell	≥ 5 Grain
Dimethylnitrosamine				
$(10^{-3}$M)	12·1	83	37·7	100
$(10^{-4}$M)	− 0·5	10	10·2	90
Diethylnitrosamine				
$(5 \times 10^{-3}$M)	19·3	92	56·8	100
$(5 \times 10^{-4}$M)	3·2	32	21·2	97
2-Acetylaminofluorene				
$(10^{-7}$M)	2·2	23	11·8	85
Benzidine				
$(10^{-6}$M)	23·5	92	41·9	99
$(10^{-7}$M)	1·6	20	8·0	90
Methylmethane sulphate				
$(10^{-4}$M)	16·7	92	18·2	93
1-Nitropyrene				
$(10^{-5}$M)	22·3	98	6·8	67
$(10^{-6}$M)	3·5	42	− 1·2	5

Source: Kornburst & Barfknecht (1984).

Summary

It is now clear that the short-term genotoxicity assays as predictors of at least animal carcinogenicity are less reliable than their most vigorous champions would propose, but certainly better than just tossing a coin. The key issue is how can they help in the safety-assessment process. The primary purpose of identification of genotoxicity early in the development process of chemicals is obvious and requires little further comment, and should be of concern to all makers, marketers and regulators of substances to which humans are exposed.

The value of the short-term tests in helping to unravel mechanisms and support the total toxicology profile of a chemical that is exposed to humans has yet to be explored to its fullest. The database must include appropriate pharmacokinetic analysis and well-designed animal studies, taking into account the confounding influences of nutrition and other stresses that are described elsewhere in this volume. Only with this attention to the details of the technical support data will safety and regulatory decisions be made from a minimal level of ignorance.

The genotoxicity tests have provided a rich data source that needs some creative and courageous analysis. This process has started and the outcome over several following years should provide us with some new insights to the appropriate use of these tests to identify potentially harmful chemicals and understand better the results of carcinogenicity tests. In the best of all worlds we could move towards a much more flexible regulatory approach that makes intelligent and reasonable use of all the data available.

References

Ames, B. N., Dunston, W. E., Yamasaki, E. and Lee. F. D., 1973, Carcinogens are mutagens: a simple test system combining liver homogenates for activation and bacteria for detection. *Proc. natn. Acad. Sci. U.S.A.*, **70**, 2281–2285.

Ames, B. N., McCann, J. and Yamasaki, E., 1975, Methods for detecting carcinogens and mutagens with the salmonella/mammalian microsomes mutagenicity test. *Mutation Res.*, **31**, 347–364.

Ashby, J., Leferre, P. A., Elliott, B. M. and Styles, J. A., 1982, An overview of chemical and biological reactivity of 4CMB and structurally related compounds: possible relevance to the overall findings of the UKEMS study. *Mutation Res.*, **100**, 417–433.

Ashby, J., de Serres, F. J., Draper, Jr., M., Ishidate, M., Margolin, B. H., Matter, B. E. and Shelby, M. D., 1985, Overview and conclusions of the IPCS collaborative study on *in vitro* assay systems. In *Evaluation of Short-term Tests for Carcinogens: Report on the International Programme on Chemical Safety's Collaborative Study on* in vitro *Assays . Progress in Mutation Research*, Vol. 5, edited by J. Ashby, F. J. de Serres, M. Draper, Jr, M. Ishidate, B. H. Margolin, B. E. Matter, and M. D. Shelby (Amsterdam: Elsevier), pp. 117–174.

Brusick, D., Ashby, J., de Serres, F., Lohman, P., Matsuhima, T., Matter, B., Mendelsohn, M. and Waters, M., 1985, Genetic toxicology of environmental chemicals. In *Proceedings of the Fourth International Conference on Environmental Mutagens* (New York: A. R. Liss).

Fleiss, J. L., 1981, *Statistical Methods for Rates and Proportions* (New York: John Wiley).

Galloway, S. M., Bloom, A. D., Resnick, M., Margolin, B. H., Nakamura, F., Archer, P. and Zeiger, E., 1985, Development of a standard protocol for *in vitro* cytogenetic testing with Chinese hamster ovary cells: comparison of results of 22 compounds in two laboratories. *Envir. Mutagenesis*, **7**, 1–51.

Kornbrust, D. J. and Barfknecht, T. R., 1984, Comparison of rat and hamster hepatocyte primary culture/DNA repair assays. *Envir. Mutagenesis*, **6**, 1–11.

Loury, D. J. and Byard, J. L., 1985, Genotoxicity of the cooked-food mutagens IQ and MelQ in primary cultures of rat, hamster, and guinea-pig hepatocytes. *Envir. Mutagenesis*, **7**, 245–254.

Purchase, I. F. H., Longstaff, E., Ashby, J., Styles, J. A., Anderson, D., Leferre, P. A. and Westwood, F. R., 1982, An evaluation of 6 short-term tests for detecting organic chemical carcinogens. *Br. J. Cancer*, **37**, 837–859.

Tennant, R. W., Stasiewicz, S. and Spalding, J. W., 1986,. Comparison of multiple parameters of rodent carcinogenicity and *in vitro* genetic toxicity. *Envir. Mutagenesis*, **8**, 205–227.

Williams, G. M., 1977, Detection of chemical carcinogens by unscheduled DNA synthesis in rat liver primary cell cultures. *Cancer Res.*, **37**, 1845–1851.

Testing procedures to define carcinogens as human cancer risks

John H. Weisburger and Gary M. Williams

American Health Foundation, Valhalla, NY 10595–1599, USA

Introduction

Cancer comprises a set of chronic diseases found in high incidence and mortality in many parts of the world. Because of its slow, yet often inexorable, progression, people fear cancer more than most other diseases. Historic events provide the basis for the public belief that chemicals are major causes of cancer, in turn, leading to public demands that these cancer risks be controlled. An example expressing these fears and the consequent political action is the Delaney Clause of the Food and Drug Act in the USA. In other countries, similar concerns have been translated into legal regulations.

This chapter presents the current means of qualitative detection and quantitative evaluation of chemicals involved in cancer causation, promotion and development. Further discussed are the major advances in our understanding of the complex carcinogenic process, leading to a classification of carcinogens into genotoxic and epigenetic categories. Finally, a new definition of what types and amounts of carcinogens are human cancer risks will be presented.

Carcinogenic process and mechanisms

Neoplastic behaviour is transmitted by a cell to its progeny and, therefore, involves a genetic abnormality. The process by which this deviation is induced by chemicals is a multi-step series of events, usually with a protracted expression time from the onset of exposure to the agent until the manifestation of a neoplasm. As the first event, most chemical carcinogens are converted to an active form through biotransformation, although a few synthetic chemicals are directly reactive. The activation reaction, mainly carried out by the cytochrome P-450 metabolic system or similar electron-withdrawing reactions, is a function of both the host and environmental conditions (Figure 1). The reactive chemical, an electrophilic reactant or a radical cation, interacts with cellular macromolecules at nucleophilic centres (Miller & Miller, 1981). Reaction with DNA, which upon cell duplication yields further gene alterations, including gene rearrangement and gene amplification, particularly the oncogene-containing codons, is one and, probably the principal, means by which a cell

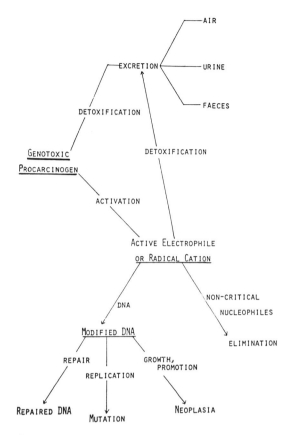

Figure 1. Schematic presentation of the diverse biochemical reactions involved in the metabolic activation and detoxification of genotoxic carcinogens. For many carcinogens, there are reactions leading to detoxified metabolites facilitating excretion. Usually only a small fraction of a dose of a carcinogen is converted, in one or more steps, to more toxic and carcinogenic metabolites, which are reactive electrophiles or radical cations. These metabolites can undergo enzymic detoxification reactions yielding excretable products, or they can react with nucleophiles that are non-critical to the carcinogenic or mutagenic process in competition with the critical nucleophiles, especially DNA. Systems *in vitro* have different ratios of activation : detoxification enzymes and distinct levels of non-critical nucleophiles, and thus account for differences found between assays *in vivo* and *in vitro*. The key reaction is with DNA, providing a parallel between mutagenesis and carcinogenesis. This lesion can be repaired, an effect that plays a role in quantitative carcinogenesis and in the specific organ primarily affected by a given carcinogen. Essential elements in the overall process towards mutation or neoplasia are a modified DNA and cell duplication, growth and promotion.

with an abnormal genome is generated. This sequence of actions is part of the genotoxic pathway (Searle, 1984; Upton *et al.*, 1984).

A neoplastic cell can remain latent, meaning that it persists and replicates, but does not manifest itself. The growth and development of the abnormal cell to form a tumour requires the participation of host factors as well as external agents operating on growth-control elements that may play a role in function and differentiation (Hecker *et al.*, 1982; Pereira, 1983; Börzsönyi *et al.*, 1984; Shubik, 1984; Berenblum, 1985). These conditions are certainly quite different from those that produce genetic alterations. Environmentally important agents acting as promoters may enhance this stage of the overall process. Promotion appears to relate to the effect of certain chemicals in modifying membranes and receptors, which, through mechanisms yet to be established, release cells from growth control. These modes of action may involve epigenetic effects on inter-cellular communication, differentiation and endocrine systems (Trosko *et al.*, 1985; Williams, 1985).

The conversion of a benign tumour to a malignant invasive neoplasm, or of a highly differentiated cancer to an anaplastic undifferentiated cancer, has been termed progression (Foulds, 1979; Shubik, 1984). The mechanisms whereby this process occurs are not known, although the operation of additional alterations of the genetic apparatus seems likely.

Carcinogen detection and safety assessment means the capability to detect agents that are genotoxic and other agents that act as promoters, or if future research indicates that progression is susceptible to external influences, to detect chemicals that affect that part of the process (Weisburger & Williams, 1984).

One direct means of carcinogen detection is the observation of cancer in humans exposed to specific chemicals, as in occupation-related cancers (Muir & Higginson, 1985). Contemporary efforts aim to determine the nature of exogenous factors bearing on the aetiology of the common human cancers. Great progress has been made along these lines by establishing that, in the main, conditions of lifestyle such as smoking, excessive alcohol use, and nutritional traditions and, in part, malnutrition are the major causes of most human cancers in the world (Hiatt *et al.*, 1977; Doll & Peto, 1981; Surgeon General Report, 1982; Schottenfeld & Fraumeni, 1982; Wynder *et al.*, 1983; Brunnemann *et al.*, 1985).

The traditional approach to carcinogen bioassay involved the administration of test chemicals to rodents. This approach was based on the fact that known human carcinogens, when so tested, usually elicited neoplasms in high incidence with a relatively short expression period. A test compound, displaying such properties typical of a potent carcinogen upon administration to several strains or species of rodents, was then construed by a human cancer risk.

More recently, large-scale animal bioassays sometimes yielded statistically significant, yet small, increases in the incidence of single types of neoplasms. Such results were interpreted as evidence of carcinogenicity, even if based on neoplasms in endocrine-sensitive tissues such as the adrenal or thyroid, sometimes in only one species. Many lifetime tests in rats and mice eventually yield an increase of neoplasms in the liver of mice, but no excess neoplasms in rats. Another situation is illustrated by butylated hydroxyanisole (BHA),

Table 1. 'Decision Point Approach' in carcinogen testing.

A. Structure of chemical
B. Short-term tests *in vitro*
    1. Bacterial mutagenesis
    2. Mammalian mutagenesis
    3. DNA repair
    4. Chromosome tests
    5. Cell transformation
Decision Point 1: Evaluation of all tests under A and B
C. Tests for promoters
    1. *In vitro*
    2. *In vivo*
Decision Point 2: Evaluation of results from stages A–C
D. Limited bioassays *in vivo*
    1. Altered foci induction in rodent liver
    2. Skin neoplasm induction in mice
    2. Pulmonary neoplasm induction in mice.
    3. Breast cancer induction in female Sprague–Dawley rats
Decision Point 3: Evaluation from the beginning plus results from any of the appropriate tests under D.
E. Long-term bioassay.
Decision Point 4: Final evaluation of all results available and application to health risk analysis. This evaluation must include data from stages A–C to provide the basis for mechanistic considerations.

---

which induced tumours only in the forestomach of rats and hamsters at high doses, but not in mice (Ito *et al.*, 1983 a, b; Ito *et al.*, 1984; Altmann *et al.*, 1985; Iverson *et al.*, 1985). High doses of saccharin, especially in two-generation tests, have induced bladder cancer in rats, but not in mice (Saccharin, 1985). It may be questioned whether chemicals with such circumscribed ability to increase the occurrence of neoplasms are actually human cancer hazards. In the absence of data on the mechanism of action, such a declaration is scientifically tenuous. For that reason, it is absolutely essential to generate detailed information on the broad toxicological properties of a suspect chemical. For this purpose, we have developed a systematic 'Decision Point Approach' to delineate a means of data acquisition and interpretation (Table 1). This approach has been evaluated, and a recent monograph on carcinogen testing by Milman and Weisburger (1985) is organized along these lines.

Short-term tests

In recognition that the early events in carcinogenesis involved an alteration of the genome, efforts have been made to develop rapid bioassays to detect DNA-reactive carcinogens (Hollaender & de Serres, 1971–83). Rosenkranz *et al.* (1980) developed indicators based on *Escherichia coli*, and Ames (Maron & Ames, 1983) evolved systems utilizing *Salmonella typhimurium* mutants, permitting tests of large series of chemicals. In addition, a number of mammalian cell systems were introduced. In contrast, however, to recently explanted cells, many of these cells have been in culture for a number of generations, and often they have only low levels of the necessary metabolic activation systems. Thus, most of the mammalian cell systems used also require an external supply of a metabolizing unit.

The procedures of Ames involved the use of a mitochondrial supernatant, including cytosol and microsomal fractions of rodent liver. This S9 fraction has found application also for the production of mutants or to secure transformation of mammalian cells with poor endogenous metabolic capability.

The S9 fraction of liver includes most of the required metabolic capability to convert procarcinogens to reactive products, but usually has quite low capabilities, in the absence of added co-factors, to produce type II conjugation reactions (Anders, 1985). Hence, tests of chemicals under these conditions may yield false-positive responses because of the absence of type II conjugation systems that usually lead to detoxification (Jakoby, 1984). For example, a number of flavones, including quercetin, are positive in prokaryotic test organisms plus a liver S9 fraction, whereas in the presence of detoxification systems, and *in vivo*, such chemicals are negative (Hirono, 1986; Williams, 1986).

Use of the S9 fraction, even though essential, constitutes an inherent potential weakness, because any test is limited by the metabolic system it utilizes. No matter which indicator DNA is employed, if the same type of S9 fraction is used in several different tests, the performance of these test systems depends on the extent of available biochemical power. When a battery of tests involves tests using indicator DNA from different organisms with comparable sensitivity in detecting altered DNA, but the tests use an identical limiting S9 fraction, this confines the value of the battery, and is clearly redundant.

It is obvious, therefore, that great care and thought is required to select a battery of tests to provide optimal information on possible genotoxicity of chemicals. Any test system has several components. One is the biochemical activation and detoxification system used to mimic as closely as possible the situation prevailing *in vivo* in experimental animals and in man. The second is the indicator DNA and genetic material. The third is the transfer of any DNA-reactive metabolite from its site of production to the indicator DNA.

Freshly explanted hepatocytes have a biochemical competence mimicking the situation *in vivo* (Croci & Williams, 1985); they are now widely utilized for studies *in vitro*. In hepatocytes the indicator DNA is in the same cell that performs the metabolic conversion. Only the nuclear membrane might then be an obstacle to the efficient transfer of reactive metabolite. In fact, in some instances, enzymes within the nucleus were found to convert a chemical to an active metabolite. The induction of DNA damage in freshly explanted hepatocytes, proposed by Williams (1977) and since validated by his laboratory and others, probably resembles most closely the overall biochemical and physiological features prevailing *in vivo*. Hepatocytes from several species, including human, have been used. Freshly explanted cells represent virtually the gamut of enzymic activities prevailing *in vivo* and include activation as well as detoxification systems (Williams *et al.*, 1983). The target DNA is in the same cell, alleviating the problem of transfer of metabolites through cellular membranes. These considerations suggest that this system should be considered an essential part of a battery of bioassay systems to detect genotoxic chemicals *in vitro*.

A number of groups have adapted the hepatocyte test systems using an *in vivo/in vitro* scheme (Ashby *et al.*, 1985). Under some conditions, such as tests of nitroaryl compounds or conjugates with a glucosidic residue such as cycasin, bacterial enzymes from the intestinal tract are needed to produce reactive intermediates or proximate carcinogens. However, the Williams test can be adapted by adding specific enzymes such as glucosidases to the medium when the chemical to be tested is a conjugate. Enzyme mixtures from bacteria can also be added *in vitro* to provide the necessary source of enzymes for other reactions such as nitro-group reduction. The *in vivo/in vitro* scheme is less economical because the test compound needs to be administered to a number of animals at several dose levels.

Further tests involve cell transformation and sister chromatid exchange (SCE) (Milman & Weisburger, 1985). Technically, cell transformation systems are much more demanding, and if epithelial cells rather than mesenchymal cells are used, the end-points are difficult to quantify. More importantly, cell transformation has been obtained with chemicals that in other tests for genotoxicity were clearly negative. Thus, cell transformation as an indicator *in vitro* only yields data on possible neoplasm-inducing properties in the broadest sense, rather than as a specific indicator of DNA reactivity. The same limitation applies to SCE. Agents that were not genotoxic have yielded positive responses, but others that were clearly genotoxic did not. SCE can be detected not only in cells from tissues but also in formed elements from blood. Thus, despite its clear limitations, SCE can be usefully extended to detect possible exposure to harmful chemicals in the workplace, provided the results are interpreted in the light of corollary supporting facts.

In the process development are immunoassays for specific carcinogen–DNA or carcinogen–protein adducts (Poirier *et al.*, 1983; Berlin *et al.*, 1984). Of interest also is a novel means of determining the existence of DNA–carcinogen adducts by the ^{32}P-postlabelling technique (Everson *et al.*, 1986). The extent of human exposure to potential genotoxic agents can be determined by examining urine for mutagenic metabolites. These techniques, of course, are of value only with current or recent intake of the agent.

Promotion and promoters

Mouse skin, the first model for studies of promotion in carcinogenesis, has been supplemented by studies in other organs such as colon, breast, liver, pancreas and urinary bladder (Pereira, 1983). Further, it seems clear that human cancer causality at specific target organs is the result of initiation, co-carcinogenesis and promotion. For example, tobacco smoke, which is the cause of several types of human cancers, contains a complex mixture of initiators, co-carcinogens and promoters (Surgeon General report, 1982). Furthermore, in nutritionally linked carcinogenesis, cancer at target sites such as breast, colon, pancreas and perhaps other organs depends to a considerable extent on promotion (Wynder *et al.*, 1983).

In the evaluation of large-scale bioassays for carcinogens, it became evident that a number of environmental chemicals, pesticides such as DDT and chlordane, and solvents such as trichloroethylene or perchloroethylene, usually led to neoplasms in the liver of the mouse strains used, but not so in rats or hamsters. These mouse strains normally display spontaneous liver cancer and a high frequency of activated oncogenes in the neoplasms (Nutrition Foundation, 1983; Fox & Watanabe, 1985; Reynolds *et al.*, 1986). When these kinds of compounds or their metabolites were tested for genotoxicity, they were overwhelmingly negative (Moriya *et al.*, 1983).

These facts suggest that such compounds induce liver cancer in mice by the phenomenon of promotion. This distinction is important because agents that are promoters need different public health action for cancer control purposes, compared with those agents that are definitely genotoxic.

Test systems to delineate promoting potential depend on the property of promoters to break gap junctions and lead to interruption of inter-cellular communication in cell culture (Trosko *et al.*, 1985; Williams *et al.*, 1985). Chemicals such as certain halogenated hydrocarbons, the antioxidant butylated hydroxytoluene (BHT) or bile acids are all positive in this system.

Limited *bioassays* in vivo

When the battery of tests used *in vitro* has provided qualitative evidence that a chemical is a genotoxic carcinogen or a promoter, validation of such properties and exploration of potency is necessary. Specific rapid tests *in vivo* based on the probable mechanisms of action, whether genotoxic or promoting, of a given chemical can be applied (Weisburger & Williams, 1984).

The tests include the induction of: (1) abnormal foci in rodent liver, (2) skin tumours in mice, (3) mammary neoplasms in Sprague–Dawley female rats, and (4) pulmonary tumours in sensitive strains of mice. Most of these tests take less than one year. They should be conducted at a number of dose levels to indicate the slope of the dose–response curve of the test compound versus the known positive control carcinogen or promoter. The test systems can be designed to delineate the potency of genotoxic carcinogens by using a variant with one or a few doses applied to target organs or delivered systemically, followed by an appropriate promoter, to provide potency data for an initiator.

For mouse skin, the usual promoter is the phorbol ester TPA, for rat or mouse liver, phenobarbital, and for mammary gland, a high-fat diet. However, phenobarbital yields liver neoplasms in mice, and therefore the time of occurrence and slope of the dose–response curve are important criteria in evaluating the comparative effect.

For tests of agents as promoters, a genotoxic carcinogen appropriate for the relevant target organ is administered, followed by the test substance at four to five dose levels. Here again, the appropriate positive control promoter at several dose levels will indicate relative potency.

With these bioassay systems *in vivo*, three end-points can be quantified: (1) per cent of animals with histopathologically validated lesions, (2) the multiplicity and size of neoplasms, and (3) the expression time from exposure to occurrence of tumour.

A key decision point is the overall evaluation of results from the battery of tests *in vitro* and the limited bioassay tests *in vivo*. Especially revealing is the series of limited bioassays performed at four to six dose levels that visualizes the potency of a chemical based on the shape of its dose–response curve. Squire (1981) and Wang (1984) have reported on a semi-quantitative rating system, in which genotoxicity is taken into account. Overall, the battery of data generated by tests *in vitro* for genotoxicity or promoting potential, and properly designed limited bioassays *in vivo*, most often will provide an adequate database, necessary to protect the public. Thus, chronic bioassays will be needed only infrequently.

Bioassays for chronic toxicity and carcinogenicity

With the advent of a better understanding of the mechanisms of cancer causation, the insight derived from the tests for genotoxicity, and the beginning of development of rapid tests for possible promoting substances, the classic long-term bioassay may no longer be essential in order to perform health risk analyses. Indeed, from the experience of the National Cancer Institute (NCI) bioassay programme, originated by the Weisburgers (Weisburger, 1983; Cameron *et al.*, 1985) and continued by the National Toxicology Program (NTP), it appears that the test results can be easily misinterpreted if the data obtained are not scrutinized with regard to the underlying mechanisms. Test results for hundreds of chemicals are now available. Some chemicals were clearly negative and some clearly positive. In a large number of cases, however, evidence of 'carcinogenicity' was based on a relatively small, yet statistically significant, incidence, compared with simultaneous controls of given neoplasms such as pheochromocytomas, thyroid adenomas or neoplastic nodules in the liver, especially in mice (without evidence of carcinomas). Such chemicals either gave no evidence of activity in bioassays *in vitro*, or else activity was seen in perhaps one specific, often not widely used, test, without a simultaneous test of known positive controls. A recent exchange of published letters discusses the implications of the finding that 85% of chemicals tested in animals were found to be 'carcinogenic' in the US bioassay series (Rosenkranz *et al.*, 1984a,b; Trosko, 1984; Wilmer, 1984; Vainio *et al.*, 1985). Do such numbers truly have meaning in relation to the actual risk of cancer for persons exposed to these chemicals? This question will be discussed later.

Such far-reaching interpretations of bioassays, with possible regulatory implications, have led to critical questions, interestingly *not* on the *interpretation* of results, *but* rather on the *procedures* used in bioassays. The concept that one dose level should be high – the maximally tolerated dose (MTD) – has been especially challenged. Yet there are good reasons for having such a dose level (Weisburger & Williams, 1984). Known human carcinogens, when tested in animal models, demonstrated their carcinogenicity best at high doses. The classic human carcinogen 2-naphthylamine led to urinary bladder cancer in hamsters at 10 000 p.p.m. but not at 1000 p.p.m. (see Weisburger & Williams, 1984). In cigarette smokers, the chronic consumption of 40 cigarettes per day clearly represents a health risk, whereas the effect of four cigarettes per day is difficult to visualize (Surgeon General Report, 1982).

The decision to do a large-scale expensive experiment, as well as working out its design, will benefit from data on the presence or absence of genotoxicity. Another key element is the likely large-scale human exposure at appreciable dose levels for extended periods of time, especially in young people. The definitive bioassay should employ four or more dose levels, including the MTD. This scheme will provide information on the shape of the dose–response curve, an essential database for health risk assessment. It is not proper, and in fact scientifically unacceptable, to perform health risk assessments based on results available at only one or two dose levels. Every chemical has specific biological properties. For some, activity is apparent over a large range of dosages as, for example, with dimethylnitrosamine (range about 100:1) or benzo[*a*]pyrene (range about 1000:1). For others, such as safrole, a sharp decrease in activity occurs as a function of dose. It is clear that the health risk formulation depends to a considerable extent on the quality of the quantitative data available.

Limited bioassays and standard chronic bioassays *in vivo* can be designed to reveal the effect of promoters on their specific target organ. Pretreating animals with an appropriate dose of a genotoxic carcinogen for that target organ, followed by a number of dose levels of the promoter, provides quantitative information on the effect of the promoter. With a sufficient number of dose levels, taking into account possible human exposure, any no-effect level (presumed to exist with promoting substances) can be pinpointed. To facilitate statistical data management, a greater number of experimental animals at lower dose levels should be used. The untreated and, where indicated vehicle-treated controls should involve the same larger number of animals as that used with the lowest dosage group.

Quantitative aspects of carcinogenesis

DNA-reactive carcinogens

The response to chemical carcinogens is dose-dependent, which is true basically for every toxicological effect. However, carcinogens of the electrophilic DNA-reactive type are distinct from other xenobiotics. Drugs, and toxic chemicals generally, exert their action rapidly. As the chemical is metabolized and excreted, the effect diminishes to vanishing point, and in most instances no residual effect persists. Subsequent exposures act anew in the same manner, without any long-lasting effects. In contrast, while the onset of the interaction between a carcinogen and the cell is fundamentally similar in that the chemical may undergo biotransformation, the key biochemically activated ultimate carcinogen reacts with tissue macromolecules, of which DNA is critical. During DNA synthesis and cell duplication, altered DNA can lead to gene or chromosomal mutations imprinting a permanent effect in the cell. Therefore, with DNA-reactive genotoxic carcinogens, an exposure, if sufficient, can result in permanent cellular abnormalities. Subsequent dosages can add to such a change. After a sufficient number of such alterations have been produced, the multiplication of abnormal cells results in a detectable lesion and eventually a neoplasm. Because the effects vary with the carcinogen and the tissue in which it exerts its action, the time required for a neoplasm to appear varies. Thus, time as well as dose are key factors in assessing the properties of chemical carcinogens. It is primarily in this way that DNA-reactive carcinogens differ from other types of toxins; a number of small doses may give no immediate evidence of their action, but in time they can yield neoplasms within the lifespan of the host. Indeed, some carcinogens of the DNA-reactive type can induce cancer in animal models with a single dose. With toxins, comparable dosages for acute effects would be likely to be completely innocuous.

In numerous experiments using appropriate quantitative parameters, detailed dose–response relationships have been demonstrated. Two effects are usually observed with potent genotoxic carcinogens: with increasing dose (1) the percentage yield and multiplicity of neoplasms increases, and (2) the time required for neoplasm appearance decreases. In most cases, the overall neoplasm yield in any specific organ is proportional to the total dose, but the speed or rate of neoplasm appearance is related to the amount in an individual dose or dose rate (Druckrey, 1967; Littlefield & Gaylor, 1985; Williams & Weisburger, 1986). In general, with many genotoxic carcinogens, the lower the dose and dose rate, the lower the incidence of specific neoplasms. However, in a few instances, such as polycyclic aromatic hydrocarbons injected subcutaneously, the same total dose, when administered as smaller doses over a longer period of time, may actually be more effective than when given as larger, yet fewer, individual doses in a shorter period of time (Hueper & Conway, 1964). In the extreme, several chemicals, such as 2-acetylaminofluorene, which are potent carcinogens when administered chronically, are not at all active when given as a single large dose (Weisburger, 1982).

A controversial issue in dose−response relationships is whether no-effect or threshold levels exist for chemical carcinogens. DNA-reactive carcinogens vary greatly in their potency. For example, among liver carcinogens, a greater than 50% incidence is produced by life-time administration of aflatoxin B_1 at 1 p.p.b, by diethylnitrosamine at 5 p.p.m., by safrole at 1000−5000 p.p.m. and by acetamide at 12 500 p.p.m. Relatively few studies have been done on the effect of dose rate or even dose response with the weaker DNA-reactive carcinogens. Shimkin *et al.* (1966) examined the potential of alkylating drugs of diverse structures to induce pulmonary tumours in mice. They found that the strong carcinogens were active over a broad dose range, whereas the weaker ones gave evidence of some carcinogenicity only at the highest, but not at lower, dose levels. Long *et al.* (1963) fed safrole in the diet to groups of 50 rats at levels of 100, 500, 1000 and 5000 p.p.m. Malignant liver cancers were obtained only at the highest dose level, and benign adenomas at the two highest, but not the lower doses. Based upon considerations of metabolism, the barriers to electrophiles in reaching critical targets in DNA, protective DNA repair processes and the like, it seems probable that for every carcinogen there must be a threshold. It may be very low for powerful carcinogens, as suggested by the two studies on 2-acetylaminofluorene (Smith, 1981) and the nitrosamines (Peto *et al.*, 1984), but seems to be correspondingly higher for weak carcinogens.

These dose−response studies on DNA-reactive carcinogens have provided the data for mathematical modelling. A number of models have been proposed (Office of Technology Assessment, 1982; Hoel *et al.*, 1985), and there is active debate as to which of these is most appropriate. One model, widely used by regulatory agencies because it is 'conservative' consists of a linear no-threshold extrapolation. As noted, it has not been demonstrated for any carcinogen that there is no threshold. To the contrary, thresholds have been observed in many studies, particularly with weak carcinogens. The assumption of linearity at low doses is also not well-founded. Indeed, even for the less complicated process of chemical mutagenesis *in vivo.*, a drop below linearity at low doses has been demonstrated (Russell *et al.*, 1982). Therefore, a 'hockey stick' shaped curve (Hoel *et al.*, 1983) probably best fits current data and concepts on carcinogenic effects at low levels of exposure.

Dose-dependent carcinogenic effects have also been observed in human exposure to carcinogens (Williams *et al.*, 1985). The most reliable quantitative data on human cancer resulting from exposure to specific carcinogens comes from the studies of occupational or therapeutic exposures. In these situations, adequate data for several carcinogens show that human cancer incidence is proportional to dose, often measured by length of employment, since there are virtually no actual data on the prevailing levels of any chemical in the industrial environment, especially in the past. The cancer incidence in workmen exposed to benzidine, vinyl chloride or bis(chloromethyl)ether indicates a general relationship between exposure and disease occurrence. Workmen engaged in uranium or asbestos mining exhibited a risk of cancer broadly related to the length of time an individual was engaged in these particular occupations. Likewise, with the drug chlornaphazine, where intake was reasonably well established, the percentage of treated patients that subsequently developed bladder cancer was proportional to the amount of drug consumed. Many of the available dose–response relationships were observed in limited populations of people exposed iatrogenically (Schmähl *et al.*, 1977). In two plants with potential exposure to bis(chloromethyl)ether, a carcinogenic effect on workmen was noted in only one of the sites, indicating that it is possible to protect staff even with highly potent carcinogens (McCallum *et al.*, 1983). This of course, should be the goal. Safety should be part of the engineering and design.

The question of whether there are thresholds in human exposure to carcinogens is controversial. This issue has great contemporary importance in the light of the capability of analytic chemists to measure accurately, at the parts per billion and even the parts per trillion level, the presence of several types of carcinogens in the food chain and in the general environment. Several chemicals such as nitrosopyrrolidine, found in bacon, can induce liver cancer in several species with appropriate higher dosages of the order of parts-per-million to parts-per-thousand. Primary liver cancer is rarely seen in populations that consume fried bacon. Is this evidence for a no-effect level? Similar questions can be raised for the trace amounts of powerfully carcinogenic mycotoxins such as aflatoxin B_1 currently permitted in food. Hepatocellular carcinoma is relatively rare in much of the Western World, even though unavoidable contamination of foods with the highly potent liver carcinogens aflatoxin and dimethylnitrosamine has occurred for decades and continues to be found. Thus, there may be practical no-effect levels even for strong carcinogens, especially in the absence of specific promoting factors. Nevertheless, it is clear that prudent policy dictates rational avoidance, wherever possible, of exposure to genotoxic carcinogens.

Such considerations are controversial; opinions abound and facts are few. It must be accepted that the issue is currently beyond the reach of exact science. Perhaps this is why decisions are often based on non-scientific considerations. The public is informed that they are being protected from cancer when, unfortunately, most of the time this is not so. Based on the current understanding of the causes of the main human cancers, effective action taken on certain lifestyle practices would lower risk for cancer and other chronic diseases, but such changes are rarely implemented, again for non-scientific reasons. Thus, real progress in general cancer control through prevention is slow because it depends chiefly on public education.

Epigenetic (non-genotoxic) carcinogens

For carcinogens that are not DNA-reactive and operate by producing other cellular effects, the carcinogenic effects might be expected to parallel the dose–response relationships for the cellular effect that underlies carcinogenicity. Unfortunately, relatively few dose–response studies have been done with carcinogens of the epigenetic type, and almost none with regard to toxicological or pharmacological effects. Data exist for the chelating agent nitrilotriacetic acid, with which kidney and bladder tumours are produced by exposures to about 75 mmol/kg diet. This effect diminishes dramatically, in a non-linear fashion, when the exposure is reduced below 50 mmol/kg diet (Andersen *et al.*, 1982; Kitahori *et al.*, 1985). The mechanistic explanation is based on the cytotoxicity of high levels of agent. A dose–response study (Schoenig *et al.*, 1985) in which saccharin was fed to large numbers of rats over two generations shows that a 37% yield of bladder carcinoma plus papilloma was induced with 7·5% dietary saccharin, 20% with 6·25%, 15% with 5%, 12% with 4%, 8% with 3%, 5% with 1% and 0·8 with 0%, the controls. Thus, the data show a sizable drop in incidence with a reduction of less than half of the dose; 3% and 1% saccharin appear to be no-effect levels.

For several types of epigenetic carcinogens, especially promoters, theoretical considerations as well as available data from experimental studies strongly support the concept and existence of no-effect levels or thresholds. When the promoting agents DDT, phenobarbital or BHA were tested by themselves for carcinogenicity in rats, an effect was evident only at the highest dose levels given in life-time studies. These observations are supported by tests for promotion, where, after an appropriate genotoxic carcinogen is administered, higher yields of neoplasms are induced in a shorter time. After exposure to the appropriate tissue-specific genotoxic carcinogens, no-effect levels have been observed in promotion assays for saccharin in bladder cancer promotion (Council on Scientific Affairs, 1985; Golberg, 1985), butylated hydroxytoluene (BHT) or phenobarbital in liver cancer promotion (Peraino *et al.*, 1977; Schulte-Hermann, 1985).

Butylated hydroxyanisole (BHA), a useful food antioxidant, has been reported to induce squamous carcinoma in the forestomach of 33/103 rats upon feeding a diet containing 2% BHA (Ito *et al.*, 1983 a). With a dose level of 0·5% BHA, only 2/101 rats had a papilloma and none had carcinoma. In appropriate tests for genotoxicity, BHA proved negative (Williams *et al.*, 1984). This behaviour is consistent with a promoting effect, which was explored by administration of a single gavage dose of the direct-acting gastric carcinogen *N*-methyl-*N'*-nitro-*N*-nitrosoguanidine (MNNG) to male rats. One week later, groups of rats were placed on diets containing 60–12 000 p.p.m. BHA for life. Gross forestomach tumours were clearly induced as a function of BHA dose. There was no enhancing effect apparent with 3000 p.p.m. and lower doses of BHA (Table 2). Ito *et al.* (1984) noted

Table 2. Promotion of stomach tumours by butylated hydroxy-anisole as a function of dose.

Treatment		Rats with gastric tumours (%)[†]
MNNG only [‡]		38
MNNG + BHA	60 p.p.m.	29
MNNG + BHA	300 p.p.m.	38
MNNG + BHA	1000 p.p.m.	33
MNNG + BHA	3000 p.p.m.	31
MNNG + BHA	6000 p.p.m.	59
MNNG + BHA	12 000 p.p.m.	80
BHA alone	12 000 p.p.m.	0
Control (no MNNG or BHA)		0

[†] $n = 30$ in each group.

[‡] Single dose of 250 mg/kg body wt. MNNG in 1 ml water at pH 5·0 was given as initiating carcinogen. One week later test diets including six dose levels of BHA ranging from 12000 p.p.m. to 60 p.p.m. and controls, were administered *ad libitum*. The experimental design calls for a life-time study. Presented in this table are the data for grossly visible tumours in rats that either died or were killed by 20 months.

promoting effects with 5000 p.p.m. BHA. These results are supported by finding increased proliferative lesions with 20 000 p.p.m. BHA, fewer with 5 000 p.p.m. and none with 2500 p.p.m. Even when feeding 20 000 p.p.m. BHA, there was reversibility one to two weeks after ceasing BHA intake (Altmann *et al.*, 1985; Iverson *et al.*, 1985). Of the two isomers present in commercial food-grade BHA, the active compound is the 3-*tert*-butyl-4-hydroxyanisole; the 2-isomer is inactive (Kurata *et al.*, 1984). Thus, the information available suggests: (1) the existence of a threshold, and (2) reversibility, as is typically expected of agents operating through epigenetic mechanisms.

　　Useful data exist for the quantitative effects of promoting agents in humans. Bile acids are demonstrated promoters for colon cancer. In high-risk populations for colon cancer in the Western World, the prevailing concentration of bile acids is 12 mg/g of faeces, stemming from the traditional high-fat low-fibre diets. In Japan with a low-fat intake, or in Finland with a high cereal fibre intake, the risk for colon cancer is low, and the concentration of faecal bile acids is about 4 mg/g, only one third of the concentration associated with high risk (Reddy *et al.*, 1980; Wynder *et al.*, 1983). Complex tobacco smoke contains relatively small amounts of genotoxic polycyclic aromatic hydrocarbons, nicotine-derived nitrosamines and certain heterocyclic amines (Surgeon General Report, 1982). The major effect of tobacco stems from the promoting effect of the acidic fraction of the smoke. It is established that an individual chronically smoking 40 cigarettes per day is at high risk, but with 10 cigarettes per day the risk is much lower, and with four cigarettes per day the risk is most difficult to evaluate accurately. These observations represent evidence that enhancing factors have steep dose–response curves in humans, as in experimental animals. Cessation of smoking reduces the risk considerably because promotion is removed (Hiatt *et al.*, 1977).

Human beings have been exposed to significant levels of a variety of epigenetic carcinogens such as certain of the organochlorine pesticides, phenobarbital and physiological levels of oestrogens without evidence of cancer causation (Clemmesen *et al.*, 1980; Hayes, 1982). Yet carcinogens that are not DNA-reactive have produced human cancer, for example, asbestos through occupational exposure and diethylstilboestrol (DES) at high pharmacological levels. These two chemicals, however, are special cases. Inhaled asbestos fibres remain in the lung; thus, there is lifelong continuing exposure of the tissue, even if the agent is no longer in the outside environment. Most lung cancers, however, are mainly caused by tobacco smoke, powerfully enhanced by asbestos (Hammond *et al.*, 1979). With high levels of transplacental DES, there appears to be permanent imprinting of the endocrine system of the foetus, which is eventually expressed at puberty as a special type of endocrine-related neoplasm, clear cell carcinoma of the vagina (Iguchi *et al.*, 1986). The negative findings with other epigenetic agents suggest that their exposure levels have been below the thresholds for cancer production and also do not involve long residence in the body at sufficient levels or imprinting on a differentiating organ.

Thus, carcinogens, both DNA-reactive and epigenetic, act in a dose-dependent fashion, although the dose–response relationships appear to be different. Thresholds have been observed for both types of carcinogens in experimental animals and humans. The thresholds for DNA-reactive carcinogens vary greatly and may be low. Those for non-genotoxic epigenetic carcinogens, particularly of the promoter class, have been fairly high and are a function of classical pharmacological and toxicological phenomena. These comments bear on the design and interpretation of carcinogen tests to delineate human risk, as discussed previously in this paper.

Which experimental carcinogens are potential human carcinogenic risks?

A chemical labelled 'carcinogen' based on bioassay results alone is in fact only an experimental carcinogen (Weisburger, 1985). How can a human carcinogenic risk be defined reliably and predictably? In addition to strict statistical considerations, it is important to consider mechanisms of action.

It has been dogma that human carcinogens are also animal carcinogens, and vice versa. The 'vice-versa' statement depends on what is an 'animal carcinogen'. The concept should be more correctly expressed as follows. Tests of virtually all human carcinogens in the customary animal models at high dose levels induce cancer in several different species, in high yield, with 80–100% of animals affected, and with a latent period that is often relatively short, of the order of 6–18 months. Human carcinogens that are genotoxic, and most of them are, reproducibly display activity in most of the short-term tests *in vitro*. The reverse is likely to be true also. Thus, a chemical that is (1) reliably active in batteries of short-term tests (not just a single test) and that can thus be concluded to be genotoxic, (2) that is definitively active (high yield of specific neoplasms, latent period less than 18 months) in several bioassay systems *in vivo*, and (3) that exhibits activity over a range of dose levels, is likely to be a human cancer risk. A chemical with such characteristics requires appropriate controls to avoid cancer risk. The human carcinogen 4-aminobiphenyl exhibits powerful carcinogenicity in several rodent species and in dogs, and demonstrates reliable activity in a number of bioassay systems *in vitro* (International Agency for Research on Cancer, 1972–85). Other genotoxic human carcinogens likewise are uniformly active in many tests *in vitro* (Waters *et al.*, 1983). The recently discovered mutagenic heterocyclic amines formed during cooking display activity in most of the bioassays *in vitro* and potent carcinogenicity in every test performed in mice and rats (Sugimura *et al.*, 1986). On the other hand, agents such as benzene (leukaemogen) or diethylstilboestrol (high-dose level, specific action on endocrine-sensitive tissue) are often negative in the tests *in vitro*, suggesting an absence of genotoxicity. There human carcinogenicity may stem from specific exposure conditions. For benzene, there were unhygienic workplaces involving high chronic exposure levels. For DES, it was also high dosages during the critical developmental and differentiating periods of the foetus (Williams *et al.*, 1985).

Activity of a test chemical in only a few or only one of the bioassays *in vitro* requires careful analysis of the positive and negative experiments before classifying it as genotoxic. The plant flavone quercetin is active in the Ames test with metabolic activation, but not in other tests *in vitro*; it is negative in the Williams hepatocyte repair assay (Williams, 1986). Careful bioassays of quercetin in mice, rats and hamsters have failed to demonstrate carcinogenicity (Hirono, 1986). High-dose-level feeding induced liver tumours in low yield (Ertürk *et al.*, 1984), consistent with a promoting rather than a carcinogenic effect. The underlying mechanism suggests that quercetin and related polyhydroxylated flavones may be positive in the Ames test because H_2O_2 or hydroxyl radicals can be generated under the conditions of the test (Troll & Wiesner, 1985). In mammalian systems, biochemical defence mechanisms protect against these reactive molecules or radicals, which would account for the fact that in mammalian systems these agents are usually negative. Hence, even a definitely positive response in a single test alone requires careful analysis as to the underlying mechanism.

A limited response in a carcinogenicity bioassay also needs evaluation of the relevant modes of action. Neoplasms in endocrine-sensitive target organs such as the adrenal, thyroid or pituitary gland may be due to the creation of hormonal imbalances, via mechanisms to be established. These, in turn, are usually highly dose-dependent and call for a multi-dose bioassay to determine the possible existence of no-effect levels. Dose–response studies are absolutely essential to determine the linearity or non-linearity of an effect (see data on BHA above).

Finally, increasingly sensitive chemical analytical techniques can detect the existence of numerous chemicals in the environment. Do the minute amounts detectable by high-resolution methods have toxicologic significance, especially in respect to cancer risks? Thus, it is vital to acquire essential data on the quantitative aspects of an effect. Quantitation is particularly indicated in the overall assessment of the causes of major types of human cancer that can involve complex interactions of genotoxic components present in relatively small amounts and promoters or enhancers that control the eventual development of cancer. For example, in nutritional carcinogenesis, the genotoxic components may be generated during the cooking of food (Sugimura *et al.*, 1986). The intake of dietary fat yields important promoting or enhancing elements at specific target organs such as breast or colon, but not in other organs such as the liver (Wynder *et al.*, 1983). Understanding of the tissue-specific promoting phenomenon accounts for the failure of the newly discovered carcinogens to induce liver cancer in man, even though high-level intake in mice and rats suggests the liver as one of the target organs, in addition to colon and breast (Sugimura *et al.*, 1986). In the absence of promoters, the liver is not affected by the small amounts consumed by man.

Thus, the database required for risk assessment and the protection of man against cancer hazards involves systematic analysis of data as follows.

A. Structure–activity relationships.
B. Biotransformation as a function of species.
C. Results from a battery of short-term *in vitro* tests yielding data that:
   1. indicate genotoxicity;
   2. indicate non-genotoxicity;
   3. are indeterminate (such as positive in one test or a few, but negative in most tests).
D. Bioassays *in vivo* indicating:
   1. high incidence of malignant neoplasms in mice, rats and/or hamsters with a relatively short latent period;
   2. evidence of non-carcinogenicity;
   3. low but statistically significant incidence with a long latent period in:
      a, endocrine-sensitive target organs:
      b, specific non-endocrine target organs;
      c, liver of select mouse strains.

The results at either extreme are clearcut, requiring little discussion: in C-1 and D-1, namely, there are genotoxicity and rapid powerful action in animal models at one end, or in C-2 and D-2, negative results exist in all bioassays *in vitro* and *in vivo*. Any environmental chemical, synthetic or naturally occurring, displaying reliably positive results could be a likely carcinogenic risk to man, provided the amount and length of exposure is sufficient. Such a chemical should be controlled, or eliminated whenever possible. Negative results are obviously do not represent direct cancer risks.

The third type of result described under test systems C and D needs detailed analysis. In most instances, chemicals with properties (*a*) (*b*) or (*c*) listed under D-3 above, displayed after systematic test series A, B, C and D, are not likely to be human cancer risks at the exposure levels prevailing in man's environment. No human carcinogen is known that has such properties.

Thus, human cancer risks are defined by tests that yield clear positive results, as per C-1 and D-1. International actions to control such substances, and especially greater efforts to lower the promoting effects associated with certain lifestyle-related parameters, would provide a focus towards the economic yet effective, control of cancer.

Final comments

It is now possible to provide the field of carcinogen bioassay and health risk analysis with procedures and recommendations that can be economically and rapidly carried out worldwide to forecast possible carcinogenic hazards. These abbreviated procedures, based on current understanding of the mechanisms of carcinogenesis, are deemed no less efficient than the former cumbersome, time-consuming and expensive chronic bioassays. In fact, because the current and future procedures will entail critical components with 'yes' or 'no' answers related to mechanisms of action, these techniques actually provide enhanced qualitative decision-making potential. Future advances in molecular biology may provide additional improvements in diagnosing potential cancer risks. Indeed, some genotoxic carcinogens have now been found to lead to activation of cellular proto-oncogenes. It is possible that this area might yield even more efficient means of determining, from a qualitative standpoint, whether or not a given product could eventually elicit cancer. Furthermore, improved knowledge in the area of the mechanism of promotion may likewise contribute to the development of additional test systems that would facilitate the detection of materials with promoting properties.

Toxicologists and those who apply toxicological research results to public protection must have much more cognition of the quantitative aspects and interactive events in carcinogenesis. The power of analytical chemistry is such that trace amounts of chemicals can be determined specifically and accurately. Claims have been made about the risk of disease associated with materials, to be found in trace amounts in air or drinking water, that were 'carcinogenic'

Table 3. Long-term goals for chronic disease prevention.

Action	Disease reduction benefit
Control smoking – less harmful cigarettes	Coronary heart disease; cancers of the lung, kidney, bladder, pancreas
Lower total fat intake	Coronary heart disease; cancers of the colon, breast, prostate, ovary, endometrium
Lower salt Na^+ intake; balance $K^+ + Ca^{2+}/Na^+$ ratio	Hypertension, stroke, cardiovascular disease
Increase natural fibre	Colorectal cancer
Avoid pickled, smoked, highly salted foods	Stomach cancer, hypertension, stroke
Increase and balance micronutrients, vitamins, minerals	Cardiovascular disease, several types of cancer
Lower intake of fried foods	Cancers of colon, breast

based on the induction of liver neoplasms in mice. It seems reasonably certain that even powerful carcinogens at those low levels are toxicologically non-significant, and certainly non-genotoxic agents that mainly induce mouse hepatomas are harmless under these conditions. Doubt is justified on the value of national or international efforts (incurred at large expense) to control such elements of questionable toxicological importance in contrast to the need to protect people from those factors that are actually causing cancer. Little official action is taken in many parts of the world on established health risks, whether this be the use of tobacco products, consuming salted and pickled foods, too much total or saturated fat in the diet, or the relative absence of cereal fibre, and related lifestyle elements. Many human cancers and other fatal or disabling chronic diseases are avoidable if the procedures described herein are applied with suitable attention paid to the interpretation of results in the light of mechanisms. Above all, it is important to control lifestyle-related factors, especially tobacco use and nutritional elements more effectively (Table 3).

References

Altmann, H. J., Wester, P. W., Mathiaschk, G., Grunow, W. and van der Heijden, C. A., 1985, Induction of early lesions in the forestomach of rats by 3-tert-butyl-4-hydroxyanisole (BHA). *Fd. Chem. Tox.*, **8**, 723–731.

Anderson, R. L., Alden, C. L. and Merski, J. A., 1982, The effects of nitrilotriacetate on cation disposition and urinary tract toxicity. *Fd Chem. Tox.*, **20**, 105–122.

Anders, M. W. (ed.), 1985, *Bioactivation of Foreign Compounds* (New York: Academic Press).

Ashby, J., Lefevre, P. A., Burlinson, B. and Penman, M. G., 1985, An assessment of the *in vivo* rat hepatocyte DNA-repair assay. *Mutation Res.*, **156**, 1–18.

Berenblum, I., 1985, Challenging problems in cocarcinogenesis. *Cancer Res.*, **45**, 1917–1921.

Berlin, A., Draper, M., Hemminki, K. and Vainio, H. (eds), 1984, *Monitoring Human Exposure to Carcinogenic and Mutagenic Agents*, IARC Scientific Publication 59, (Lyon: International Agency for Research on Cancer).

Börzsönyi, M., Day, N. E., Lapis, K. and Yamasaki, H. (eds), 1984, *Models, Mechanisms and Etiology of Tumour Promotion*, IARC Scientific Publication 56, (Lyon: International Agency for Research on Cancer).

Brunnemann, K. D., Genoble, L. and Hoffman, D., 1985, *N*-nitrosamines in chewing tobacco: an international comparison. *J. Agric. Fd Chem.*, **33**, 1178–1181.

Cameron, T. P., Hickman, R. L., Kornreich, M. R. and Tarone, R. E., 1985, History, survival and growth patterns of B6C3F1 mice and F344 rats in the National Cancer Institute Carcinogenesis Testing Program. *Fund. appl. Tox.*, **5**, 526–538.

Clemmesen, J., Conning, D. M., Henschler, D. and Oesch, F. (eds), 1980, Quantitative aspects of risk assessment in chemical carcinogenesis. *Archs Tox.* (Suppl. 3) 1–330.

Council on Scientific Affairs, American Medical Association, 1985, Saccharin. Review of safety issues. *J. Am. Med. Assoc.*, **254**, 2622–2624.

Croci, T. and Williams, G. M., 1985, Activities of several phase I and phase II xenobiotic biotransformation enzymes in cultured hepatocytes from male and female rats. *Biochem. Pharmac.*, **34**, 3029–3035.

Doll, R. R. and Peto, R., 1981, The causes of cancer: quantitative estimates of avoidable risks of cancer in the United States today. *J. natn. Cancer Inst.*, **66**, 1191–1308.

Druckrey, H., 1967, Quantitative aspects in chemical carcinogenesis. *UICC Monogr.*, **7**, 60–77.

Ertürk, E., Hatcher, J. F., Nunoya, T., Pamukcu, A. M. and Bryan, G. T., 1984, Hepatic tumours in Sprague–Dawley (SD) and Fischer 344 (F) female rats chronically exposed to quercetin (Q) or its glycoside rutin (R). *Proc. Am. Assoc. Cancer Res.*, **25**, 95.

Everson, R. B., Randerath, E., Santella, R. M., Cefalo, R. C., Avitts, T. H. and Randerath, K., 1986, Detection of smoking-related covalent DNA adducts in human placenta. *Science*, **231**, 54–57.

Foulds, L., 1979, *Neoplastic Development* (New York: Academic Press).

Fox, T. R. and Watanabe, P. G., 1985, Detection of a cellular oncogene in spontaneous liver tumours of B6C3F1 mice. *Science*, **228**, 596–597.

Golberg, L. (ed.), 1985, Saccharin: current status. *Fd Chem. Toxicol.* **23**, 417–546.

Hammond, E. C., Selikoff, I. J. and Seidman, H., 1979, Asbestos exposure, cigarette smoking and death rates. *Ann. N.Y. Acad. Sci.*, **330**, 474–490.

Hayes Jr, W. J., 1982, *Pesticides Studied in Man* (Baltimore: Williams and Wilkins).

Hecker, E., Fusenig, N. E., Kunz, W., Marks, F. and Thielmann, H. W., 1982, Cocarcinogenesis. and biological effects of tumor promoters. In *Carcinogenesis—A Comprehensive Survey*, Vol. 7 (New York: Raven Press).

Hiatt, H. H., Watson, J. D. and Winsten, J. A. (eds), 1977, *Origins of Human Cancer* (Cold Spring Harbor, NY: Cold Spring Harbor Laboratory).

Hirono, I., 1986, Carcinogenicity of plant constituents: pyrrolizidine alkaloids, flavonoids, bracken fern. In *Genetic Toxicology of the Diet. Progress in Clinical and Biological Research*, Vol. 206, edited by I. Knudsen (New York: Alan R. Liss), pp. 45–54.

Hoel, D. G., Kaplan, N. L. and Anderson, M. W., 1983, Implication of nonlinear kinetics on risk estimation in carcinogenesis. *Science*, **219**, 1032–1037.

Hoel, D. G., Merrill, R. A., and Perera, F. P. (eds), 1985, *Risk Quantitation and Regulatory Policy. Banbury Report*, 19 (Cold Spring Harbor, NY: Cold Spring Harbor Laboratory).

Hollaender, A. and de Serres, F. (eds), 1971–83, *Chemical Mutagens, Principles, and Methods for Their Detection*, Vols 1–8 (New York: Plenum Press).

Hueper, W. C. and Conway, W. D., 1964, *Chemical Carcinogenesis and Cancers* (Springfield, IL: Charles C. Thomas).

International Agency for Research on Cancer, 1972–85, IARC *Monographs on the Evaluation of the Carcinogenic Risk of Chemicals to Humans, Suppl. 4. Chemicals, Industrial Processes and Industries Associated with Cancer in Humans.* IARC Monographs Vols 1–29 (Lyon: International Agency for Research on Cancer).

Iguchi, T., Takase, M. and Takasugi, N., 1986, Development of vaginal adenosis-like lesions and uterine epithelial stratification in mice exposed perinatally to diethylstilbestrol. *Proc. Soc. exp. Biol. Med.*, **181**, 59–64.

Ito, N., Fukushima, S., Hagiwara, A., Shibata, M. and Ogiso, T., 1983a, Carcinogenicity of butylated hydroxyanisole in F344 rats. *J. natn. Cancer Inst.*, **70**, 343–352.

Ito, N., Fukushima, S., Imaida, K., Sakata, T. and Masui, T., 1983b, Induction of papilloma in the forestomach of hamsters by butylated hydroxyanisole. *Gann*, **14**, 459–461.

Ito, N., Fukushima, S., Tsuda, H., Shirai, T., Tatematsu, M. and Imaida, K., 1984, Modification of chemical carcinogenesis by antioxidants. In *Cellular Interactions by Environmental Tumor Promoters*, edited by H. Fujiki, E. Hecker, R. E. Moore, T. Sugimuara and I. B. Weinstein (Tokyo: Japan Scientific Society Press), pp. 381–389.

Iverson, F., Lok, E., Nera, E., Karpinski, K. and Clayson, D. B., 1985, A 13-week feeding study of butylated hydroxyanisole: the subsequent regression of the induced lesions in male Fischer 344 rat forestomach epithelium. *Toxicology*, **35**, 1–11.

Jakoby, W. B., (ed.), 1984, *Metabolic Basis of Detoxification: Metabolism of Functional Groups* (New York: Academic Press).

Kitahori, Y., Konishi, N., Shimoyama, T. and Hiasa, Y., 1985, Dose-dependent promoting effect of trisodium nitrilotriacetate monohydrate on urinary bladder carcinogenesis in Wistar rats pretreated with N-butyl-N-(4-hydroxybutyl)nitrosamine. *Jap. J. Cancer Res.*, (*Gann*), **76**, 818–822.

Kurata, Y., Ikawa, E., Mera, Y. and Fukushima, S., 1984, Induction of forestomach hyperplasia by crude butylated hydroxyanisole, a mixture of 3-tert and 2-tert isomers, in Syrian Golden hamsters is due to 3-tert-butylated hydroxyanisole. *Gann*, **75**, 471–474.

Littlefield, N. A. and Gaylor, D. W., 1985, Influence of total dose and dose rate in carcinogenicity studies. *J. Tox. envir. Hlth*, **15**, 545–550.

Long, E. L., Nelson, A. A., Fitzhugh, O. G. and Hansen, W. H., 1963, Liver tumors produced in rats by feeding safrole. *Archs Path.*, **75**, 595–604.

Maron, D. M. and Ames, B. N., 1983, Revised methods for the *Salmonella* mutagenicity test. *Mutation Res.*, **113**, 173–215.

McCallum, R. I., Woolley, V. and Petrie, A., 1983, Lung cancer associated with chloromethyl methyl ether manufacture: an investigation at two factories in the United Kingdom. *Br. J. Ind. Med.*, **40**, 384–389.

Miller, E. C. and Miller, J. A., 1981, Mechanisms of chemical carcinogenesis. *Cancer*, **47**, 1055–1064.

Milman, H. A. and Weisburger, E. K. (eds), 1985, *Handbook of Carcinogen Testing* (Park Ridge, NJ: Noyes Publ.).

Moriya, M., Ohta, T., Watanabe, K., Miyazawa, T., Kato, K. and Shirasu, Y., 1983, Further mutagenicity studies on pesticides in bacterial reversion assay systems. *Mutation Res.*, **116**, 185–216.

Muir, C. S. and Higginson, J., 1985, In *Handbook of Carcinogen Testing*, edited by H. A. Milman and E. K. Weisburger (Park Ridge, NJ: Noyes Publ.), pp. 28–56.

Nutrition Foundation, 1983, *The Relevance of Mouse Liver Hepatoma to Human Carcinogenic Risk. A Report of the International Expert Advisory Committee to the Nutrition Foundation* (Washington, DC: The Nutrition Foundation).

Office of Technology Assessment, 1982, *Cancer Risk: Assessing and Reducing the Dangers in Our Society* (USA: Westview Press).

Peraino, C., Fry, R. J. M., Staffeld, E and Christopher, J. P., 1977, Enhancing effects of phenobarbitone and butylated hydroxytoluene on 2-acetylaminofluorene-induced hepatic tumorigenesis in the rat. *Fd Cosmet. Tox.*, **15**, 93–96.

Pereira, M. A. (ed.), 1983, International symposium on tumor promotion. *Envir. Hlth Perspect.*, **50**, 3–330.

Peto, R., Gray, R., Brantom, P. and Grasso, P., 1984, *Nitrosamine Carcinogenesis in 5120 Rodents: Chronic Administration of Sixteen Different Concentrations of NDEA, NDMA, NPYR and NPIP in the Water of 4440 Inbred Rats, with Parallel Studies on NDEA Alone of the Effect of the Age of Starting (3, 6, or 20 weeks) and of the Species (Rats, Mice or Hamsters)*. IARC Scientific Publication No. 57 (Lyon: International Agency for Research on Cancer), pp. 627–665.

Poirier, M. C., Nakayama, J., Perera, F. P., Weinstein, I. B. and Yuspa, S. J., 1983, Identification of carcinogen-DNA adducts by immunoassays. In *Application of Biological Markers to Carcinogen Testing*, edited by H. A. Milman and S. Sell (New York: Plenum Press), pp. 427–440.

Reddy, B. S., Cohen, L. A., McCoy, G. D., Hill, P., Weisburger, J. H. and Wynder, E. L., 1980, Nutrition and its relationship to cancer. *Adv. Cancer Res.*, **32**, 237–345.

Reynolds, S. H., Stowers, S. J., Maronpot, R. R., Anderson, M. W. and Aaronson, S. A., 1986, Detection and identification of activated oncogenes in spontaneously occurring benign and malignant hepatocellular tumors of the B6C3F1 mouse. *Proc. natn. Acad. Sci. U.S.A.*, **83**, 33–37.

Rosenkranz, H. S., Karpinsky, G., and McCoy, E. C. (1980). Microbial assays: evaluation and application to the elucidation of the etiology of colon cancer. In Short-Term Test Systems for Determining Carcinogens, edited by K. Norpoth and R. C. Garner, pp. 19–57. (Berlin, Heidelberg: Springer-Verlag).

Rosenkranz, H. S., Klopman, G., Chankong, V., Pet-Edwards, J. and Haimes, Y. Y., (1984a), Prediction of environmental carcinogens: a strategy for the mid 1980's. *Environ. Mutagen.* **6**, 231–258.

Rosenkranz, H. S., Pet-Edwards, J., Chankong, V. and Haimes, Y. Y. (1984b), Reply to letter to editor. *Environ. Mutagen.* **6**, 631–632.

Russell, W. L., Hunsicker, P. R., Raymen, G. D., Steele, M. H., Stelzner, K. F., and Thompson, H. M., (1982). Dose response for ethylnitrosurea-induced specific-locus mutagens in mouse spermatogonia. *Proc. Natn. Acad. Sci.* **73**, 3589–3591.

Schmähl, D., Thomas, C., and Auer, R., 1977, *Iatrogenic Carcinogenesis* (Berlin, Heidelburg: Springer-Verlag).

Schoenig, G. P., Goldenthal, E. I., Geil, R. G., Frith, C. H., Richter, W. R. and Carlborg, F. W., 1985, Evaluation of the dose response and *in utero* exposure to saccharin in the rat. *Fd Chem. Tox.*, **23**, 475–490.

Schottenfeld, D. and Fraumeni Jr, J. F., 1982, *Cancer Epidemiology and Prevention* (Philadelphia: Saunders and Co.)

Schulte-Hermann, R., 1985, Tumor promotion in the liver. *Archs Tox.*, **57** 147–158.

Searle, C. E. (ed.), 1984, *Chemical Carcinogens*, 2nd edn, ACS Monograph 182 (Washington, DC: American Chemical Society).

Shimkin, M. B., Weisburger, J. H., Weisburger, E. K., Gubareff, N., and Suntzeff,

V., 1966, Bioassay of 29 alkylating chemicals by the pulmonary-tumor response in strain A mice. *J. natn. Cancer Inst.*, **36**, 915–935.

Shubik, P., 1984, Progression and promotion. *J. natn. Cancer Inst.*, **73**, 1005–1011.

Smith, J., 1981, Re-examination of the ED01 study. Overview. *Fund. Appl. Tox.*, **1**, 28–128.

Squire, R. A., 1981, Ranking animal carcinogens: a proposed regulatory approach. *Science*, **214**, 877–880.

Sugimura, T., Sato, S., Ohgaki, H., Takayama, S., Nagao, M. and Wakabayashi, K., 1986, Overview: mutagens and carcinogens in cooked food. In *Genetic Toxicology of the Diet. Progress in Clinical and Biological Research.*, Vol. 206, edited by I. Knudsen (New York: Alan R. Liss), pp. 85–107.

Surgeon General Report, 1982, The health consequences of smoking. *Cancer*, US Government Publication No. DHHS (PHS) 82-50179 (Washington, DC: Superintendent of Documents, US Government Printing Office), Chap. 5.

Troll, W. and Wiesner, R., 1985, The role of oxygen radicals as a possible mechanism of tumor promotion. *Ann. Rev. Pharmac. Tox.*, **25**, 509–528.

Trosko, J. E., 1984, A new paradigm is needed in toxicology evaluation. *Envir. Mutagen.*, **6**, 767–769.

Trosko, J. E., Jone, C., Aylsworth, C. and Chang, C. C., 1985, *In vitro* assay to detect inhibitors of intercellular communication. In *Handbook of Carcinogen Testing* edited by H. A. Milman and E. K. Weisburger (Park Ridge, NJ: Noyes Publ.), pp. 422–437.

Upton, A. C., Clayson, D. B., Jansen, J. D., Rosenkranz, H. S., and Williams, G. M., 1984, Report of ICPEMC Task Group No. 5 on the differentiation between genotoxic and non-genotoxic carcinogens. *Mutation Res.*, **133**, 1–49.

Vainio, H., Hemminki, K. and Wilbourn, 1985, Data on the carcinogenicity of chemicals in the IARC Monographs programme. *Carcinogenesis*, **6**, 1653–1665.

Wang, G. M., 1984, Evaluation of pesticides which pose carcinogenicity potential in animal testing. 1. Developing a tumor data evaluation system. *Regul. Toxic. Pharmac.*, **4**, 355–360.

Waters, M. D., Garrett, N. E., Covone-de Serres, C. M., Howard, B. E. and Stack, H. F., 1983, Genetic toxicology of some known or suspected human carcinogens. In *Chemical Mutagens, Principles and Methods for Their Detection*, Vol. 8, edited by F. J. de Serres (New York: Plenum Press), pp. 261–342.

Weisburger, E. K., 1982, *N*-2-Fluorenylacetamide and derivatives. In *Carcinogens in Industry and the Environment*, edited by J. Sontag (New York: Marcel Decker), pp. 583–666.

Weisburger, E. K., 1983, History of the bioassay program of the National Cancer Institute. *Progr. exp. Tumor Res.*, **26**, 187–201.

Weisburger, J. H., 1985, Definition of a carcinogen as a potential human carcinogenic risk. *Jap. J. cancer Res.*, (*Gann*), **76**, 1244–1246.

Weisburger, J. H. and Williams, G. M., 1984, Bioassay of carcinogens: *in vitro* and *in vivo* tests. In *Chemical Carcinogens*, Vol. 2, edited by C. E. Searle (Washington, DC: American Chemical Society), pp. 1323–1373.

Williams, G. M., 1977, The detection of chemical carcinogens by unscheduled DNA synthesis in rat liver primary cell culture. *Cancer Res.*, **37**, 1845–1851.

Williams, G. M., 1985, Types of enhancement of carcinogenesis and influences on human cancer. *Carcinogen.-Comp. Surv.*, **8**, 447–457.

Williams, G. M., 1986, Food-borne carcinogens. In *Genetic Toxicology of the Diet. Progress in Clinical Biological Research*, Vol. 206, edited by I. Knudsen (New York: Alan R. Liss), pp. 73–81.

Williams, G. M. and Weisburger, J. H., 1986, Chemical carcinogens. In *Casarett and*

Doull's Toxicology. The Basic Science of Poisons, 3rd edn, edited by J. Doull, C. D. Klaassen and M. O. Amdur (New York: Macmillan), pp. 99–173.

Williams, G. M., Dunkel, V. C. and Ray, V. A. (eds), 1983, Cellular systems for toxicity testing. *Ann. N.Y. Acad. Sci.*, Vol. 407 (New York: N.Y. Academy of Sciences).

Williams, G. M., Shimada, T., McQueen, C., Tong, C. and Ved Brat, S., 1984, Lack of genotoxicity of butylated hydroxyanisole (BHA) and butylated hydroxytoluene (BHT). *Toxicologist*, **4**, 104.

Williams, G. M., Reiss, B. and Weisburger, J. H., 1985, A comparison of the animal and human carcinogenicity of environmental, occupational and therapeutic chemicals. In *Advances in Modern Environmental Toxicology, Vol. XII. Mechanisms and Toxicity of Chemical Carcinogens and Mutagens*, edited by W. G. Flamm and R. J. Lorentzen (Princeton, NJ: Princeton Scien. Publ.) pp. 207–248.

Wilmer, J. L., 1984, On the carcinogenicity of aniline. *Envir. Mutagen.*, **6**, 629–630.

Wynder, E. L., Leveille, G. A., Weisburger, J. H. and Livingston, G. E. (eds), 1983, *Environmental Aspects of Cancer: The Role of Macro and Micro Components of Foods* (Westport, CT: Food and Nutrition Press), pp. 1–295.

Risk assessment considerations for the reproductive and developmental toxicity of oestrogenic xenobiotics

John. A. McLachlan[1], Retha R. Newbold[1], Kenneth S. Korach[1] and Michael D. Hogan[2]

Developmental Endocrinology and Pharmacology Section, Laboratory of Reproductive and Developmental Toxicology[1] and Biometry and Risk Assessment[2], National Institute of Environmental Health Sciences, National Institutes of Health, Research Triangle Park, NC 27709, USA

Oestrogenic xenobiotics: an introduction

Oestrogens are chemicals which stimulate proliferation and differentiation in target tissues, including the mammary gland and female genital tract. Many compounds of diverse chemical structure express oestrogenic activity (Duax & Weeks, 1980). Thus, this class of chemicals is defined more by the biological function than the structure of its members. The expression of hormonal activity by chemicals other than those having a steroid nucleus is apparently unique to oestrogens. The potency of oestrogenic chemicals varies widely, but the presence of a phenolic group in the molecule seems to be a necessary, but not always sufficient, requirement for high biological activity.

As seen in Figure 1, exposure to environmental oestrogens may involve a variety of chemicals. There are many naturally occurring oestrogenic substances in plants (e.g., coumestrol and equol), and some fungi produce oestrogenic mycotoxins (zearalenone). Another source of oestrogens in the environment arises from synthetic processes. In some cases, an environmental oestrogen is made and used as a hormone (e.g., diethylstilboestrol or DES), whereas in others, the products are synthesized for non-hormonal purposes but have oestrogenic activity (e.g., kepone or DDT). In the latter case, metabolism of these compounds from hormonally inactive (prohormone) to more active forms may become an important factor. In fact, the role of metabolism in the activity and toxicity of xenobiotic oestrogens is probably four-fold:

1. In some cases, chemicals may be metabolized from less to more active oestrogens. This usually involves the addition or unmasking of a hydroxyl group; hydroxylation of benz[a]anthracene to 3,9-dihydroxybenz[a]anthracene (Schneider *et al.*, 1976) increases its oestrogenic potency 50-fold;

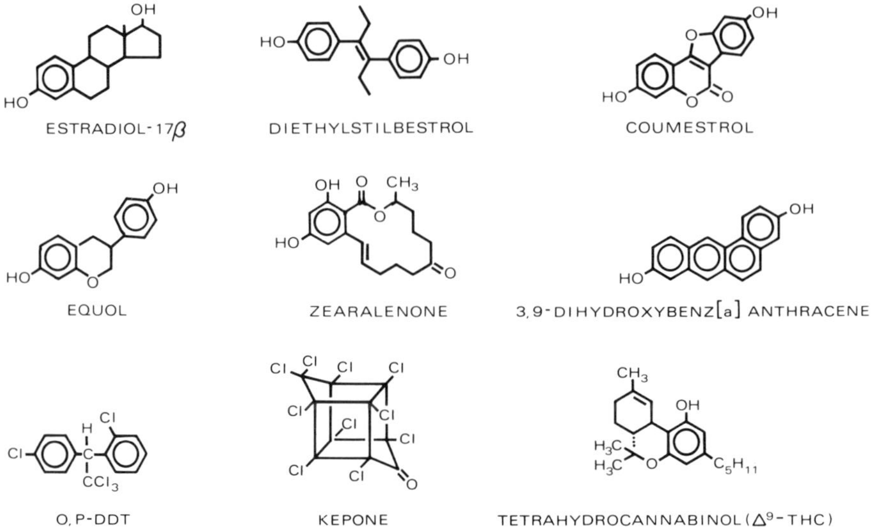

Figure 1. Chemicals reported to be oestrogenic. Selected references include: oestradiol and diethylstilboestrol (Korach *et al.*, 1978); coumestrol and equol (Setchell, 1985); zearalenone (Wilson & Hagler, 1985); 3,9-dihydroxybenz[*a*]anthracene (Schneider *et al.*, 1976); *o,p*-DDT (Kupfer & Bugler, 1980); kepone (Eroschenko & Palmiter, 1980); tetrahydrocannabinol (Rawitch *et al.*, 1977)

likewise, hydroxylation of the chlorinated hydrocarbon, DDT, is considered important for binding to the oestrogen receptor (Kupfer and Bulger, 1980).

2. Conversely, potent oestrogens can be metabolized to much less hormonally active compounds; DES is metabolized, in most species, to *z,z*-dienoestrol, a very weak oestrogen (Korach *et al.*, 1978).

3. In some rare cases, potent oestrogenic chemicals are metabolized to anti-oestrogens which possess good receptor binding activity but poor biological activity. The metabolic conversion of DES to pseudo-DES is an example (Korach *et al.*, 1979).

4. In each case, metabolism may result in reactive intermediates which may contribute to the toxicities associated with these compounds. For example, when DES is metabolized to the inactive oestrogen, *z,z*-dienoestrol, it proceeds along a pathway involving the generation of phenoxy free radical and para-quinone; both of these compounds are chemically reactive towards cellular macromolecules (Metzler & McLachlan, 1978).

Developmental and reproductive toxicology of xenobiotic oestrogens

The developing reproductive system is especially sensitive to long-term modifications by oestrogenic xenobiotics (McLachlan *et al.*, 1981). It has been shown that peri-natal treatment of laboratory animals with hormonally active compounds such as clomiphene (McCormack & Clark, 1979), methoxychlor (Harris *et al.*, 1974) or kepone (Eroschenko & Palmiter, 1980) results in irreversible alterations in the structure and function of the reproductive system. Of the compounds studied, DES has received the most thorough attention.

Adult female mice which have been exposed pre-natally to DES exhibit structural (Newbold *et al.*, 1983b) and functional (Maier *et al.*, 1985) alterations in their genital tracts; developmentally oestrogenized mice also show a dose-related decrease in fertility (McLachlan *et al.*, 1982) and increase in genital tract neoplasia (McLachlan *et al.*, 1980). In mouse foetuses exposed transplacentally to radiolabelled DES, unconjugated radioactivity accumulated in the developing genital tract (Shah & McLachlan, 1976). Moreover, the foetal mouse genital tract has been shown to metabolize DES along pathways involving reactive intermediates (Maydl *et al.*, 1983) and to express molecular lesions which persist into later life (Newbold *et al.*, 1984). Thus, the study of mechanisms underlying the formation of differentiation defects and their later manifestations in the reproductive system of developmentally oestrogenized laboratory animals starts to provide a basis for a comparison with similarly exposed humans.

Relationship between developmentally oestrogenized experimental animals and humans

Female mice or humans exposed pre-natally to DES share several structural and functional reproductive tract defects (Table 1). Some of these lesions (such

Table 1. Comparable reproductive tract lesions reported in mice or women exposed pre-natally to DES.

Site of lesion	Report of pre-natal exposure	
	Mouse	Human
Vagina		
Adenosis	Newbold & McLachlan (1982)	Stafl *et al.* (1974)
Adenocarcinoma	McLachlan *et al.* (1980) Newbold & McLachlan (1982)	Herbst *et al.* (1971)
Uterus		
Structural abnormality	McLachlan *et al.* (1980)	Haney *et al.* (1979)
Oviduct		
Structural malformation	McLachlan *et al.* (1980) Newbold *et al.* (1983a,b)	DeCherney *et al.* (1981)
Salpingitis isthmica nodosa	Newbold *et al.* (1983a,b, 1984)	Shen *et al.* (1983)
Ovary		
Paraovarian cysts (mesonephric origin)	Newbold *et al.* (1983a)	Haney *et al.* (1986)

as oviductal malformation) are apparently teratogenic effects since, at least in the mouse, they are apparent at birth. Others (such as salpingitis isthmica nodosa, a proliferative lesion of the oviductal epithelium, or vaginal adenocarcinoma) are apparently progressive in nature, although the cellular defect may exist at birth. In both species, developmental exposure to oestrogens results in disruption of the normal integrative function of the reproductive system with subsequent deficits in reproductive function.

The cohort of women exposed pre-natally to DES represents a unique resource for testing the hypotheses underlying risk assessment in reproductive and developmental toxicology. The population is one with well documented exposure data, in terms of both dose and time. Moreover, several cohorts of high or low exposures have been followed longitudinally over time with appropriately matched controls. When compared to the well-characterized animal models for developmental oestrogenization, qualitative relationships such as shown in Table 1 can be established and utilized as clinical guidelines and, since animals can be thoroughly studied for pathobiology, aetiological indicators. Due to the integrative nature of the reproductive process, such studies still require whole animals.

Of equal or, perhaps, greater interest is to utilize the developmentally oestrogenized animal models and human cohorts to ask questions about quantitative relationships which test our assumptions of species extrapolations in reproductive toxicology and teratology. For example, in an early attempt to apply those principles, we have compared the relative potencies for DES in the induction of vaginal adenosis, a cellular lesion seen in both laboratory animals and women exposed developmentally to this synthetic oestrogen, calculated either as total gestational exposure or that dose which was given during the comparable developmental period for vaginal cellular development in each species. As seen in Table 2, the relative potency index is close to unity when determined with the underlying developmental biology in mind (Hogan *et al.*,

Table 2. Relative potency ratios for reproductive tract abnormalities associated with pre-natal exposure to DES.

Comparison	Relative potency index (animal/human) for:	
	Total gestation†	Comparable developmental period‡
Vaginal adenosis in:		
Mouse vs. human	4·19	1·00
Monkey vs. human	3·45	0·93

Modified from Hogan *et al.*, (submitted).
† Average dose of DES ($mg\ kg^{-1}\ d^{-1}$) throughout gestation.
‡ Average dose of DES ($mg\ kg^{-1}\ d^{-1}$) during that portion of the comparable developmental period in which exposure occurred.

1987). Hopefully, studies will be done utilizing these populations, which will begin to yield new models with which to assess risk for reproductive and developmental toxicities. The pertinence of such studies, especially with oestrogenic xenobiotics, was recently underlined by reports of premature sexual development in young girls in Puerto Rico (Haddock *et al.*, 1985); no aetiological basis for these clinical observations yet exists. Certainly, the application of evolving notions of the structural biology of hormonally active environmental chemicals to the, as yet, embryonic discipline of reproductive risk assessment is the necessary first step in this important area of environmental health.

References

DeCherney, A. H., Cholst, I. and Naftolin, F., 1981, Structure and function of the fallopian tubes following exposure to diethylstilbestrol (DES) during gestation. *Fert. Steril.*, **36**, 741–745.

Duax, W. L. and Weeks, C. M., 1980, Molecular basis of estrogenicity: x-ray crystallographic studies. In *Estrogens in the Environment.*, edited by J. A. McLachlan (New York: Elsevier/North Holland), pp. 11–32.

Eroschenko, V. P. and Palmiter, R. D., 1980, Estrogenicity of kepone in birds and mammals. In *Estrogens in the Environment*, edited by J. A. McLachlan (New York: Elsevier/North Holland), pp. 305–326.

Haddock, L., Lebron, G., Martinez, R., Cordero, J. F., Freni-Titulaer, Carrion, F., Cintron, C. and Gonzalez, L., 1985, Premature sexual development in Puerto Rico: background and current status. In *Estrogens in the Environment II: Influences on Development*, edited by J. A. McLachlan (New York: Elsevier/North Holland), pp. 358–379.

Haney, A. F., Hammond, C. B., Soules, M. R. and Creasman, W. T., 1979, Diethylstilbestrol-induced upper genital tract abnormalities. *Fert. Steril.*, **31**, 142–146.

Haney, A. F., Newbold, R. R., Fetter, B. F. and McLachlan, J. A., 1986, Hyperplastic paraovarian cysts associated with prenatal diethylstilbestrol exposure: comparison between human and mouse. *Am. J. Path.*, **124**, 405–411.

Harris, S. J., Cecil, H. C. and Bitman, J., 1974, Effect of several dietary levels of technical methoxychlor on reproduction in rats. *J. Agric. Fd. Chem.*, **22**, 969–973.

Herbst, A. L., Ulfelder, J. and Poskanzer, D. C., 1971, Adenocarcinoma of the vagina: association of maternal stilbestrol therapy with tumor appearance in young women. *New Engl. J. Med.*, **284**, 878–881.

Hogan, M. D., Newbold, R. R. and McLachlan, J. A., 1987, The extrapolation of teratogenic responses from experimental animals to humans: DES as an illustrative example. (Submitted).

Korach, K. S., Metzler, M. and McLachlan, J. A., 1978, Estrogenic activity *in vivo.* and *in vitro* of some metabolites and analogs of diethylstilbestrol. *Proc. natn. Acad. Sci. U.S.A.*, **75**, 468–471.

Korach, K. S., Metzler, M. and McLachlan, J. A., 1979, Diethylstilbestrol metabolites and analogs: new probes for the study of hormone action. *J. biol. Chem.*, **254**, 8963–8968.

Kupfer, D. and Bulger, W. H., 1980, Estrogenic properties of DDT and its analogs.

In *Estrogens in the Environment*, edited by J. A. McLachlan (New York: Elsevier/North Holland), pp. 239–264.

Maier, D. B., Newbold, R. R. and McLachlan, J. A., 1985, Prenatal diethylstilbestrol exposure alters murine uterine responses of prepubertal estrogen stimulation. *Endocrinology*, **116**, 1878–1887.

Maydl, R., Newbold, R. R., Metzler, M. and McLachlan, J. A., 1983, Diethylstilbestrol metabolism by its target tissue, the fetal genital tract. *Endocrinology*, **113**, 146–152.

McCormack, S. A. and Clark, J. H., 1979, Clomid administration to the pregnant rat causes abnormalities of the reproductive tract in offspring and mothers. *Science*, **204**, 629–631.

McLachlan, J. A., Newbold, R. R. and Bullock, B. C., 1980, Long-term effects on the female mouse genital tract associated with prenatal exposure to diethylstilbestrol. *Cancer Res.*, **40**, 3988–3999.

McLachlan, J. A., Newbold, R. R., Korach, K. S., Lamb IV, J. C., and Suzuki, Y., 1981, Transplacental toxicology: prenatal factors influencing postnatal fertility. In *Developmental Toxicology*, edited by C. A. Kimmel, and J. Buelke-Sam (New York: Raven Press), pp. 213–232.

McLachlan, J. A., Newbold, R. R., Shah, H. C., Hogan, M. and Dixon, R. L., 1982, Reduced fertility in female mice exposed transplacentally to diethylstilbestrol. *Fert. Steril.*, **38**, 364–371.

Metzler, M. and McLachlan, J. A., 1978, Peroxidase-mediated oxidation, a possible pathway for metabolic activation of diethylstilbestrol. *Biochem. biophys. Res. Commun.*, **85**, 874–884.

Newbold, R. R. and McLachlan, J. A., 1982, Vaginal adenosis and adenocarcinoma in mice transplacentally exposed to diethylstilbestrol. *Cancer Res.*, **42**, 2003–2011.

Newbold, R. R., Bullock, B. C. and McLachlan, J. A., 1983a, Exposure to diethylstilbestrol during pregnancy permanently alters the ovary and oviduct. *Biol. Reprod.*, **28**, 735–744.

Newbold, R. R., Tyrey, S., Haney, A. F. and McLachlan, J. A., 1983b, Developmentally arrested oviduct: a structural and functional defect in mice following prenatal exposure to diethylstilbestrol. *Teratology*, **27**, 417–426.

Newbold, R. R., Carter, D. B., Harris, S. E. and McLachlan, J. A., 1984, Molecular differentiation of the mouse genital tract: altered protein synthesis following prenatal exposure to diethylstilbestrol. *Biol. Reprod.*, **30**, 459–470.

Rawitch, A. B., Schultz, G. S., Ebner, K. E. and Vardaris, R. M., 1977, Competition of Δ^9-tetrahydrocannabinol with estrogen in rat uterine estrogen receptor binding. *Science*, **197**, 1189–1191.

Schneider, S. L., Alks, V., Morreal, C. E., Sinha, D. K. and Dao, T. L., 1976, Estrogenic properties of 3,9-dihydroxybenz[a]anthracene, a potential metabolite of benz[a]anthracene. *J. natn. Cancer Inst.*, **57**, 1351–1355.

Setchell, K. D. R., 1985, Naturally occurring non-steroidal estrogens of dietary origin. In *Estrogens in the Environment II: Influences on Development*, edited by J. A. McLachlan, (New York: Elsevier/North Holland), pp. 69–85.

Shah, H. C. and McLachlan J. A., 1976, The fate of diethylstilbestrol in the pregnant mouse. *J. Pharmac. exp. Ther.*, **197**, 687–696.

Shen, S. C., Bansal, M., Purrazella, R., Malviya, V. and Strauss, L., 1983, Benign glandular inclusions in lymph nodes, endosalpingiosis and salpingitis isthmica nodosa in a young girl with clear cell adenocarcinoma of the cervix. *Am. J. Surg. Path.*, **7**, 293–300.

Stafl, A., Mattingly, R. F., Foley, D. V. and Fetherston, W. C., 1974, Clinical diagnosis of vaginal adenosis. *Obstet. Gynec.*, **43**, 118–128.

Wilson, M. E. and Hagler Jr, W. M., 1985, Metabolism of zearalenone to a more estrogenically active form. In *Estrogens in the Environment II: Influences on Development*, edited by J. A. McLachlan (New York: Elsevier/North Holland), pp. 238–250.

Selection of animals for reproductive toxicology studies: An evaluation of selected assumptions in reproductive toxicity testing and risk assessment

Donald R. Mattison and Peter J. Thomford

Division of Reproductive Pharmacology and Toxicology, Department of Obstetrics and Gynecology, University of Arkansas for Medical Sciences, Little Rock, AR, USA.

and

Division of Reproductive and Developmental Toxicology, National Center for Toxicological Research, Jefferson, AR, USA

Introduction

The past decade has seen a growing concern for adverse reproductive effects following occupational, environmental or drug exposures. The National Institute for Occupational Safety and Health (NIOSH) has identified disorders of reproduction, infertility, spontaneous abortion and teratogenesis as areas of concern for work-related diseases and injuries (NIOSH, 1985a). Some of the compounds identified as reproductive toxins by NIOSH in a recent survey of industrial exposures are listed on Table 1 (NIOSH, 1985b).

Environmental exposures also cause concern with respect to reproductive toxicity. Table 2 lists the number of priority hazardous waste sites throughout the USA. Even a seemingly pristine state like Arkansas has seven high-priority toxic-waste dumpsites. Some of the compounds in these toxic-waste dumpsites are reproductive toxins in animals and man, and include benzene and polychlorinated biphenyls which are associated with oestrus cycle disturbances in animals, and menstrual disorders in humans (Barlow & Sullivan, 1982). Polychlorinated biphenyls have also been associated with pregnancy-related disorders, including low birthweight, high perinatal mortality and skin discolouration. It is important to note that occupational and environmental exposures are not the only exposures associated with reproductive dysfunction. Individuals may also be taking medications or recreational drugs which can produce adverse reproductive effects.

Table 3 lists the effects of a group of selected medications on female reproduction. Alpha-methyldopa, an anti-hypertensive agent, has been

Table 1. NIOSH reproductive toxins.†

Compound	Male	Female	Pregnancy
Chloroprene			X
Ethylene oxide			X
Ethylene dibromide	X		X
Ethylene dichloride			X
Glycidyl ethers	X		
2-Methoxyethanol		X	X
2-Ethoxyethanol	X	X	
2,3,7,8-Tetrachlorodibenzo-*p*-dioxin			X
1,3-Butadiene			X
Methyl chloride			X
Dinitrotoluene	X		

† This table lists compounds identified by NIOSH as having potential for adverse reproductive effects. Based on available data we have classified these putative reproductive toxins by susceptible reproductive event. The classification of only two as female reproductive toxins reflects lack of data rather than invulnerability.
Data from NIOSH (1985b).

Table 2. High priority hazardous waste dumpsites†

State	Dumpsites (no.)	State	Dumpsites (no.)
Alabama	9	Missouri	15
Alaska	0	Nebraska	4
Arkansas	7	Nevada	0
Arizona	6	New Hampshire	11
California	60	New Jersey	95
Colorado	14	New Mexico	4
Connecticut	6	New York	58
Delaware	9	North Carolina	7
District of Columbia	0	North Dakota	1
Florida	35	Ohio	28
Georgia	5	Oklahoma	4
Hawaii	6	Oregon	5
Idaho	4	Pennsylvania	49
Illinois	22	Rhode Island	7
Indiana	21	South Carolina	10
Iowa	6	South Dakota	1
Kansas	7	Tennessee	8
Kentucky	9	Texas	25
Louisiana	6	Utah	9
Maine	6	Vermont	2
Maryland	6	Virginia	10
Massachusetts	21	Washington	23
Michigan	6	West Virginia	6
Minnesota	34	Wisconsin	23
Mississippi	2	Wyoming	1

† This table lists the number of toxic-waste dumpsites identified as high priority by the USEPA.

Table 3. Effects of selected medications on female reproduction.

Medication	Effects
Alpha-methyldopa	Decreased libido, impaired arousal, loss of orgasm
Anticholinergics	Impaired sexual arousal, decreased vaginal lubrication
Antihistamines	Decreased libido, decreased vaginal lubrication
Barbiturates	Irregular menses, inhibition of luteinizing hormone/follicle stimulating hormone (LH/FSH), decreased libido, decreased orgasm
Benzodiazepines	Menstrual irregularities, decreased ovulation
Haloperidol	Increased prolactin levels, irregular menses
Phenothiazines	Increased prolacting levels, decreased LH/FSH, blocked ovulation, decreased libido
Prazosin	Decreased libido
Reserpine	Decreased libido, increased prolactin levels
Spironolactone	Breast tenderness, irregular menses

Modified from Mattison (1984).

associated with impaired libido and altered sexual response. Anticholinergic agents and antihistamines are associated with altered sexual response and impaired vaginal lubrication during sexual arousal. Barbiturates are associated with irregular menses, inhibition of the release of luteinizing hormone and altered sexual response. Benzodiazepines, major tranquilizers, are also associated with menstrual irregularities and altered ovulatory response (Mattison, 1984).

This broad range of reproductive toxins demonstrates the heterogeneous nature of reproductive toxicology. Successful risk assessment in reproductive toxicology requires a multidisciplinary approach utilizing epidemiology, reproductive biology, genetics, pharmacology, toxicology, developmental biology, clinical reproduction and development, and industrial and environmental hygiene. Because of the heterogeneous nature of reproductive toxicology, reproductive toxicologists often interact with scientists who use different vocabularies. As a result, it is necessary to pay special attention to definitions and not assume that colleagues in other sciences understand our jargon.

This review will begin by suggesting a working definition for reproductive toxins, then focus on some assumptions used in reproductive toxicology risk assessment. Specific areas will be pointed out in which the use of these assumptions has resulted in toxic exposures to humans, producing adverse reproductive outcomes. Then suggestions will be offered for interpreting reproductive hazards in a way which will preserve human reproductive health through appropriate risk assessment. Finally, a brief description will be given of one approach to developing methods for reproductive risk assessment in human populations based on our understanding of the regulation of fecundity and fertility.

Definition of a reproductive toxin

As shown in a simplified form in Figure 1, reproduction results from a relatively complex series of interrelated events. If any one of these events fails, reproduction will be impaired. This figure also suggests one of the unique characteristics of the reproductive system compared to other systems – that it does not function continuously. Hepatic, pulmonary, renal and cardiovascular systems function continuously throughout the life of an individual – intermittent function is not appropriate in these systems. Because the cost of reproductive function is high, both economically and metabolically, humans and nature have devised a series of controls which result in intermittent rather than continuous expression of this function (Overstreet & Blazak, 1983; Takizawa & Mattison, 1983). Some of these factors include age, season and availability of nutrients.

Before puberty, and after menopause, or reproductive senescence, animals are reproductively incompetent. In addition, reproductive competence varies as a function of age (Federation CECOS *et al.*, 1982). Nutritional factors also play a major role in regulating reproductive function in humans (Yen, 1978) and animals (van Tienhoven, 1968). Humans also go to great lengths to further regulate the intermittent expression of reproduction with the use of contraceptives. Therefore, we have defined 'successful reproduction' as the ability to produce structurally and functionally healthy offspring at the *appropriate time*

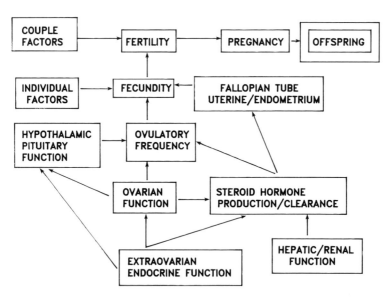

Figure 1. Male fecundity, female fecundity, frequency of intercourse and spontaneous abortion rate are all involved in successful reproduction. Male fecundity is influenced in part by sperm production and function. Female fecunidity is influenced in part by ovulatory frequency, fallopian tube, endometrial and uterine function.

in the life of a couple. Additionally, because of the intermittent nature of reproduction it is also necessary to provide *effective contraception* when reproduction is not appropriate or desirable. By this definition, a reproductive toxin is any compound which:

(*a*) impairs fertility, either by effects on gametes or hormonal integration of the reproductive system;

(*b*) produces structurally or functionally abnormal offspring, or

(*c*) impairs the effectiveness of contraceptives.

Current testing systems place great emphasis on the identification of xenobiotics which impair fertility or produce structurally abnormal offspring, with a growing concern for functional abnormality. Unfortunately, testing systems presently in use do not identify compounds which decrease the effectiveness of oral contraceptives. This is not a trivial concern; Table 4 lists a series of drugs that have been suggested to decrease the effectiveness of oral contraceptives (Mattison, 1984). These compounds impair oral contraceptive effectiveness by one of two mechanisms: increasing hepatic clearance or decreasing enterohepatic circulation.

Part of the efficacy of the recently introduced low-dose formulations of oral contraceptives derives from gastrointestinal bacterial cleavage of the large polar conjugated moiety on the synthetic oestrogen, followed by reabsorption of that oestrogen. Antibiotics that sterilize or partially deplete the gut of bacteria which serve this important role in enterohepatic circulation will decrease oestrogen reabsorption. Lower levels of oestrogen will increase the likelihood of breakthrough ovulation and fertilization.

Table 4. Drugs that decrease the effectiveness of oral contraceptives.

Increase hepatic clearance:

Antibiotic
  Rifampin (Rifadin, Rifamate, Rimactane)
Anticonvulsants
  Aminopyrine
  Phenobarbital (Antrocol, Isordil, Isuprel, Primatene)
  Phenytoin (Dilantin)
  Primidone (Mysoline, Primidone)

Decrease enterohepatic circulation:
Antibiotics
  Ampicillin (Amcill, Ampicillin, Omnipen, Polycillin)
  Chloramphenicol (Chloromycetin, Chloromyxin)
  Neomycin (Cortisporin, Mycolog, Mytrex, Neosporin, Neo-synalar)
  Phenoxymethylpenicillin
  Sulphamethoxypyridazine

Modified from Mattison (1984). Names in parenthesis are tradenames of the indicated drugs.

Mechanisms of reproductive toxicity

One of the critical issues in reproductive toxicology for risk assessment is the identification of the site and mechanism of action of compounds which alter reproductive function (Mattison, 1983, 1984). Table 5 provides one approach for characterizing reproductive toxins by mechanism of action. Reproductive toxins are divided into two major categories, direct and indirect acting. Those that are direct acting do so by either chemical reactivity or structural similarity to endogenous molecules. Those that are indirect acting do so by either altering hormonal control of the reproductive system or are metabolized to a direct-acting reproductive toxin.

Table 5. Mechanisms of action of reproductive toxins.

Mechanism	Compounds
Direct-acting reproductive toxins	
Structural similarity	Steroid hormones
	Cimetidine
	Diethylstilboesterol
	Azathioprine
	6-Mercaptopurine
	Halogenated polycyclic hydrocarbons
Chemical reactivity	Alkylating agents
	Cadmium
	Boron
	Lead
	Mercury
Indirect-acting reproductive toxins	
Metabolic activation	Diethylstilboesterol
	Ethanol
	Chlorcyclizine
	Dibromochloropropane
	Polycyclic aromatic hydrocarbons
	Cyclophosphamide
	Ethylene dibromide
Disrupted homeostasis	Salicylazosulphapyridine
	Halogenated polycyclic hydrocarbons
	Anticonvulsants
	Ethanol

Modified from Mattison (1983, 1984).

Assumptions in reproductive toxicity risk assessment

In most risk assessment settings, the compound identified as a reproductive hazard is evaluated in more than one species of experimental animal, a no-effect level is determined, and then a safety factor is applied to that no-effect level assuming the animal models are as, or more sensitive than, the human. We think that assumption may not be valid.

Humans are more sensitive than the animal model

One example of a reproductive toxin for which humans are more sensitive than animal models is dibromochloropropane (DBCP). We will not review DBCP as that has been done in the past (Whorton & Foliart, 1983). We believe that DBCP is an example of an adult testicular toxin, in which animals appear less sensitive than humans. DBCP was identified as a testicular toxin in a range of animals including mouse, rat, rabbit and guinea-pig in 1961 (Torkelson *et al.*, 1961). In spite of that study, there was no reproductive monitoring of workers exposed to this compound. In the mid-1970s, a group of workers complaining of infertility went to a urologist in northern California, and that began a series of clinical studies which culminated in the identification of DBCP as a human testicular toxin (Whorton *et al.*, 1977; Whorton & Foliart, 1983). Although this is an example in which animal data suggested the necessity for human monitoring, unfortunately this was not done. Subsequently, comparison of the testicular effects in animals and in humans suggests that humans are *more sensitive* than the animal models.

Another example of a testicular toxin for which the available data suggests that humans are more susceptible than animals is ethylene dibromide (EDB). EDB is of interest because it is produced in Arkansas, and because OSHA has recently considered changing the short-term exposure limit and time-weighted average. The major use for EDB historically has been as a lead scavenger in gasoline. It is presently used for fumigation of fruit before shipping (Ter Haar, 1980).

There have been several studies evaluating the reproductive effects of EDB in experimental animals, and in some studies conducted in workers exposed to EDB in the USA (Wong *et al.*, 1979). A well designed study is being conducted by NIOSH among workers exposed to EDB during fruit fumigation in Hawaii, unfortunately the data have not been published. We will review one study by Short, which evaluates the effect of EDB on male and female reproductive function in rats and mice exposed to three different doses in air (Short *et al.*, 1979). It is clear from these studies that both male and female animals exposed to 89 p.p.m. EDB have suppression of reproductive function (Table 6, Figure 2). Those exposed to 39 p.p.m. EDB have minimal suppression of reproductive function. This data suggests that the no-effect level appears to be 19–20 p.p.m., until recently the permissible exposure limit for humans.

How does this level defined in an animal model compare to reproductive effects observed among individuals exposed to EDB in an occupational setting? Tables 7 and 8 demonstrate sperm counts obtained from EDB workers in Magnolia, Arkansas (Ter Haar, 1980). Table 7 shows sperm counts for workers in the plant in 1977 and 1978, and suggests that from one year to the

Table 6. Fertility of male rats exposed to EDB for 10 weeks.

	EDB exposure (p.p.m.)			
Fertility parameters	0	19	39	89
Rats exposed (no.)	9	10	10	9
Rats impregnated (no.)	9	9	10	0
Pregnant rats (no.)	16	15	14	0
Implants/dam (no.)	13 ± 1	14 ± 1	11 ± 1	n.p.
Viable implants	12 ± 1	13 ± 1	10 ± 1	n.p.

Data from Short *et al.* (1979). n.p., Not pregnant.

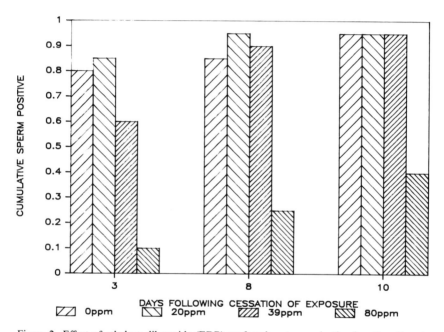

Figure 2. Effect of ethylene dibromide (EDB) on female rat reproductive function. Female rats were exposed to EDB in air in concentrations ranging from 0 to 80 p.p.m. for three weeks. EDB exposure was then discontinued and the females were mated with untreated male rats. Female reproductive function was assessed by determining the number of female animals with sperm in vaginal smears. Note that exposure of female rats for three weeks was sufficient to impair ovarian function. Data from Short *et al.* (1979).

next, with continued exposure, there is a doubling in the number of workers whose sperm counts are below 2×10^7 sperms/ml. Evaluating sperm counts among workers in 1977 as a function of estimated levels of exposure (Table 8), there is a preponderance of workers (42%) in the 0·5–5·0 p.p.m. exposure range with sperm counts less than 4×10^7 sperm/ml, whereas only 20% of those with estimated exposure of less than 0·59 p.p.m. have sperm counts less

Table 7. Sperm count of EDB workers.

Sperm counts (no/ml)	Percentage of workers evaluated	
	1977 (59)	1978 (24)†
$0-2 \times 10^7$	11·9‡	20·8
$2 \times 10^7-4 \times 10^7$	15·3	12·5
$4 \times 10^7-10^8$	49·1	37·5
$>10^8$	23·7	29·2

From Ter Haar (1980).
† Numbers in parentheses are number of workers evaluated. Eighteen of the workers were evaluated both in 1977 and 1978.
‡ One zero count.

Table 8. Effect of EDB on sperm count.

Estimated EDB exposure	Percentage of workers evaluated at various sperm counts (no./ml)			
	(<20) million/ml	(20–40) million/ml	(40–60) million/ml	>60 million/ml
$<0·5$ p.p.m. (40)†	10	10	55	25
$0·5-5·0$ p.p.m. (19)†	16	26	37	21

From Ter Haar (1980).
† Numbers in parentheses are numbers of workers evaluated.

than 2×10^7 sperm/ml. These data suggest time- and dose-dependent suppression of spermatogenesis in the range of $0·5-5·0$ p.p.m. In animal models the no-effect level occurred at about 20 p.p.m. in both males and females. Comparable human data from women have not been published, but the data from men suggest that exposures in the range of $0·5-5·0$ p.p.m. *are* suppressing spermatogenesis. The no-effect level for EDB testicular toxicity in humans is below that observed in experimental animals.

The assumption in reproductive toxicity risk assessment under evaluation is that animal models are as sensitive as humans. This assumes that a no-effect level in animals can be translated into a safe level for humans. Based on the data for DBCP and EDB this assumption is false. This suggests that a conservative approach would assume that *all* reproductive toxins are more toxic to humans than to experimental animals. Hazard identification in experimental animals conveys the obligation for *careful* monitoring of exposed human populations. Even with a conservative safety factor, it may be necessary to assume that adverse reproductive effects may be observed in humans until surveillance demonstrates human reproductive safety.

Genotoxins destroy germ cells

Another assumption common in reproductive toxicity testing has to do with damage to germ cells. It has generally been assumed that if a compound is toxic to germ cells they will be destroyed or become non-functional. There are two examples which suggest that this assumption is incorrect. The first is from the dominant lethal mutation literature (Generoso *et al.*, 1979), and the second from studies which demonstrate that sperms and oocytes possess DNA repair capabilities (Lee & Dixon, 1978; Pedersen & Mangia, 1978, Lee, 1983).

In assessing for dominant lethal mutations, male or female animals are treated with a compound, then bred and the number of resorptions ascertained. Of interest for this assumption is the study by Generoso which explored whether different strains of female mice could handle mutagenized sperm differentially. He used the $(C3H \times 101)F_1$ heterozygote males and four separate strains of females: $(C3H \times C57BL)F_1$, $(C3H \times 101)F_1$, $(SEC \times C57BL)F_1$, and T-stock. The compounds evaluated were: benzo[*a*]-

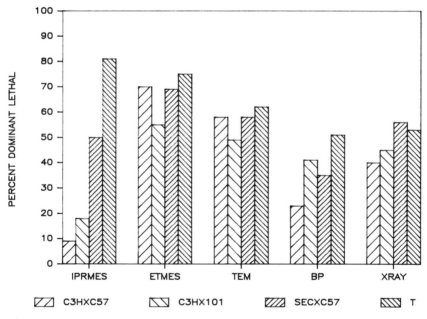

Figure 3. Expression of dominant lethal mutations in different female mice. Heterozygote male mice (either $(101 \times C3H)F_1$ or $(C3H \times 101)F_1$) were treated with isopropylmethane sulphonate (i.p., 65 mg/kg, IPRMES), ethyl methanesulphonate (i.p., 200 mg/kg, ETEMES), triethylenemelamine (i.p., 0·2 mg/kg, TEM), benzo[*a*]pyrene (i.p., 500 mg/kg, BP) or ionizing radiation (500 R, X-ray). The males were then mated with female mice of the indicated type and dominant lethal mutations determined. The heterozygote female mice used in this experiment were $(C3H \times C57BL)$ F_1 abbreviated C3H × C57, $(C3H \times 101)$ F_1 abbreviated C3H × 101, $(SEC \times C57BL)$ F_1 abbreviated SEC × C57, and T-stock abbreviated T. Data from Generoso *et al.* (1979).

pyrene (BP), triethylenemelamine (TEM), isopropyl methane sulphonate (IPRMES) and ethyl methane sulphonate (ETMES) (Figure 3). Treatment of males with TEM produces dominant lethals at about the same level in all of the female mice (50–60%). This is also true for ETMES with 55–75% dominant lethals in the tested female mice. Notice, however, that when the mutagen is IPRMES, there is substantial difference in the expression of dominant lethals in the females – less than 10% to more than 80%. This suggests that females of different strains can handle mutagenized sperm differently. These data have been interpreted by some as suggesting differential capabilities for repair of sperm DNA damage in the oocyte.

Pedersen & Mangia (1978) have also reported an experiment which lends credence to the suggestion that oocytes have DNA repair capability as suggested by the experiments of Generoso (Generoso *et al.*, 1979). Pedersen harvested oocytes from mice, exposed them to ultraviolet radiation in doses ranging from 0 to 60 J/m^2, and then assessed unscheduled oocyte DNA synthesis by uptake of tritiated thymidine (Figure 4). This experiment demonstrates that mature oocytes have the capability of repairing thymidine dimers. These experiments by Pedersen and Generoso suggest that germ cell responses to mutagens are not 'all or none'.

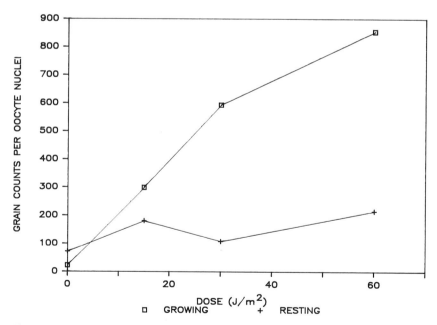

Figure 4. Unscheduled DNA synthesis in rodent oocytes as measured by incorporation of [^{3}H]thymidine. Oocytes were harvested from mice, exposed to ultraviolet light and then incubated with [^{3}H]thymidine. Following autoradiography grains over oocyte nuclei were counted. Data from Pedersen & Mangia (1978).

We have also been studying germ cell death following exposure to a broad range of mutagens. The results of our studies, summarized elsewhere, suggest that there is a striking relationship between potency of the mutagen and oocyte death (Mattison *et al.*, 1983a; Takizawa *et al.*, 1985). Others have also demonstrated that these mutations may not be repaired in all cases, and may be expressed. Preconception exposure to mutagens may actually produce heritable congenital malformations or tumours. In summary, the range of germ cell responses to mutagens appears remarkably similar to the responses observed in somatic cells: cell death, incorporation and repair of mutation, or incorporation and expression of mutation.

Comparison of ovarian toxicity in primates and rodents: cyclophosphamide

At this point it is useful to focus on the comparative reproductive toxicity of cyclophosphamide (CTX) in primates, subhuman primates and rodents. CTX is an indirect-acting alkylating agent (Table 5) which has extensive clinical use in the treatment of a variety of neoplastic and non-neoplastic diseases. One interesting observation has been the age-dependent decrease in dose required to produce human ovarian failure. For example, Table 9 demonstrates that the dose of CTX required to produce menopause decreases as a function of age. This data is from a group of women who were being treated with CTX for breast cancer (Koyama *et al.*, 1977). We have data from patients treated with CTX for autoimmune diseases which demonstrates a similar effect (Kay and Mattison, unpublished data). These data suggest that there are age-dependent factors that control the susceptibility of the ovary to this indirect-acting alkylating agent.

We have explored the age-dependent difference in ovarian response to CTX using a rodent model (Mattison *et al.*, 1983b; Shiromizu *et al.*, 1984). Mice at

Table 9. Dose of cyclosphosphamide required to produce human ovarian failure.

Age (years)	Dose of CTX (g)
20–29	20·4
30–39	9·3
40–49	5·2

Data were collected from patients treated with CTX for breast cancer (Koyama *et al.*, 1977).

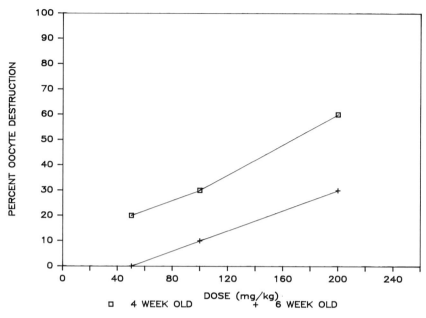

Figure 5. Dose response for primordial oocyte destruction in four week old and six week old C57BL/6N mice. Data from Mattison *et al.* (1983b).

four and six weeks of age were treated with one of three doses of CTX (50, 100 and 200 mg/kg) and dose–response curves calculated (Figure 5). There is an age-dependent difference, but in the mouse model it is reversed from that observed in women – younger animals are more sensitive than older animals. One explanation for this phenomena is shown in Figure 6: as animals mature the levels of glutathione, which are important in protecting the ovary by detoxifying reactive metabolites, increase. This may provide a partial explanation for the age-dependent difference in mice, however it does not explain the reverse age-dependent difference observed in women.

Because of this difference, we have evaluated the effects of CTX on ovarian function in cynomolgus monkeys. Figure 7 summarizes some of the events that occur in the female reproductive system during follicular development and ovulation. Because there is a broad range of rapid changes taking place in the ovary during the ovarian cycle, we have evaluated endocrine sensitivity to CTX before and after ovulation in the non-human primate, to determine if there were differences in ovarian response to treatment at different stages of the cycle (Mattison, 1985).

Table 10 indicates the number of animals treated with CTX (i.v., 1 g/m^2) on the indicated day of the ovarian cycle, and the outcome of the treatment. Animals treated four to six days before ovulation (-4 to -6) all have complete disruption of the ovarian cycle. Animals treated from one to three days

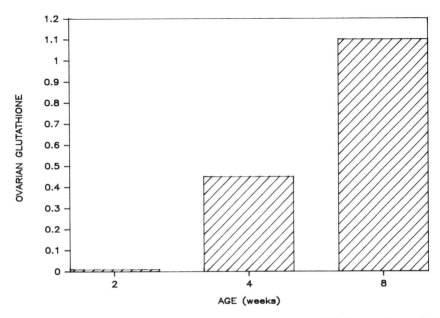

Figure 6. Ovarian glutathione (GSH) in C57BL/6N mice. Mice were killed at two, four and eight weeks of age and reduced ovarian GSH concentration (μg/mg wet weight) in a minimum of eight mice assayed individually. Data from Mattison *et al.*, (1983b).

before ovulation (-1 to -3) are for the most part normal or appear to be somewhat less sensitive than animals treated earlier in the cycle. Animals treated on the day of, or following, ovulation have no endocrine disturbances following CTX treatment. This suggests that in primates the timing of exposure relative to the menstrual cycle has an impact on the reproductive

Table 10. Effect of cyclophosphamide on menses.

Day of cycle	Phase of cycle	Response
-6 to -4	Follicular	6 Abnormal 0 Normal
-3 to -1	Follicular	1 Abnormal 4 Normal
0	Ovulation	0 Abnormal 1 Normal
$2+$ to $+6$	Luteal	0 Abnormal 4 Normal

Adult cycling cynomolgus monkeys were treated with cylophosphamide (i.v., 1 g./m^2) on the indicated day of their menstural cycle. Day 0 is the day on which ovulation occurs. D. R. Mattison and D. L. Pfeiffer, unpublished data).

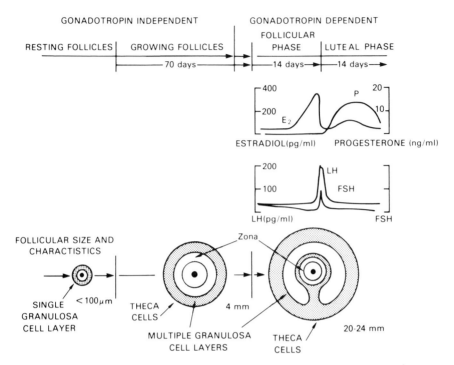

Figure 7. The female reproductive cycle. Ovulation in the sexually mature female requires a complex interaction between the hypothalamus, pituitary and ovary. This figure illustrates ovarian production of oestradiol (E₂) and progesterone (P) and peripheral levels of luteinizing hormone (LH) and follicle stimulating hormone (FSH). During the follicular phase of the ovarian cycle one follicle is selected to ovulate from the many growing follicles available. Those growing follicles not selected to ovulate undergo atresia. Reproduced from Mattison (1985) with permission.

effects observed. This puts an additional constraint on risk assessment from hazard evaluation in animals like rodents, where the control of reproductive function is different to that in primates.

Simulating human fertility

One area of recent concern has been ways in which to improve reproductive risk assessment. This concern arises from the importance of establishing a firm basis for the methods used in reproductive risk assessment. We have been evaluating reproductive risk assessment from the perspective of human reproductive function. Figure 1 is a simple fertility model developed as a first approximation for the evaluation of risk-assessment techniques for human reproduction (Mattison & Torres, 1985). We will share some of our early results using this model to explore the effects of two couple-mediated factors on fertility, frequency of intercourse and frequency of abortion (Barrett & Marshall, 1969; Bongaarts, 1975; 1982).

The first approximation for fertility simulation is quite simple, with two assumptions: (i) pregnancy results *only* when intercourse occurs on the day of ovulation, and (ii) none of the pregnancies are aborted. The first assumption is incorrect – there is a five to seven day 'window' in which fertilization can occur (Barrett & Marshall, 1969). The second assumption is also not accurate, approximately 75% of all conceptions are aborted (Wilcox, 1983; Lasley *et al.*,1985; Wilcox *et al.*, 1985). Using these assumptions if a couple is having daily intercourse, all of the women will become pregnant within the first cycle (Figure 8). Half of the couples having intercourse on an alternate-day basis will become pregnant on the first cycle and so on. The whole group will not become pregnant for seven to eight cycles. There are similar decrements in fertility as the frequency of intercourse decreases (Barrett, 1971).

If two patients were studied, one becoming pregnant within the first menstrual cycle and another taking eight menstrual cycles to become pregnant following cessation of contraception, most physicians would assume that there were differences in fecundity or fertility in those individuals. This very simple model suggests this may not be the case. The difference may simply reflect the intermittent nature of the expression of reproductive function.

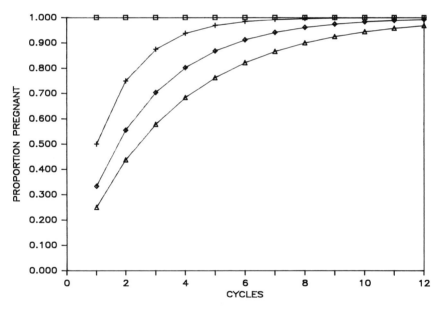

Figure 8. Effect of the frequency of intercourse on cumulative fertility rates. In this model women and men are assumed to have a fecundity of 1, and the abortion rate is 0. The frequency of intercourse is 1 (daily), □; 0·5 (every other day), +; 0·33 (every third day), ◇; 0·25 (every fourth day), △ represented by triangles.

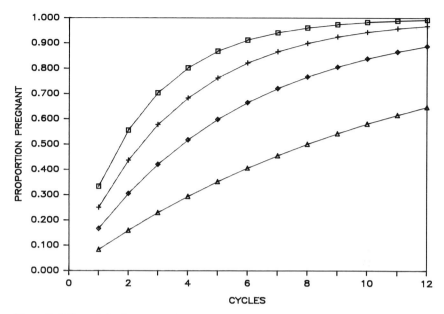

Figure 9. Effect of the frequency of spontaneous abortion on cumulative fertility rates. In this model women and men are assumed to have perfect fecundity (1·0). The frequency of intercourse is 0·33, every third day. The abortion rate is 0, □; 0·25, +; 0·50, ◇; 0·75, △.

Next a slightly higher degree of sophistication is added to this model, spontaneous abortions. Two assumptions were used to evaluate the effect of spontaneous abortion on fertility: (i) abortion, if it does occur, will occur in the cycle in which conception took place and, (ii) those women who abort will be fully fertile in a subsequent cycle. This model also generates a series of cumulative fertility curves at slightly lower levels than those in the first model (Figure 9). These and other models may form a basis for evaluating human populations exposed to putative reproductive toxins. The use of fertility models in conjunction with animal response data may help the development of a more rational basis for proceeding from hazard identification to risk assessment, and finally provide methods for surveillance of exposed human populations.

Conclusions

Exploration of two assumptions commonly used in reproductive risk assessment, (i) equal sensitivity of humans and animals and (ii) destruction of germ cells by mutagens, suggests that it is necessary to adopt a conservative approach. It is necessary to assume, until proven otherwise, that humans are more susceptible to adverse reproductive effects following xenobiotic exposure than the animal used. It is essential to critically re-evaluate safety factors used in extrapolating from animal models to human exposure limits for reproductive toxins. In addition, it is no longer possible to assume that exposures which damage an oocyte or a sperm will make that gamete non-functional. In some cases those exposures will alter oocyte or sperm DNA and those mutations will be expressed. It is important to define the effect of species differences in reproduction on risk assessment. Human exposures at different times in the menstrual cycle are going to produce entirely different results in terms of reproductive impairment. Finally, it is useful to develop mathematical models of human reproduction. The models will allow gedanken experiments exploring the effects of alterations in male or female fecundity or reproductive behaviour on fertility.

References

Barlow, S. M. and Sullivan, F. M., 1982, *Reproductive Hazards of Industrial Chemicals* (New York: Academic Press).

Barrett, J. C., 1971, Fecundability and coital frequency. *Population Stud.*, **25**, 309–313.

Barrett, J. C. and Marshall, J., 1969, The risk of conception on different days of the menstrual cycle. *Population Stud.*, **23**, 455–461.

Bongaarts, J., 1975, A method for the estimation of fecundability. *Demography*, **12**, 645–660.

Bongaarts, J., 1982, The fertility inhibiting effects of the intermediate fertility variables. *Stud. Fam. Plan.*, **13**, 179–189.

Federation CECOS, Schwartz, D. and Mayaux, M. J., 1982, Female fecundity as a function of age. *New Engl. J. Med.*, **306**, 404–406.

Generoso, W. M., Cain, K. T., Krishna, M. and Hufts, S., 1979, Genetic lesions induced by chemicals in spermatozoa and spermatids of mice are repaired in the egg. *Proc. natn. Acad. Sci. U.S.A.*, **76**, 435–437.

Koyama, H., Wada, T., Nishizawa, Y. Iwanaga, P., Aoki, Y., Terasawa, T., Kosaki, G., Yamamoto, T. and Wada, A., 1977, Cyclophosphamide-induced ovarian failure and its therapeutic significance in patients with breast cancer. *Cancer*, **39**, 1403–1409.

Lasley, B. L., Stabenfeld, G. H., Overstreet, J. W., Hanson, F. W., Czekala, N. and Munro, C., 1985, Urinary hormone levels at the time of ovulation and implantation. *Fert. Steril.*, **43**, 861–867.

Lee, I. P., 1983, Adaptive biochemical repair response toward germ cell DNA damage. *Am. J. ind. Med.*, **4**, 135–148.

Lee, I. P. and Dixon, R. L., 1978, Factors influencing reproductive and genetic toxic effects on male gonads. *Envir. Hlth. Perspect*, **24**, 117–127.

Mattison, D. R., 1983, The mechanisms of action of reproductive toxins. *Am. J. ind. Med.*, **4**, 65–79.

Mattison, D. R., 1985, Clinical manifestations of ovarian toxicity. In *Reproductive Toxicology*, edited by R. L. Dixon (New York: Raven Press), pp. 109–130.

Mattison, D. R., 1984, How everyday drugs can affect reproduction. *Contemp. Obstet. Gynec.*, **24**, 92–108.

Mattison, D. R. and Torres, S., 1985, Human fertility simulation using PASCAL. *Comput. Patient Care*, **4**, December.

Mattison, D. R., Shiromizu, K. and Nightingale, M. S., 1983a, Oocyte destruction by polycyclic aromatic hydrocarbons. *Am. J. ind. Med.*, **4**, 191–202.

Mattison, D. R., Shiromizu, K., Pendergrass, J. A. and Thorgeirsson, S. S., 1983b, Ontogeny of ovarian glutathione and sensitivity to primordial oocyte destruction by cyclophosphamide. *Pediat. Pharmac.*, **3**, 49–55.

NIOSH, 1985a, Leading work-related diseases and injuries – United States: disorders of reproduction. *Morbidity Mortality Week. Rep.*, **34**, 537–540.

NIOSH, 1985b, NIOSH Current Intelligence Bulletins: Summaries. *Morbidity Mortality Week. Rep.* (Suppl. 2S), **34**, 33S–51S.

Overstreet, J. W. and Blazak, W. F., 1983, The biology of human male reproduction: an overview. *Am. J. ind. Med.*, **4**, 5–15.

Pedersen, R. A. and Mangia, F., 1978, Ultraviolet light induced unscheduled DNA synthesis by resting and growing oocytes. *Mutation Res.*, **49**, 425–429.

Shiromizu, K., Thorgeirsson, S. S. and Mattison, D. R., 1984, Effect of cyclophosphamide on oocyte and follicle number in Sprague–Dawley rats, C57BL/6N and DBA/2N mice. *Pediat. Pharmac.*, **4**, 213–221.

Short, R. D., Winston, J. M., Hong, C. B., Minor, J. L., Lee, C. C. and Seifler, J., 1979, Effects of ethylene dibromide on reproduction in male and female rats. *Toxic. appl. Pharmac.* **49**, 97–105.

Takizawa, K. and Mattison, D. R., 1983, Female reproduction. *Am. J. ind. Med.*, **4**, 17–30.

Takizawa, K., Yagi, H., Jerina, D. M. and Mattison, D. R., 1985, Experimental ovarian toxicity following intraovarian injection of benzo(*a*)pyrene or its metabolites in mice and rats. In *Reproductive Toxicology*, edited by R. L. Dixon (New York: Raven Press), pp. 69–94.

Ter Haar, G., 1980, An investigation of possible sterility and health effects from exposure to ethylene dibromide. In *Banbury Report 5. Ethylene Dichloride: A Potential Health Risk*, edited by B. Ames, P. Infante, and R. Reitz (Cold Spring Harbor, NY: Cold Spring Harbor Press), pp. 167–185.

Torkelson, T. R., Sadek, S. E., Rowe, V. K., Kodama, J. A., Anderson, H. H., Loquvam, G. S. and Hine, C. H., 1961, Toxicological investigation of 1,2-dibromo-3-chloropropane. *Toxicol. appl. Pharmac.*, **3**, 545–559.

van Tienhoven, A., 1968, Effects of nutrition on reproduction. In *Reproductive Physiology of Vertebrates*, edited by A. van Tienhoven (Philadelphia: W. B. Saunders), pp. 355–387.

Whorton, M. D. and Foliart, D. E., 1983, Mutagenicity, carcinogenicity, and reproductive effects of dibromochloropropane (DBCP). *Mutation Res.*, **123**, 13–30.

Whorton, D., Krauss, R. M., Marshall, S., and Milby, T. H., 1977, Infertility in male pesticide workers. *Lancet*, **2**, 1259–1261.

Wilcox, A. J., 1983, Surveillance of pregnancy loss in human populations. *Am. J. ind. Med.*, **4**, 285–291.

Wilcox, A. J., Weinberg, C. R., Wehmann, R. E., Armstrong, E. G., Canfield, R. E. and Nisula, B. C., 1985, Measuring early pregnancy loss: laboratory and field methods. *Fert. Steril.*, **44**, 366–374.

Wong, O., Utidgian, H. M. D. and Karten, V. S., 1979, Retrospective evaluation of reproductive performance of workers exposed to ethylene dibromide (EDB). *J. occup. Med.*, **21**, 98–102.

Yen, S. S. C., 1978, Chronic anovulation. In *Reproductive Endocrinology*, edited by S. S. C. Yen and R. B. Jaffe (Philadelphia: W. B. Saunders), pp. 341–372.

PART 5

Pharmacogenetic and human monitoring considerations in animal selection

Section editor
W. E. Ribelin

Pharmacogenetic considerations in the selection of appropriate animal models in teratology

Stephen P. Spielberg

University of Toronto, Division of Clinical Pharmacology, The Hospital for
Sick Children, Toronto, Ontario, Canada

Introduction

The problem of extrapolation of animal teratogenicity data to human pre-natal toxicity risk was brought sharply into focus by the thalidomide tragedy (Lenz, 1961; McBride, 1961). The failure to detect the teratogenic potential of this drug in the rat led to widespread use of the drug in humans during pregnancy with obvious disastrous outcomes. Subsequently, it was found that the drug could produce phocomelia in rabbits and primates. Part of the differences in species susceptibility may relate to species differences in metabolism of the drug to a foetotoxic metabolite (Gordon *et al.*, 1981). In a practical sense, experience with animal testing has often led to incorrect data with respect to human teratogenicity risk (Blake, 1982). Often, adverse effects on animal foetuses occur only at extremely high concentrations of drugs, far beyond normal human therapeutic exposures, and in the face of drug-induced illness in the maternal animal. There are species differences in placentation, in the rates of the development of different organ systems, and in the ontogeny and genetic regulation of enzyme systems critical in metabolizing drugs. Any of these can act as confounders, leading to false-positive or false-negative results in a specific animal species compared with humans. Some additional differences between experimental animals and humans are outlined in Table 1. It is clear that from both an environmental and genetic point of view, the human population differs markedly from the animal models which are commonly used to assess human birth defect risk.

Perhaps even more important in considering the role of animal testing in predicting human reproductive outcomes, however, is the very nature of the epidemiology of human drug-induced birth defects. Fortunately, few drugs carry a risk of birth defects that is anywhere near as high as thalidomide. An example of a drug with a high risk of defects is Isotretinoin (13-*cis*-retinoic acid). Isotretinoin has recently been reported to be a significant human teratogen causing cardiovascular anomalies, microtia or absent ears,

Table 1. Some differences between experimental animals and humans in drug toxicity testing

	Animals	Humans
Genetics:	Homogeneous	Heterogeneous
Diet:	Defined	Variable
Environment:	Defined	Variable
Disease	Free	Ill
Exposures	None	Drugs, cigarettes, alcohol

craniofacial abnormalities, microphthalmia, and a variety of severe CNS abnormalities (Rosa, 1983; Fernhoff & Lammer, 1984; Lott *et al.*, 1984; Stern *et al.*, 1984). In early studies, it appeared that the vast majority of foetuses exposed will either be miscarried or end up with major malformations. Subsequent prospective studies indicate that perhaps 40% of foetuses exposed to Isotretinoin during pregnancy will have birth defects (Lammer *et al.*, 1985). This compares to a background rate of malformalities of 4.5% for all defects, and 2.8% of children having major defects requiring medical or surgical intervention (Heinonen *et al.*, 1977). For most drugs which have been labelled as human teratogens, however, the relative risk for birth defects associated with the use of the drug rarely is greater than two- or three-fold over the unexposed population. Thus, the vast majority of human foetuses exposed to the compounds will not develop birth defects. Even in the case of valproic acid, which is associated with a marked increase in lumbosacral meningomyelocele, only 1–2% of exposed foetuses will develop neural tube defects (Bjerkedal *et al.*, 1982; Robert & Guibaud, 1982; Robert & Rosa, 1983; Lindhout & Meinardi, 1984).

With these considerations in mind, we may in fact be asked the wrong question with our animal studies. The question is generally framed in the context: "Is drug 'X' a human teratogen and to what extent do animal studies help in deciding?". If, however, there are marked differences in susceptibility within the human population to drug-induced developmental toxicity, we should instead be asking: (1) Is the risk of developing specific drug-induced birth defects evenly distributed in the population? (2) If not, what are the mechanisms involved, and to what extent do genetic differences in the handling of our response to the drug determine outcome? (3) If not, can individual risk of adverse effects of drug exposure be assigned to specific patients? In other words, consideration of the possibility of 'idiosyncratic teratogenesis' should make us focus on the use of animal studies to help define mechanisms of dysmorphogenesis and to help determine mechanisms of individual differences in susceptibility. For those women who must take drugs during pregnancy, the issue is not what the population risk as a whole may be, but what is the individual risk to that mother–foetal pair. Abnormal pre-natal outcomes with a specific compound in a specific animal species may perhaps raise a 'red flag' with respect to some undefined risk in the human population, but such studies cannot help us deal with individual risk unless specific mechanisms of drug-induced developmental toxicity are established. In the remainder of this chapter, we will focus on two situations where understanding of basic mechanisms in animal studies has contributed towards understanding differences in susceptibility to drug-induced birth defects in the human population.

Susceptibility to polycyclic aromatic hydrocarbon-induced birth defects

Predisposition to a variety of idiosyncratic toxicities including hepatic damage, aplastic anaemia, and carcinogenesis may be generally determined (Nebert & Jensen, 1979; Nebert, 1981). Many such toxicities are mediated not by the parent compounds, but rather by highly reactive unstable metabolites capable of covalently interacting with cell macromolecules resulting in cell death or mutation. Genetic differences within and among species in the balance of rates of formation and detoxification of some metabolites may determine the amount of metabolites bound and the extent of toxicity. Such mechanisms have increasingly been implicated in the developmental toxicity of several compounds.

The role of genetics in toxic metabolite-mediated teratogenesis has been studied most extensively in inbred mouse strains. Particular attention has been focused on the genetic regulation of cytochromes P-450 inducibility. The cytochrome P-450 mono-oxygenases are a group of enzymes which oxidize many different substrates, often with the production of reactive electrophilic intermediates. In the mouse, inducibility of one class of such enzymes (aryl hydrocarbon hydroxylase, AHH) is controlled by a single genetic locus (Nebert & Jensen, 1979). High inducibility of this enzyme is inherited as an autosomal dominant trait. Susceptibility of inbred mice to benzo[a]pyrene (BP)-induced birth defects correlates with high inducibility of AHH (Lambert & Nebert, 1977). Similarly, there is a good correlation between AHH inducibility, birth defects, and the ability of foetal liver homogenates to convert BP to a mutagenic metabolite as assayed in the Ames test (Blake *et al.*, 1979).

The above experiments suggest that genetically regulated rates of formation of toxic metabolites may, in part, determine the likelihood of birth defects resulting from certain chemical exposures. Shum & co-workers (1979) used inbred mouse strains with high and low AHH inducibility to expand on this hypothesis. Using selective matings, they produced pregnancies with an equal mixture of foetuses with high or low inducibility in mothers with low enzyme activity. Under these circumstances, exposure to BP led to more binding of BP metabolites, more foetal resorptions, more birth defects, and poorer growth in high inducibility foetuses. In other matings, the same mixture of foetal genotypes was present in mothers with high AHH inducibility. In this situation, maternal metabolism of BP overwhelmed the differences between the high- and low-activity foetuses. Thus, the genotype and phenotype of both the mother and the foetus, as well as exposure to specific compounds, determined the ultimate foetal outcomes.

In humans, cigarette smoking increases the risk of spontaneous abortion, premature delivery, foetal growth retardation, and perhaps also increases the risk of certain birth defects (Ericson *et al.*, 1979; Landsman-Dwyer & Emmanuel, 1979; Kline *et al.*, 1980). Based on concepts developed in the animal models of AHH inducibility, Manchester & co-workers undertook a study examining the role of increased AHH activity in human placentas in determining foetal outcome from exposure to polycyclic aromatic hydrocarbons present in cigarette smoke (Manchester *et al.*, 1984). They hypothesized that increased placental AHH activity might metabolize BP and prevent it from reaching the foetus. They found that in pregnancies where AHH activity was high in the placenta, umbilical vein endothelium from these same placentas had low AHH activity. When the endothelial cells were cultured *in vitro*, however, their AHH activity was inducible by polycyclic aromatic hydrocarbons. The results suggest that high enzyme activity in the placenta prevents potentially toxic compounds from entering foetal circulation and thus protects the foetus from potential adverse effects of exposure to certain environmental chemicals. AHH activity, in turn, may be determined by both genetic regulation of inducibility as well as environmental variables such as previous exposure to inducing agents. While the precise consequences of inducibility of AHH in human maternal, placental and foetal tissues are not yet fully elucidated, the above experiments provide an interesting example of how data obtained on mechanisms of adverse effects of drugs in animal models may lead to specific hypotheses. These hypotheses can then be tested and examined in humans, with the ultimate goal being the determination of individual differences in risk from environmental exposures such as cigarette smoke in specific maternal–foetal pairs.

Phenytoin-induced birth defects

The precise role of phenytoin in causing birth defects is uncertain. The term 'foetal hydantoin syndrome' has been applied to a pattern of congenital abnormalities of variable expressivity, including minor craniofacial and other dysmorphic features, developmental delay, and major malformations (Hanson & Smith, 1975; Hanson *et al.*, 1976; Andermann, *et al.*, 1982; Dansky, *et al.*, 1982; Kelly, 1984). There appears to be perhaps a two- to three-fold increased risk of major defects, including congenital heart disease and orofacial clefts, associated with the use of the drug by epileptic mothers, and up to 40% of offspring exposed to the drug may have some feature of the syndrome. Discordance in outcome of heteropaternal twins simultaneously exposed to phenytoin *in utero* has been reported (Phelan *et al.*, 1982). Thus, similar to the situation with most drugs considered to be human teratogens, the majority of foetuses exposed to phenytoin *in utero* do not have significant birth defects, and genetic differences might contribute to altered susceptibility. Animal studies similarly have resulted in variable patterns and incidences of abnormalities associated with phenytoin exposure (Finnell & Chernoff, 1984; Gupta *et al.*, 1984). Again, the primary question is how animal studies can contribute to our understanding of differences in susceptibility of adverse outcomes of human pre-natal phenytoin exposure.

Phenytoin is metabolized by cytochrome P-450 mono-oxygenases to several oxidized products (Eadie & Tyrer, 1980). Arene oxides, reactive electrophilic compounds, are intermediates in such oxidative reactions (Jerina & Daly, 1974). Martz & co-workers (1977) have demonstrated covalent binding of such metabolites to rat foetal macromolecules. When they disrupted the balance between the rate of formation and detoxification of such reactive metabolites by inhibiting the detoxification enzyme, epoxide hydrolase, they found an increase in covalent binding of metabolites in foetal macromolecules and a coincident increase in the incidence of malformations in the foetuses. Epoxide hydrolase activity is normally low in the developing foetus (Pacifici & Rane, 1982). Thus, genetic abnormalities in phenytoin arene oxide detoxification might further alter the critical balance between production and detoxification of metabolites, leading to an increased foetal toxicity risk (Spielberg, 1982).

We have found a human genetic defect in the detoxification of arene oxide metabolites of phenytoin which predisposes patients to hepatotoxicity and bone-marrow aplasia (Spielberg *et al.*, 1981; Gerson *et al.*, 1983). Lymphocytes from patients who have experienced adverse reactions to the drug exhibit increased toxicity from metabolites generated by a microsomal metabolizing system *in vitro*. Cells from family members of the patients show abnormal phenytoin metabolite detoxification with a pattern suggesting an autosomal co-dominant inheritance. Therefore, it was wondered if such a human genetic polymorphism in the detoxification of phenytoin metabolites might predispose certain foetuses to abnormal outcomes of exposure *in utero*.

We studied 24 children from 16 families who were exposed to phenytoin *in utero* throughout pregnancy, along with their parents (Strickler *et al.*, 1985). Subjects were examined for the presence of major and minor birth defects. Blood samples were obtained for analysing cell detoxification capacity of phenytoin arene oxide metabolites. The cell studies were performed randomly without knowledge of the findings of the physical examinations of the patients. Patients whose cell response to phenytoin metabolites showed a significant increase in cell death over baseline were defined as having a 'positive response' to phenytoin metabolite challenge. As can be seen in Figure 1, those children who had a positive cell challenge with phenytoin metabolites were far more likely to have major birth defects than were those with a negative assay.

	NEGATIVE										POSITIVE													
	1	2	3	4	5	6	7	8	9	10	11	12	13	14	15	16	17	18	19	20	21	22	23	24
CARDIAC											■					■	■						■	■
CLEFT LIP	■																							
CLEFT LIP/PALATE																■							■	
GENITO-URINARY																								■
MICROCEPHALY (1)	■																	■	■					
MICROCEPHALY (2)											■					■						■		
MACROCEPHALY															■									
EYE											■				■	■								
HIP																							■	
FEET									■		■	■				■								

Figure 1. Correlation of major birth defects with 'negative' and 'positive' phenytoin metabolite toxicity assays *in vitro*. Filled-in squares represent positive findings. Specific defects include the following. Cardiac: ventriculo-septal defect (patients 11, 16, 23); tetralogy of Fallot (24); hypertrophic cardiomyopathy with endocardial fibroelastosis and conduction defect (15). Genito-urinary: hypospadias, urethral stenosis, undescended testes (24). Microcephaly (1): head circumference greater than 2 standard deviations below the mean. Microcephaly (2): head circumference between 1·3 and 2·0 standard deviations below the mean, and greater than 2 standard deviations from the mean of the ratio of head circumference to length. Macrocephaly: head circumference 2 standard deviations above the mean. Eye: strabismus (11, 14); congenital nystagmus (15). Hip: congenital dislocation. Feet: club foot requiring casting or bracing. From Strickler *et al.*, (1985) with permission.

Results were highly statistically significant for an increase in cardiac defects, microcephaly, and the presence of more than one major defect, more than two major defects, and more than three major defects among subjects with positive *in vitro* assays. In contrast, however, as can be seen in Figure 2, there was no correlation between a positive or negative cell assay and minor anomalies. Each child with a positive assay had one or the other parent with a positive assay. There were an equal number of positive assays among fathers and mothers of the patients. No patient had both parents with an abnormal assay and minor birth defects. The extent of the abnormality appears to be consistent with cell responses of parents of patients with overt hepatotoxicity, that is, an intermediate pattern suggesting possible heterozygosity. This normally does not predispose adult patients to hepatotoxicity from the drug; the mothers of patients who were taking the drug did not develop phenytoin toxicity. *In utero*, where epoxide hydrolase activity is already low, this genetic defect might sufficiently alter the critical balance between the production and detoxification of phenytoin metabolites to lead to increased covalent binding and increased major birth defects. The results are consistent with the data obtained in the animal studies where epoxide hydrolase was inhibited with resultant increased covalent binding and an increased incidence of major birth defects (Martz *et al.*, 1977).

The difference in the association of a positive test *in vitro* with major birth defects, as opposed to minor anomalies, suggests that the ultimate outcome of

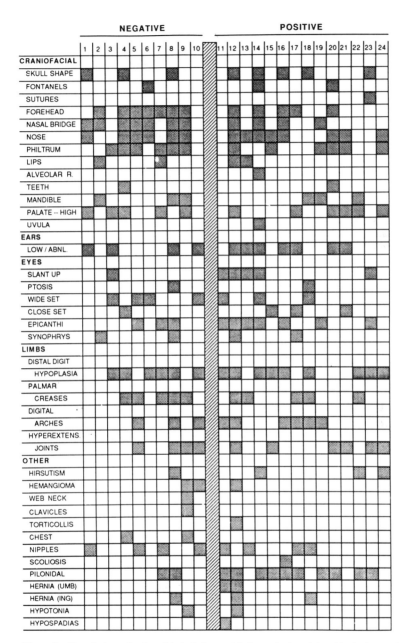

Figure 2. Correlation of minor birth defects with 'negative' and 'positive' phenytoin metabolite toxicity assays *in vitro*. Filled-in squares represent abnormal findings. From Strickler *et al.*, (1985) with permission.

foetuses exposed to phenytoin during gestation in mothers with seizure disorders is in all likelihood multifactorial (Dansky *et al.*, 1982). Maternal epilepsy *per se* may be a risk factor for foetal anomalies (Heinonen *et al.*, 1977). Other factors which might have an impact on outcome are shown in Figure 3. Maternal factors including the cause of the epilepsy (e.g., metabolic disease as opposed to head trauma), other drugs, diet, habits (e.g., cigarette smoking and alcohol), and genetically determined differences in tissue response to phenytoin or its metabolites may all have an impact on outcome. There may also be specific genetic predispositions to specific types of congenital anomalies within specific families. Under these circumstances, exposure to a drug which might further disrupt processes leading to such malformations may lead to an increased risk of those specific types of defects. The results from these studies, based on animal experiments into mechanisms of toxicity, however, demonstrate that a pharmacogenetic defect in the detoxification of a specific metabolite of phenytoin is correlated with an increased risk of major birth defects. The present assay system is somewhat too cumbersome to use as a general population screening device. In the future, as the specific biochemical genetic defect causing this abnormality is elucidated, it may become possible to use pre-natal screening techniques to aid in assigning specific estimates of risk for specific patients. Thus, instead of counselling patients based on epidemiological considerations in the population as a whole, it may ultimately be possible to provide individualized counselling based on assessment of individual differences in risk for drug-induced birth defects.

Recently, it has been noted that the pattern of malformations in inbred mouse strains exposed to phenytoin varies considerably (Finnell & Chernoff, 1984). Here is an example where initial knowledge of mechanism derived from animal studies, subsequent epidemiological and now pharmacological studies in humans, can then lead back to exploring mechanisms in depth in the animal model. Differences in susceptibility among and within species may now be ap-

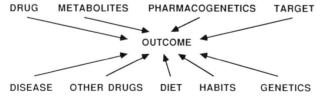

Figure 3. Interacting variables in the pathogenesis of drug-induced birth defects.

proached similarly to the way the differences in susceptibility have been approached in humans to pursue biochemical mechanisms in depth.

Conclusions

The above discussion and the considerations presented in Table 1 and Figure 3 suggest the complexity and multifactorial nature of foetal outcomes in humans. Present animal screening for teratogenic potential may provide a 'red flag' for further in-depth investigation. However, such studies cannot address the issue of how great the risk is within the human population in general, nor help define what subpopulations are at increased risk. In order for clinicians and patients to have safe and effective therapeutic agents available to treat diseases during pregnancy, we need to know far more about the mechanisms of possible foetal effects of drugs and how to determine polymorphisms in the human population with respect to those mechanisms. Perhaps one of the best uses of animal experiments will be to generate hypotheses which can be tested in human epidemiological and pharmacological (pharmacogenetic) studies to define risk factors for susceptibility to drug-induced birth defects. Similarly, animal models may be useful in testing hypotheses generated from human exposure data at a biochemical and cellular level. Such approaches will ultimately achieve the goal of individualized counselling of drug toxicity risk for patients and the choice of the safest drug for specific maternal–foetal pairs when therapy is required during pregnancy.

References

Andermann, E., Dansky, L., Andermann, F., Loughnan, P. M. and Gibbons, J., (1982), Minor congenital and dermatoglyphic alterations in the offspring of epileptic women: a clinical investigation of the teratogenic effects of anticonvulsant medications. In *Epilepsy, Pregnancy, and the Child*, edited by D. Janz, M. Dam and A. Richens (New York: Raven Press), pp. 235–249.

Blake, D. A., 1982, Requirements and limitations in reproductive and teratogenic risk assessment. In *Drug Use in Pregnancy*, edited by J. P. Niebyl (Philadelphia: Lea and Febiger), pp. 1–8.

Blake, D. A., Martz, F., Gery-Martz, A., Gordon, G. B. and Mellits, E. D., 1979, Fetal tissues from various strains of induced mice metabolize benzo(*a*)pyrene to mutagenic metabolites. *Teratology*, **20**, 377–382.

Bjerkedal, T., Czeizel, A., Goujard, J., Kallen, B., Mastroiacova, P., Nevin, N., Oakley Jr, G. and Robert, E., 1982, Valproic acid and spina bifida. *Lancet*, **2**, 1096.

Dansky, L., Andermann, E. and Andermann, F., 1982, Major congenital malformations in the offspring of epileptic patients: genetic and environmental risk factors. In *Epilepsy, Pregnancy and the Child*, edited by D. Janz, M. Dam and A. Richens (New York: Raven Press), pp. 223–234.

Eadie, M. J. and Tyrer, J. H., 1980, *Anticonvulsant Therapy: Pharmacologic Basis and Practice*, 2nd edn. (New York: Churchill Livingstone), pp. 45–132.

Ericson, A., Kallen, B. and Westerholm, P., 1979, Cigarette smoking as an etiologic factor in cleft lip and palate. *J. Pediat.*, **135**, 348.

Fernhoff, P. M. and Lammer, E. J., 1984, Craniofacial features of isotretinoin embryopathy. *J. Pediat.*, **105**, 595–597.

Finnell, R. H. and Chernoff, G. F., 1984, Variable patterns of malformation in the mouse fetal hydantoin syndrome. *Am. J. med. Genet.*, **19**, 463–471.

Gerson, W. T., Fine, D. G., Spielberg, S. P. and Sensenbrenner, L. L., 1983, Anticonvulsant-induced aplastic anemia: increased susceptibility to toxic drug metabolites *in vitro*. *Blood*, **61**, 889–893.

Gordon, G. B., Spielberg, S. P., Blake, D. A. and Balasubramanian, V., 1981, Thalidomide teratogenesis: evidence for a toxic arene oxide metabolite. *Proc. natn. Acad. Sci. U.S.A.*, **78**, 2545–2548.

Gupta, C., Katsumata, M. and Goldman, A. S., 1984, H-2 influences phenytoin binding and inhibition of prostaglandin synthesis. *Immunogenetics*, **20**, 667–676.

Hanson, J. W., Myrianthopoulous, N. C., Harvey, M. A. S. and Smith, D. W., 1976, Risks to the offspring of women treated with anticonvulsants, with emphasis on the fetal hydantoin syndrome. *J. Pediat*, **89**, 662–668.

Hanson, J. W. and Smith, D. W. 1975, The fetal hydantoin syndrome. *J. Pediat*, **87**, 285–290.

Heinonen, O. P., Slone, D. and Shapiro, S., 1977, *Birth Defects and Drugs in Pregnancy* (Littleton, Mass.: Publishing Sciences Group).

Jerina, D. M. and Daly, J. W., 1974, Arene oxides: a new aspect of drug metabolism. *Science*, **185**, 573–582.

Kelly, T. E., 1984, Teratogenicity of anticonvulsant drugs: review of the literature. *Am. J. Med. Genet.*, **19**, 413–434.

Kline, J., Stein, Z., Susser, M. and Warburton, D., 1980, Environmental influences on early reproductive loss in a current New York City study. In *Human Embryonic and Fetal Death*, edited by I. H. Porter and E. B. Hood (New York: Academic Press), p. 225.

Lambert, G. H. and Nebert, D. W., 1977, Genetically mediated induction of drug-metabolizing enzymes associated with congenital defects in the mouse. *Teratology*, **16**, 147–153.

Lammer, E. J. Chen, D. T., Hoar, R. M., Agnish, N. D., Benke, P. J., Braun, J. T., Curry, C. J., Fernhoff, P. M., Grix Jr, A. W., Lott, I. T. Richard, J. M. and Sun, S. C., 1985, Retinoic acid embryopathy. *New Engl. J. Med.*, **313**, 837–841.

Landesman-Dwyer, S. and Emmanuel, I., 1979, Smoking during pregnancy. *Teratology*, **19**, 119.

Lenz, W., 1961, Kindliche Missabildungen nach Medikament während der Gravidität. *Dt. med. Wschr.*, **86**, 2555–2558.

Lindhout, D. and Meinardi, H., 1984, Spina Bifida and *in utero* exposure to valproate. *Lancet*, **2**, 396.

Lott, I. T., Bocian, M., Pribram, H. W. and Leitner, M., 1984, Fetal hydrocephalus and ear anomalies associated with maternal use of isotretinoin. *J. Pediat.*, **105**, 597–600.

Manchester, D. K., Parker, N. B. and Bowman, C. M., 1984, Maternal smoking increases xenobiotic metabolism in placenta but not umbilical vein endothelium. *Pediatr. Res.*, **18**, 1071–1075.

Martz, F., Failinger III, C., and Blake, D. A., 1977, Phenytoin teratogenesis: correlation between embryopathic effect and covalent binding of putative arene oxide metabolite in gestational tissue. *J. Pharmac. exp. Ther.*, **203**, 231–239.

McBride, W. G., 1961, Thalidomide and congenital malformations. *Lancet*, **2**, 1358.

Nebert, D. W., 1981, Genetic differences in susceptibility to chemically induced myelotoxicity and leukemia. *Envir. Hlth. Perspect.*, **39**, 11–22.

Nebert, D. W. and Jensen, N. M., 1979, The *Ah* Locus: genetic regulation of the metabolism of carcinogens, drugs and other environmental chemicals by cytochrome P-450 mediated monooxygenases. *CRC Crit. Rev. Biochem.*, **6**, 401–437.

Pacifici, G. M. and Rane, A., 1982, Metabolism of styrene oxide in different human fetal tissues. *Drug. Metab. Disp.*, **10**, 302–305.

Phelan, M. C., Pellock, M. M. and Nance, W. E., 1982, Discordant expression of fetal hydantoin syndrome in heteropaternal dizygotic twins. *New Engl. J. Med.*, **307**, 99–102.

Robert, E. and Guibaud, P., 1982, Maternal valproic acid and congenital neural tube defects. *Lancet*, **2**, 937.

Robert, E. and Rosa, F., 1983, Valproate and birth defects. *Lancet*, **2**, 1142.

Rosa, F. 1983, Teratogenicity of isotretinoin. *Lancet*, **2**, 513.

Shum, S., Jensen, N. M. and Nebert, D. W., 1979, The *Ah* Locus: *in utero* toxicity and teratogenesis associated with genetic differences in benzo-*a*-pyrene metabolism. *Teratology*, **20**, 365–376.

Spielberg, S. P., 1982, Pharmacogenetics and the fetus. *New Engl. J. Med.*, **307**, 115–116.

Spielberg, S. P., Gordon, G. B., Blake, D. A., Goldstein, D. A. and Herlong, H. F., 1981, Predisposition to phenytoin hepatotoxicity assessed *in vitro*. *New Engl. J. Med.*, **305**, 722–727.

Stern, R. S., Rosa, F. and Baum, C., 1984, Isotretinoin and pregnancy. *J. Am. Acad. Dermatol.*, **10**, 851–854.

Strickler, S. M., Dansky, L. V., Miller, M. A., Seni, M. H., Andermann, E. and Spielberg, S. P., 1985, Genetic predisposition to phenytoin-induced birth defects. *Lancet*, **2**, 746–749.

Pharmacogenetic differences humans and laboratory implications for modelling

Elliot S. Vesell

Department of Pharmacology, The Pennsylvania State University,
College of Medicine, Hershey, PA 17033, USA

Many examples of genetically controlled variations in drug response have been described in both laboratory animals and humans. There probably exist other, as yet undiscovered, genetically determined differences in drug response. Recently the pace of discovery has accelerated, due to introduction and widespread use of convenient rapid, highly sensitive H.P.L.C. methods to measure the principal metabolites of numerous drugs.

Pharmacogenetic conditions are traditionally divided into those that affect the kinetic properties of a drug and those that influence its dynamic properties (Table 1; Vesell, 1973). Approximately 60 pharmacogenetic entities have been described in humans, whereas in laboratory animals even more have been reported (Meier, 1963; Nebert & Felton, 1976).

The term pharmacogenetics is usually restricted to conditions involving a protein that functions directly, rather than indirectly, in drug response. The principles that underlie pharmacogenetics have evolved over the past 20 years for drugs and apply as well to environmental chemicals (Kalow, 1984). For drugs, as well as other environmental chemicals, large inter-individual variations occur in both the type and extent of toxicological response, even though exposure of all subjects is to the same dose, by the same route.

For obvious ethical reasons, environmental pollutants cannot be given purposefully to human subjects. Therefore, less precise and sensitive epidemiological studies in humans have had to suffice. The results of such epidemiological investigations have frequently been equivocal, which is not surprising since often the doses and routes of chronic exposure to the environmental chemicals, or even the number and chemical nature of the pollutants, are ill-defined. Therefore, laboratory animals have been used as surrogates for man to establish the nature and mechanisms of genetic variations in toxicological response. At least in laboratory animals the investigator can rigidly control the dose, route, time of exposure and chemical nature of pollutants. Nevertheless, in this field the proper studies for mankind must ultimately involve man because of the numerous marked, yet not entirely

Table 1. Genetic conditions, probably transmitted as single factors, that alter drug response.

Condition	Aberrant enzyme and location	Mode of inheritance†	Agent provoking response
Altering the way the body acts on drugs			
Acatalasia	Catalase in erythrocytes	AR	Hydrogen peroxide
Suxamethonium sensitivity or atypical cholinesterase	Cholinesterase in plasma	AR	Suxamethonium or succinylcholine
Slow inactivation of isoniazid	Isoniazid acetylase in living	AR	Isoniazid, sulphamethazine, sulphamaprine, procainamide, phenelzine, dapsone, and hydralazine
Acetophenetidin-induced methaemoglobinaemia	? Mixed-function oxidase in liver microsomes that deethylates acetophenetidin	AR	Acetophenetidin
Deficient N-glucosidation of amobarbital	? Mixed-function oxidase in liver microsomes that N-glucosidates amobarbital	AR	Amobarbital
Polymorphic hydroxylation of debrisoquine	Mixed-function oxidase in liver microsomes that 4-hydroxylates debrisoquine	AR	Debrisoquine
Polymorphic hydroxylation of mephenytoin	Mixed-function oxidase in liver microsomes that 4-hydroxylates S-mephenytoin	AR	Mephenytoin

Altering the way drugs act on the body

Warfarin resistance	? Altered receptor or enzyme in liver with increased affinity for vitamin K	AD	Warfarin
Inability to taste phenylthiourea or phenylthiocarbamide	Unknown	AR	Drugs containing $N - C = S$ group such as phenylthiourea, methyl and propylthiouracil
Glucose 6-phosphate dehydrogenase deficiency, favism, or drug-induced haemolytic anaemia	Glucose 6-phosphate dehydrogenase	XL incomplete co-dominant	Various analgesics (acetanilide, acetylsalicylic acid, acetophenetidin [phenacetin], antipyrine, aminopyrine [Pyramidon]), sulphonamides and sulphones (sulphanilamide, sulphapyridine, N^2-acetylsulphanilamide, sulphacetamide, sulphisoxazole [Gantrisin], thiazosulphone, salicylazosulphapyridine [Azulfidine], sulphoxone, sulphamethoxypyridazine [Kynex]); antimalarials (primaquine, pamaquine, pentaquine, quinacrine [Atabrine]); nonsulphonamide anti-bacterial agents (furazolidone, nitrofurantoin [Furadantin], chloramphenicol, *p*-aminosalicylic acid); and miscellaneous drugs (naphthalene, vitamin K, probenecid, trinitrotoluene, methylene blue, dimercaprol [BAL], phenylhydrazine, quinine, and quinidine)

† AR, Autosomal recessive; AD, autosomal dominant.

predictable, differences between laboratory animals and man in pharmaco-kinetics, pharmacodynamics, genetics and environment. Moreover, each human being should be considered unique because of the particular constellation of host factors that influence his or her own response to environmental chemicals. Therefore, ideally, toxicological risk should be evaluated not in a population or group as a whole, but rather for each person, based on a knowledge of the precise dose, route of exposure and individual host factors that affect responsiveness in that particular subject (Golberg, 1985). At the present time this ideal seems to be light years away.

Most pharmocogenetic entities were discovered clinically in humans as a result of an unusual, generally toxic, response to a drug. Often, toxicity that is developed due to drug accumulation is attributable to the presence in the patient of a mutant form of an enzyme directly involved in the metabolism of that drug (*see Altering the way the body acts on drugs*, Table 1). Compared to the normal constitutive form, the mutant form of the enzyme exhibited markedly reduced affinity for the drug. Therefore, in affected subjects biotransformation of the pharmacologically active drug to its pharmacologically inactive metabolite(s) was retarded. Even after low doses, the active parent drug accumulated to high, often toxic, concentrations.

In pharmacogenetics, the potential contribution of animal models closely resembling the human condition lies in the opportunities that such models afford to investigate and elucidate the basic biochemical defect in the protein, as well as its pharmacological consequences, and also to evolve new therapies. For these purposes, useful animal models of the human pharmacogenetic condition are needed, but few are available as yet, probably because of the many impediments to their development. For example, the hepatic metabolism of many drugs is exceedingly complex, dependent on numerous enzymes, isozymes, co-factors, and modulating host factors of an environmental nature. When investigators sought animal models of human pharmacogenetic entities involving isozymes of cytochrome P-450, they encountered appreciable differences between rodents and humans in the nature and function of the system. For example, while the DA rat superficially appears to provide a valid model for the human deficiency in debrisoquine hydroxylation, the DA rat exhibits sex differences in the deficiency of the specific cytochrome P-450 isozyme that hydroxylates debrisoquine and several other drugs, whereas the human does not (Kahn *et al.*, 1985). These and additional differences have impeded progress in developing animal models that replicate the salient molecular and clinical features of the human pharmacogenetic condition. Nevertheless, depending on the objective of the model, some use could be made of animal models that diverge slightly from the human syndrome, since few, if any, drugs behave identically in humans and rodents with respect to their hepatic metabolism. Therefore, differences between humans and laboratory animals arise in such pharmacokinetic values as clearance, half-life and area under curve (AUC). The theme of this paper is the frequent occurrence of large pharmacokinetic variations among humans. Such variations arise from both genetic and environmental factors. Thus, even within a single outbred species, uniformity of response to a drug or environmental chemical should not be expected. Rather than being an exception, differences in response appear to be the rule.

It needs to be stressed that therapeutic and fundamental mechanistic advances have emerged from the availability of several well-recognized animal models of human genetic conditions. For example, successful application has been made of the following animal models: diabetes mellitus in rats, gout in Dalmatian coach hounds, malignant hyperthermia in Landrace pigs, warfarin resistance in rats, low aryl hydrocarbon hydroxylase inducibility in certain mouse strains (Lang & Vesell, 1976).

For traits controlled by multiple genetic loci, as opposed to monogenically controlled conditions, a special strategy, called selective breeding, has been successfully employed to develop a rodent model. Selection involves breeding for 10 to 15 generations according to the phenotype of an animal with respect to a particular quantitative genetically transmitted trait. Animals characterized by high quantitative values for a particular trait are mated. Animals with low values are also mated. Ultimately, after many generations of such matings of like to like, two contrasting strains emerge that differ only with respect to a single trait. One strain is characterized by very high values, the other by very low. These two strains then serve as experimental tools to define the biological nature of the quantitative difference in the particular trait and to develop and test therapy. This approach has been used to produce alcohol-preferring strains of rats and mice as a basis for an animal model of human alcoholism (Li & Lumeng, 1984).

In pharmacogenetic research, animal models of recent interest have been developed for acetylation (Weber & Hein, 1985) and for debrisoquine polymorphisms (Kahn *et al.*, 1985). Much effort has gone into this work; these animal models have revealed some interesting information, but no fresh insights into the nature of the human genetic polymorphisms. Nevertheless, they are now available for that purpose. Because animal models of these human polymorphisms have been described recently in detail, I shall not review them further here, but rather relate our experience with animal models of more general pharmacogenetic interest.

Where the biotransformation of drugs involves multiple hepatic isozymes of cytochrome P-450, man and laboratory animals appear to differ markedly in pharmacogenetic properties. Two reasons can be offered. First, there appears to be more heterogeneity associated with the genetic loci of these isozymes and their expression in man compared to laboratory animals. Hence, in humans there is greater inter-individual variation in the structural forms and amounts of these isozymes than in laboratory animals. Secondly, in practice the environmental range of factors that actually affects the activities of these isozymes is much wider in man than is permitted by the usual restricted set of

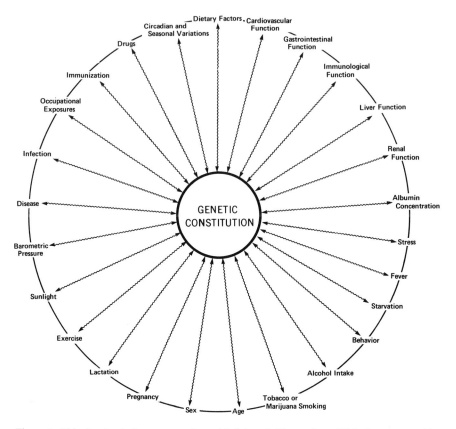

Figure 1. This circular design suggests the multiplicity of either well-established or suspected host factors that may influence antipyrine elimination in man. A line joins all such factors in the outer circle to indicate their close interrelationship. Arrows from each factor in the outer circle are wavy to indicate that effects of each host factor may occur at multiple sites and through different processes. Arrows also go from the centre circle to each host factor to indicate the potential role of genetic factors in modulating the expression of environmental and developmental factors. (Reproduced with permission from Vesell, 1982.)

conditions under which most laboratory animals are kept. Figure 1 shows that in man numerous host factors are capable of causing pharmacokinetic variations. Furthermore, these host factors can and often do interact dynamically and at many levels, producing large inter-individual variations (Figure 1 and Table 2). Probably some differences exist between humans and rodents in both the number and type of genetic loci that control cytochrome P-450 isozymes, thereby explaining why man and laboratory animals rarely resemble one another closely with respect to magnitude and nature of inter-individual pharmacokinetic variations.

A specific example of this principle may be useful. The objective of these studies was to identify the causes and establish the magnitude of inter-

Table 2. Inter-individual variations in plasma half-lives of drugs metabolized by hepatic detoxifying enzymes

Drug	Plasma half-life (h)	Fold variation	Individuals investigated (no.)
Aminopyrine	1·1–4·5	4	12
Amobarbital	1·4–6·4	5	14 pairs of twins
Antipyrine	5–35	7	33
Carbamazepine	18–55	3	6
Dicoumarol	7–74	11	14 pairs of twins
Diazepam	9–53	6	22
Phenytoin	10–42	4	
Indomethacin	4–12	3	15
Nortriptyline	15–90	6	25
Phenylbutazone	1·2– 7·3 d	6	14 pairs of twins
Primidone	3·3–12·5	4	
Theophylline	4–18	5	45
Tolbutamide	3–27	9	50
Warfarin	15–70	5	40

Reproduced from Vesell & Penno (1983).

individual variations in hepatic oxidative drug metabolism. Table 3 shows that, for hexobarbital metabolism, rates of hepatic oxidative metabolism in 11 strains of mice are similar (Vesell, 1968). Within each strain, the 24 mice investigated showed similar values as indicated by the small standard deviations for both sleeping time and hepatic hexobarbital oxidase activity.

Table 3. Sleeping time, hexobarbital oxidase activity and brain hexobarbital level on awakening in various strains of male mice.

Strain[†]	Sleeping time (min ± s.d.)	Hexobarbital oxidase (μmol/g liver/ 15 min ± s.d.)	Brain hexobarbital level (μg/gram)
AL/N	86 ± 16	0·20 ± 0·01	45 ± 6
BALB/C	46 ± 6	0·34 ± 0·02	46 ± 4
C3H/HeN	41 ± 7	0·34 ± 0·02	53 ± 5
C57BL/6N	73 ± 13	0·23 ± 0·01	52 ± 5
DBA/2N	85 ± 17	0·21 ± 0·01	48 ± 4
STR/N	47 ± 6	0·36 ± 0·01	49 ± 4
CAF$_1$	72 ± 10	0·24 ± 0·02	46 ± 4
CDF$_1$	58 ± 9	0·28 ± 0·02	54 ± 5
NIH	37 ± 5	0·32 ± 0·03	48 ± 4
CFW/N	40 ± 7	0·37 ± 0·02	46 ± 3
GP	42 ± 8	0·37 ± 0·03	52 ± 5

Reproduced from Vessell (1968).
Differences in sleeping time and liver hexobarbital oxidase activity between AL/N, DBA/2N, C57BL/6N, CAF$_1$ and CdF$_1$ mice and other strains are significant ($P < 0·05$).
† 24 animals used for each strain of mice.

Inter-strain variations in mean values for both sleeping time and hexobarbital oxidase activity were also small. Most strains were surprisingly similar to one another in such mean values. The largest inter-strain differences attained were only two-fold. Breeding experiments between strains at the extremes for these measurements produced an F_1 generation intermediate between parental values. These results were compatible with polygenic control of the inter-strain variations, but backcross matings essential to establish firmly this genetic hypothesis were not performed (Vesell, 1968).

By contrast to these results in mice on inter-strain variations in hexobarbital metabolism, the magnitude of inter-individual variation in rate of hepatic drug oxidation was much larger in normal humans, as shown in Table 2. The extent of inter-individual pharmacokinetic variations among normal subjects under carefully controlled uniform environmental conditions ranged from three-fold to 11-fold, depending both on the particular drug and subjects studied. These large variations occurred among normal subjects, despite similar environmental conditions, so that differences among subjects could not be attributed to any environmental factor acting either alone or in combination with other factors.

In twins and families carefully selected to be under such uniform environmental conditions, large inter-individual pharmacogenetic variations appeared to be caused primarily by genetic factors (Vesell, 1973, 1984). This conclusion does not imply that many environmental factors are incapable of altering markedly a subject's pharmacokinetic values. Clearly, they can (Figure 1) when they are differentially activated and operative. However, in the absence of appreciable environmental differences among subjects, large inter-individual pharmacokinetic variations persist, and these variations are genetically controlled. Thus, as Figure 1 suggests, pharmacokinetic variations can arise from many sources: multiple environmental factors can produce them, but so too can genetic factors. When subjects are studied under uniform environmental conditions, the genetic factors can be identified and demonstrated to exert their influence. In the real world, genetic and environmental factors interact dynamically, particularly in disease states, to produce fluctuation in a given subject's capacity to metabolize drugs and other environmental chemicals.

Compared to humans living under such highly variable diverse environmental conditions, laboratory animals exist under restricted uniform environmental conditions. This difference probably contributes appreciably to the more extensive inter-individual pharmacokinetic variations in humans compared to laboratory animals. In addition, humans also exhibit greater genetic heterogeneity in their cytochrome P-450 isozymes than do inbred laboratory-housed rodents.

References

Golberg, L. 1985, Complexities of evaluating the toxicological risk to humans. In *Toxicity Testing – New Approaches and Applications in Human Risk Assessment*, edited by A. P. Li (New York: Raven Press), pp. 3–13.

Kahn, G. C., Rubenfield, M., Davies, D. S., Murray, S. and Boobis, A. R., 1985, Sex and strain differences in hepatic debrisoquine 4-hydroxylase activity of the rate. *Drug Metab. Disp.*, **13**, 510–516.

Kalow, W., 1984, A pharmacologist looks at ecogenetics. In *Banbury Report No. 16* (Cold Spring Harbor, NY: Cold Spring Harbor Laboratory), pp. 15–30.

Lang, C. M. and Vesell, E. S., 1976, Environmental and genetic factors affecting laboratory animals: impact on biomedical research. *Fed. Proc.*, **35**, 1123–1165.

Li, T. K. and Lumeng, L., 1984, Alcohol preference and voluntary alcohol intakes in inbred rat strains and the NIH heterogeneous stock of rats. *Alcoholism clin. exp. Res.*, **8**, 485–487.

Meier, H., 1963, *Experimental Pharmacogenetics* (New York: Academic Press).

Nebert, D. W. and Felton, J. S., 1976, Importance of genetic factors influencing the metabolism of foreign compounds. *Fed. Proc.*, **35**, 1133–1141.

Vesell, E. S., 1968, Factors altering the responsiveness of mice to hexobarbital. *Pharmacology*, **1**, 81–97.

Vesell, E. S., 1973, Advances in pharmacogenetics. In *Progress in Medical Genetics*, Vol. 9, edited by A. T. Steinberg and A. G. Bearn (New York: Grune and Stratton), pp. 291–367.

Vesell, E. S., 1982, On the significance of host factors that affect drug disposition. *Clin. Pharmac. Ther.*, **31**, 1–7.

Vesell, E. S., 1984, Pharmacogenetic perspectives: genes, drugs and disease. *Hepatology*, **4**, 959–965.

Vesell, E. S. and Penno, M. B., 1983, Assessment of methods to identify sources of interindividual pharmacokinetic variations. *Clin. Pharmacokin.*, **8**, 378–409.

Weber, W. W. and Hein, D. W., 1985, *N*-Acetylation pharmacogenetics. *Pharmac. Rev.*, **37**, 25–79.

Studies of cellular reaction to toxicity in human cells and tissues: extrapolation of animal data to man

James H. Resau and Benjamin F. Trump†

Department of Pathology, University of Maryland School of Medicine,
Baltimore, MD 21201, USA

and

†Maryland Institute for Emergency Medical Services Systems (MIEMSS),
Baltimore, MD 21201, USA

Introduction

It has become evident that an understanding of the mechanisms of acute and chronic toxicity, including carcinogenesis in humans, must involve studies of human cells and tissues (Trump & Harris, 1979; Autrup & Harris, 1983; Harris, 1983). Variability between species based on genetic and other factors can be extreme, especially when one compares humans to experimental models. While it is important to develop models *in vitro* and *in vivo* using animal cells and tissues, ultimately the assessment of disease mechanisms and disease prevention in humans must rely on studies of human cells and tissues. In the present paper, we will first summarize data showing how it is possible to conduct such studies at the morphological, biochemical and physiological levels and then summarize some of our findings. These concepts are illustrated in Figures 1 (Harris & Trump, 1983) and 2 (Harris *et al.*, 1984). The overall strategy of our programme is to compare animal studies to those of human tissues *in vivo*, make observations *in vitro* and thereby optimize the extrapolation of conclusions on mechanisms of disease from animal data to man. Such experiments have permitted the assessment of a variety of toxic and carcinogenic compounds on human tissues and on the transformation of human epithelial cells *in vitro* (Yoakum *et al.*, 1985).

Obtaining tissues

Human tissues can be obtained for study in a variety of ways, including immediate, intermediate and routine autopsies; surgical biopsies; surgical resections; and organ donation/transplantation. At the present time these

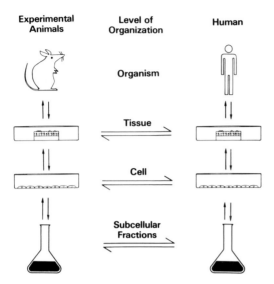

Figure 1. Extrapolation of carcinogenesis data. At different levels of biological organization, models can be used *in vitro* to compare responses between humans and experimental animals. Reprinted with permission from Harris & Trump (1983).

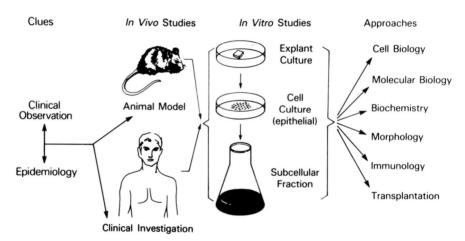

Figure 2. Human tissues in biomedical research. *In vitro* models provide a link between studies using animal models and clinical investigations. Reprinted with permission from Harris *et al.* (1984).

methods are only beginning to be utilized; there is acknowledged regret that human tissues not needed for diagnosis or transplantation are being wasted in vast quantities. Programmes such as ours could lead to major steps forward in research and provide tools for characterization of environmental and other agents on human cells and tissues.

The immediate autopsy is the most successful procedure for optimizing the availability of human tissue (Trump *et al.*, 1975, 1978; Cowley *et al.*, 1979). Most human tissues and cells survive for relatively long periods of time after somatic death. If tissues could be obtained within these time-limits, a variety of morphological and biochemical studies could be conducted that include long-term culture and xenotransplantation. Therefore, some years ago, in collaboration with Dr R. Adams Cowley of the Maryland Institute for Emergency Medical Services System (MIEMSS) and Dr Russell Fisher, then Chief Medical Examiner for the State of Maryland, we developed a programme to initiate autopsy procedures within 30 min or less following death, predominantly on shock trauma victims. This programme has yielded significant new data on the effects of shock on a variety of organs, including the liver, pancreas and kidney, and also provided a source of tissue to investigate the effects of toxic agents *in vitro*. The concept of tissue resuscitation has been very important in this work. That is, tissues obtained at immediate autopsy often show reversible changes resulting from the ischaemic period following cessation of heart beat. In previous papers (Trump *et al.*, 1975; Cowley *et al.*, 1979), we characterized the progression of cellular events following total ischaemia and concluded that the changes occurring in the tissues at the time of autopsy were probably totally reversible. Culture for as little as 24 h often resulted in complete reversal of the morphological changes.

To set up such a programme requires collaboration between the pathologist and researcher and the surgical or other teams caring for the patient. The personnel and logistical support required for this procedure is difficult to overestimate. We have chosen to set up teams of liaison personnel to interact with MIEMSS and have developed detailed protocols for the initiation culture or other studies with the tissues as soon as they are obtained, which is often in the middle of the night. Our experience in the collection of human tissue for research purposes has many parallels to the early observation of Cowley *et al.* (1979) when they established the 'shock trauma' programme. In order to collect the tissues in time for the ischaemic changes to be reversed, the team must be ready, in the unit and must have all the instruments, kits, solutions, 'on hand' and prepared for use. One cannot have everyone on call and expect to get ready in time. The programme should be able to waste a certain amount of material as it reaches its expiration date. Personnel must be willing, in theory as well as practice, to be there at a moment's notice and have as their primary interest and oal the study of human disease in human tissue. Dr Cowley realized he had to have the surgeons in the unit and not on call, and also be willing to absorb some of the costs of having these people on duty when the unit was in between cases. However, he quickly showed that once it became obvious that more lives could be saved with the team present in the unit, the 'slack' time between cases decreased rapidly. This means that such programmes are relatively expensive in terms of professional effort and require significant dedication on the part of both professional and technical personnel.

Surgical specimens are also very useful in this type of study. Such specimens are obtained at the time of biopsy or surgical resection, often from the 'normal' tissues beyond the margins of a neoplasm. Such collection efforts are similar to the immediate autopsy programme described above in that they require collaboration between the pathologist and the surgeon but, in addition, require close collaboration with the surgical pathologist responsible for the diagnosis. This is needed to preclude any interference with the histopathological diagnosis of the lesion (i.e., interference with the tumour or resection margins). The advantage of this type of specimen is that tissues can often be obtained with relatively short ischaemic intervals and under closer technical control than in routine autopsy. The disadvantages include the important possibility that, in studies of malignant transformation *in vitro*, it may be impossible to determine whether the so-called 'normal' areas are, in fact, initiated and have occult or pre-neoplastic lesions. Such tissues can be quite useful as short-term toxicological studies (e.g., cyanide anoxia, etc.) and may serve as models or pilot material for the development and/or evaluation of culture procedures.

The fears of the surgical pathologist that the tissue sample he gives up to the research group will compromise the diagnostic integrity of the specimen can be relieved by the knowledge, professionalism and dependability of the research group. In our experience, we have often been able to assist in the histopathological diagnosis. Tumour and uninvolved tissue are collected from nearly all the surgical cases in our hospital. Tissue samples are fixed and/or frozen for such techniques as electron microscopy, immunocytochemistry and culture; accurate records are maintained of all cases. Further help is available from the team by making the information obtained in the research protocols available to the physician. The determination of carcinoma or sarcoma has been helped through the information from keratin staining in the pieces of tissue received for research (McDowell *et al.*, 1983). If a research group can provide this kind of information, and help in specific diagnostic situations (e.g., electron microscopy, cytochemistry), then the degree of trust between research and diagnostic teams can only become increased.

One of the principal advantages of surgical specimens in studying neoplastic diseases is that they often provide pre-neoplastic lesions which can be used for the study of culture potential, transplantability and presence of putative tumour markers (Banks-Schlegel, 1982; Purnell *et al.*, 1982; Valerio *et al.*, 1982; McDowell *et al.*, 1983; Banks-Schlegel *et al.*, 1984).

Epidemiological profile

It is essential for every tissue that is obtained to be accompanied by an epidemiological profile of the patient which is as complete as possible. This profile is obtained from the patient records, interviews with the patient and/or the next of kin and also includes a variety of biochemical data including debrisoquine metabolism, presence of mutagens in the urine, and evaluation of DNA from the patient's leukocytes. This information can become especially useful when genetic factors in neoplastic or pre-neoplastic lesions need be considered or the effects these factors may have on the metabolism of toxic compounds (Harris & Cerutti, 1982; Blattner *et al.*, 1983). All of our studies require and have the approval of the University Human Volunteers Research/Protocol Review Committee.

Tissue transport

Detailed studies have been performed on the problems of transporting tissue between laboratories as this information is essential for collaboration between laboratories and for the transporting of tissue from the autopsy room or surgical suite to the laboratory. For many of our studies the transport medium is L-15 tissue-culture medium maintained at 0–4°C. L-15 (GIBCO) is a complete medium that is PO_4-buffered and is not affected by atmospheric CO_2 concentrations. In this medium, many human tissues survive for a few days, but some survive for one week or more. This is particularly important when transporting tissues across the country, as this can now be readily accomplished with the currently available rapid mail or delivery services. In some cases, there has been success in freezing pieces of tissue and then in thawing the tissues and obtaining significant cellular outgrowth. For freezing preservation dissociated cells are frozen or the outgrowth collected from culture dishes is frozen.

Culture

Epithelial cultures are accomplished in two principal ways: cell culture and explant culture. Each has its advantages and disadvantages. Explant culture maintains the differentiated histo-architecture of the tissues for long periods of time and potentially maintains the epithelial stromal interactions (Jones *et al.*, 1981; Shamsuddin & Trump, 1981). On the other hand, it is difficult to quantitate the changes occurring within the cultured tissue (Cottrell & Resau, 1985). Cell cultures, on the other hand, are readily quantitated (Banks-Schlegel, 1985), but often do not maintain the differentiation characteristic of the tissue of origin (Jones *et al.*, 1981).

Most of our experience with explant culture involves the bronchus, oesophagus, prostate, pancreatic duct and colon which are cultured in CMRL 1066 medium with or without serum and containing insulin, hydrocortisone, vitamin A and antibiotics (Barrett *et al.*, 1980; Jones *et al.*, 1981; Sanefuji *et al.*, 1982; Autrup & Harris, 1983; Autrup & Williams, 1983; Vocci *et al.*,

1983; Resau *et al.*, 1985a,b). Using such methodology, for example, differentiated bronchial explants can be maintained for up to one year *in vitro*.

Epithelial cell cultures can be initiated in two ways, by enzymic dissociation and plating, or by the collection of epithelial outgrowth from explants. The explant method is often used to obtain epithelia from bronchi, colon, oesophagus and pancreatic duct, while dissociation of cells by enzyme perfusion, followed by plating, is typically used for solid epithelial organs such as the liver or kidney (Klaunig *et al.*, 1982). Changes in individual explants have been followed by preparing cytological smears and returning the explants to culture. This has allowed explant cultures to be maintained for longer periods, while still enabling evaluation of their morphological state (Resau & Albright, 1986). A variety of culture media have been used for both types of cultures, and the effects of growth factors, hormones, and other substances that control proliferation are being studied. Lechner has developed several approaches to the long-term culture of human epithelium (Lechner & Laveck, 1985). These cells and explants can be easily evaluated cytologically with imprint/contact smears (Papanicolaou) and allowed to remain in culture (Resau & Albright, 1986).

Xenografts

Another technique that is very useful for studying the effects of xenobiotic compounds in human cells and tissue is to xenograft such tissues into anatomical sites of the nude mouse (Table 1; Valerio *et al.*, 1982). Various types of xenotransplant configurations have been utilized and this methodology is under rapid development in many laboratories. Explant

Table 1. Culture and xenotransplantation of normal epithelial tissues and cells.

Epithelium	Explant culture (months)	Epithelial cell culture	Xenotransplantation into athymic nude mice
Breast	3	+	+
Bronchus	12	+	+
Colon	0·8	+	+
Prostate	3	+	+
Oesophagus	3	+	+
Bladder	4	+	+
Skin	3	+	+
Gall bladder	1	+	+
Pancreatic duct	6	+	+
Uterus, cervix	4	+	+
Liver	0·8	+	+

+, Successful establishment of cell cultures, or tissues.

cultures of epithelial tissues such as the bronchus are often placed sub-cutaneously. After vascularization, these human epithelial cells at the cut edge of the explant enter the mitotic cycle, as in a repairing wound, line a spherical cyst, and then differentiate into a pseudostratified columnar epithelium. The same type of phenomenon occurs with colon, oesophagus or pancreatic duct explants, each of which differentiates into the phenotype characteristic of the parent organ. Cell suspensions, such as those of hepatocytes, can be sub-cutaneously transplanted into the anterior chamber of the eye, or into other locations such as beneath the capsule of the kidney or into the spleen. Klein-Szanto and associates (Obara *et al.*, 1986) have developed a novel method for culturing epithelia which line ducts or tubes, first by transplantation of denuded rat tracheas subcutaneously, followed by intra-luminal injection of cell suspensions such as those of bronchial epithelium, trachea or kidney. These cells proceed to divide, lining the tracheal tube, and finally differentiate into the phenotype characteristic of the parent tissue. Such methods could greatly facilitate comparative studies in the future. For example, using such a system, one could simultaneously compare the effects of an agent on rat, hamster and human proximal tubular epithelium on bronchial epithelium simultaneously in a nude mouse (Trifillis *et al.*, 1985).

Results

As indicated above, this general approach has been utilized to answer a number of questions regarding effects of toxic and carcinogenic agents on human tissues, their relationship to comparable animal studies, and their ap-plication to human carcinogenesis studies such as biochemical epidemiology. Examples of some of the major categories of studies that have been under-taken so far follow. Space precludes detailed referencing, but access to the literature can be found in the several reviews cited (Trump & Harris, 1979; Harris, 1983; Trump *et al.*, 1984).

Mechanism of acute toxicity in a variety of epithelia

In these studies, reversible and irreversible events following cell injury have been investigated. Emphasis has been placed on agents that interfere with cell membrane integrity and/or permeability and agents that modify energy metabolism. These studies have utilized a variety of biochemical and morpho-logical methods, most recently fluorescent probes that delineate readily detected ion movements. It is evident from these studies that ion deregulation plays an important role in the early events following cell injury and that these events involve modification of cell membrane and cytoskeletal function. Par-ticularly important in the early effects of cell injury are movements of protons and ionized calcium. The latter may be an important early determinant of the effects of injury and may, in many cases, trigger irreversible damage to cell membranes. It is now evident that studies on human cells can be at least equal in sophistication to the studies of cells from experimental animals (Trump *et al.*, 1981, 1984).

Activation of procarcinogens to metabolites that form adducts

Several chemical classes of carcinogens are enzymically activated to metabolites that bind to the DNA of cultured human tissues explants. These compounds include the polyaromatic hydrocarbons, nitrosamines, natural products such as aflatoxin B_1, and aromatic amides such as 2-acetylaminofluorene. In a number of cases the DNA adducts isolated from cultured human tissues have been identified for several procarcinogens. In the cases studied so far, the characteristics of the DNA adducts formed are identical to those observed in experimental animals exposed to the same carcinogens (Autrup *et al.*, 1982a,b; Groopman *et al.*, 1982; Harris *et al.*, 1982; Harris & Cerutti, 1982).

Pathways of activation and deactivation

These pathways are under study in many laboratories and it is clear that the rate-limiting enzymic reactions responsible for activation could differ greatly among human cells and tissues. Harris *et al.* (1982) have reviewed this subject and have suggested that clues could be obtained from measurements of aryl hydrocarbon hydrolase (AHA) and epoxide-hydrolase activities. Using this approach, individual tissues vary greatly in their AHA activities, and there is significant variation between individuals (Fornace *et al.*, 1983). The greatest inter-individual variation (several hundred-fold) is seen in the placenta, whereas there is 20-fold or less variation in the bronchus, skin and kidney. The mechanism responsible for this variation is not known at the moment. In contrast, epoxide hydrolase has significantly lower tissue and inter-individual variation, possibly because of greater substance specificity and fewer isoenzymes.

Pathways and rates of DNA repair

It is evident that following the formation of carcinogen–DNA adducts the processes of DNA repair may remove them at varying rates and fidelity (Haugen *et al.*, 1982; Harris *et al.*, 1984). Little detail is known yet of the effects of carcinogens or tumour promoters; however, there does appear to be significant person-to-person differences in some key enzymes such as uracil-DNA glycosolase and 06-alkylguanine DNA transalkylase. It also appears from some studies that humans have significantly higher rates of DNA repair compared to laboratory rodents, perhaps relating to the difficulty of chemically induced transformation of human epithelia *in vitro*. Such compounds as formaldehyde may, at the same time, induce DNA damage and interfere with DNA repair; they may also act as tumour promoters.

Inter-species, inter-individual and inter-cell variations in toxin and carcinogen metabolism

There is considerable variation between individuals in toxin and carcinogen metabolism in the human population, perhaps not surprising in view of pharmacokinetic studies done with identical twins. This variation in activation is tissue dependent and may or may not be correlated with risk of carcinogenesis. Furthermore, the variation in metabolism also applies to inter-species comparisons. Inter-individual variation can also be observed in tissue-mediated mutagenesis assays, as shown by Hsu *et al.* (1978). This system utilizes human cells as mediators and V79 cells as targets. In the case of the bronchus, there was wide variation in mediated frequencies of both ouabain resistance and sister chromatid exchanges. Furthermore, a significant correlation was observed between mutation frequency in the V79 cells and the amount of carcinogen–DNA adducts observed in human bronchial epithelium.

Implications for epidemiological investigations

From the section above, it follows that significant variations in activation, deactivation, DNA repair, and levels of activity of tumour promoters exist between species and individuals. This has significant implications for human risk assessment in terms of epidemiological studies. Accordingly, another important area of human disease investigation involves the validation of risk versus carcinogen or tracer drug metabolism in human populations. Among the approaches that are now being mounted in this area is whether marker drugs such as debrisoquine, that are subject to genetic polymorphisms, are metabolized differently in control individuals versus individuals at high risk of cancer (Idle *et al.*, 1979; Evans *et al.*, 1980; Ayesh *et al.*, 1984). Other important aspects of the approach requiring careful study include: the correlation between DNA repair enzymes and tumour risk; whether exposure results in increased DNA adducts in white blood cells or in urine; and whether examination of DNA obtained from leukocytes or other samples can be analysed in a way to estimate risk. Such studies are now under way in a variety of institutions and may result in improved evaluation of the study of chronic disease epidemiology.

The mechanism of tumour promotion

Much of the risk of human cancer may relate to enhancers or promoters as opposed to initiating agents (McDowell *et al.*, 1983). For example, cigarette smoke contains a variety of carcinogens but also a variety of putative tumour promoters that induce a variety of effects, including cell injury, cell death and induction of terminal differentiation. The mechanism of tumour promotion is poorly understood. One current hypothesis states that promoters act by exerting a differential toxic or differentiating effect on normal as opposed to initiated cells. Such effects have now been demonstrated in a variety of situations, especially *in vitro*. It has been shown, for example, in murine culture models that in keratinocytes the level of calcium in the culture medium exerts a differential effect on normal versus carcinogen-treated cells. In cultures of normal tissues, the physiological levels of calcium (approximately 1 mM) induce terminal differentiation, whereas in initiated cells such levels of calcium in the suspending media are permissive to cell growth. Similar effects have been reported in the human bronchus by Lechner & Laveck (1985); moreover, it has been noted that serum (probably because of TGF-β) induces terminal differentiation in normal bronchial epithelium as compared to tumour cell lines.

Some of these phenomena may relate to autocrine growth factors produced from initiated cells. Such factors may exert permissive or stimulatory effects on initiated as compared to non-initiated cells. It is quite clear at the present time that the classical definitions of initiation and promotion in the mouse skin need to be thoroughly examined in many other important human models.

Human epithelia transformed *in vitro*

In our laboratories work has been performed for some time on chemical carcinogen-transformation of human cells *in vitro*. These results may be very significant from the standpoint of extrapolation from animal data to man, especially the reliance on *in vitro* transformation tests of fibroblasts for animal–human extrapolation. Observations suggest that the transformation of human epithelium is extremely difficult. Only one significant paper has appeared on the tumourigenic transformation of human epithelia. This is the work by Parsa *et al.* (1981) in which carcinogen treatment was applied to explant cultures of human pancreatic ducts. These resulted in the production of tumourigenic nodules in nude mice.

Efforts to reproduce this effect on bronchus, prostate, kidney and oesophagus, have yielded negative results so far. A variety of factors could explain this negative result, including the efficacy of activation and/or repair, selection by culture media, and limitations of the nude mouse tumourigenesis assay.

At the same time, Yoakum *et al.* (1985) have reported that the transformation of human bronchial epithelium using a new method of transfection (to avoid the calcium-induced effect on terminal differentiation) can result in the induction of tumourigenic bronchial carcinomas. The transfection assay suggests that genomic changes may be critical to human transformation and that prolonged treatment with chemicals may be necessary in order to achieve similar results.

Acknowledgements

This study was supported in part by NIH grants nos NO1CP-31008, NO1CP-51000, AM-15440, and American Cancer Society (MD Affiliate) 1985–86.

References

Autrup, H. and Harris, C. C., 1983, Metabolism of chemical carcinogens by cultured human tissues. In *Human Carcinogenesis*, edited by C. C. Harris and H. Autrup (New York: Academic Press), pp. 169, 194.

Autrup, H. and Williams, G. M., 1983, *Experimental Colon Carcinogenesis* (Boca Raton: CRC Press), pp. 95–106.

Autrup, H., Grafstrom, R. C., Brugh, M., Mechner, J. F., Haugen, A., Trump, B. F. and Harris, C. C., 1982a, Comparison of benzo(*a*)pyrene metabolism in bronchus, esophagus, colon, and duodenum from the same individual. *Cancer Res.*, **42**, 934–938.

Autrup, H., Lechner, J. F. and Harris, C. C., 1982b, The use of human tissues and cells in carcinogen metabolism and toxicity studies. In *Safety, Evaluation and Regulation of Chemicals*, edited by F. Hamburger (Basel: S. Karger), pp. 151, 159.

Ayesh, R., Idle, J. R., Ritchie, J. C., Crothers, M. J. and Hetzel, M. R., 1984, Metabolic oxidation phenotypes as markers for susceptibility to liver cancer. *Nature*, **312**, 169–170.

Banks-Schlegel, S. P., 1985, Isolation, activation and characterization of normal human esophageal epithelial cells. *J. Tissue Culture Methods*, **9**, 95–106.

Banks-Schlegel, S. P., 1982, Keratin alterations during embryonic epidermal differentiation: a presage of adult epidermal maturation. *J. cell Biol.*, **93**, 551–559.

Banks-Schlegel, S. P., McDowell, E. M., Wilson, T. S., Trump, B. F. and Harris, C. C., 1984, Keratin proteins in human lung carcinomas. Combined use of morphology, keratin immunocytochemistry, and keratin immunoprecipitation. *Am. J. Path.*, **114**, 273–286.

Barrett, L. A., McDowell, E. M., Hill, T. A., Pyeatte, J. C., Harris, C. C. and Trump, B. F., 1980, Induction of atypical squamous metaplasia with benzo(*a*)pyrene in cultured hamster trachea. *Path. Res. Pract.*, **168**, 134–145.

Blattner, W. A., Greene, M. H., Goedert, J. J. and Mann, D. L., 1983, Interdisciplinary studies in the evaluation of persons at high risk of cancer. In *Human Carcinogenesis*, edited by C. C. Harris and H. A. Autrup (New York: Academic Press), pp. 913–939.

Cottrell, J. R. and Resau, J. H., 1985, A method to determine the viability of explant tissue in organ culture. *J. Tissue Culture Methods*, **9**(4), 191–192.

Cowley, R. A., Mergner, W. J., Fisher, R. S., Jones, R. T. and Trump, B. F., 1979, The subcellular pathology of shock in trauma patients: studies using the immediate autopsy. *Am. Surg.*, **45**, 255–269.

Evans, D. A., Mahgoub, A., Sloan, T. P., Idle, J. R. and Smith, R. L., 1980, A family and population study of the genetic polymorphism of debrisoquine oxidation in a white British population. *J. med. Genet.*, **17**, 102–105.

Fornace Jr., A. J., Lechner, J. F., Grafstrom, R. C. and Harris, C. C., 1983, Detection of DNA single-strand breaks during the repair of UV damage in xeroderma pigmentosum cells. *Radiat. Res.*, **93**, 107–111.

Groopman, J. D., Haugen, A., Goodrich, G. R., Wogan, G. N. and Harris, C. C., 1982, Quantitation of aflatoxin B1-modified DNA using monoclonal antibodies. *Cancer Res.*, **42**, 3120–3124.

Harris, C. C., 1983, Carcinogenesis studies using cultured human tissues and cells. *Cancer Res.*, **43**, 1880–1883.

Harris, C. C. and Trump, B. F., 1983, Human tissues and cells in biomedical research. *Surv. Synth. Path. Res.*, **1**, 165–171.

Harris, C. and Cerutti, P. A., 1982, *Mechanisms of Chemical Carcinogenesis. ICN–UCLA Symposia on Molecular and Cellular Biology* (New York: Alan R. Liss), pp. 419–427.

Harris, C. C., Yolken, R. H. and Hsu, I. C., 1982, Enzyme immunoassays: applications in cancer research. In *Methods in Cancer Research*, Vol. 20, edited by H. Busch and L. C. Yeoman (New York: Academic Press), pp. 213, 242.

Harris, C. C., Autrup, H., Vahakangas, K. and Trump, B. F., 1984, Interindividual variation in carcinogen activation and DNA repair. In *Banbury Report No. 16. Genetic Variability in Responses to Chemical Exposure* (Cold Spring Harbor, NY: Cold Spring Harbor Laboratory), pp. 145, 154.

Haugen, A., Schafer, P. W., Lechner, J. F., Stoner, G. D., Trump, B. F. and Harris, C. C., 1982, Cellular ingestion, toxic effects, and lesions observed in epithelial tissues and cells cultured with asbestos and glass fibers. *Int. J. Cancer*, **30**, 265–272.

Hsu, I. C., Stoner, G. D., Autrup, H., Trump, B. F., Selkirk, J. K. and Harris, C. C., 1978, Human bronchus-mediated mutagenesis of mammalian cells by carcinogenic polynuclear aromatic hydrocarbons. *Proc. natn. Acad. Sci. U.S.A.*, **75**, 2003–2007.

Idle, J. R., Sloan, T. P., Smith, R. L. and Wakile, L. A., 1979, The application of the phenotypical panel approach to the detection of polymorphisms of drug oxidation in man. *Br. J. Pharmac.*, **66**, 430–440.

Jones, R. T., Hudson, E. A. and Resau, J. H., 1981, A review of *in vitro* and *in vivo* culture techniques for the study of pancreatic carcinogenesis. *Cancer*, **47**, 1490–1496.

Klaunig, J. E., Goldblatt, P. J., Hinton, D. E., Lipsky, M. M., Knipe, S. M. and Trump, B. F., 1982, Morphologic and functional studies of mouse hepatocytes in primary culture. *Anat. Rec.*, **204**, 231–243.

Lechner, J. F. and Laveck, M. A., 1985, A serum free method for culturing normal human bronchial cells at clonal density. *J. Tissue Culture Methods*, **9**, 43–48.

McDowell, E. M., Harris, C. C. and Trump, B. F., 1983, Histogenesis and morphogenesis of bronchial neoplasms. In *Morphogenesis of Lung Cancer*, edited by T. Shimosato, M. Melamed and R. Nettesheim (New York: CRC Press), pp. 1–36.

Obara, T., Conti, C. J., Baba, M., Resau, J. H., Trifillis, A. L., Trump, B. F. and Klein-Szanto, A. J. P., 1986, Rapid detection of xenotransplated human tissues using *in situ* hybridization. *Am. J. Path.*, **122**, 386–391.

Parsa, I., Marsh, W. H. and Sutton, A. L., 1981, An *in vitro* model of human pancreas carcinogenesis: effects of nitroso compounds. *Cancer*, **47**, 1543–1551.

Purnell, D. M., Hillman, E. A., Heatfield, B. M. and Trump, B. F. 1982, Immunoreactive prolactin in epithelial cells of normal and cancerous human breast and prostate detected by the unlabeled antibody peroxidase–antiperoxidase method. *Cancer Res.*, **42**, 2317–2324.

Resau, J. H. and Albright, C. A., 1986, Explant/organ culture cytopathologic characterization. *Virchows Arch.* [Cell Path.], B. Cell Pathology., **52**, 15–24.

Resau, J. H., Cottrell, J. R., Hudson, E. A. Trump, B. F. and Jones, R. T., 1985a, Studies on the mechanisms of altered exocrine acinar cell differentiation and ductal metaplasia following nitrosamine exposure using hamster pancreatic explant organ culture. *Carcinogenesis*, **6**, 29–35.

Resau, J. H., Marzella, L., Jones, R. T. and Trump, B. F., 1985b, What's new in *in vitro* studies of exocrine pancreatic cell injury? *Path. Res. Pract.*, **179**, 576–588.

Sanefuji, H. Heatfield, B. M., Trump, B. F. and Young Jr. J. D., 1982, Studies on carcinogenesis of human prostate. II. Long-term explant culture of normal prostate and benign prostatic hyperplasia: light microscopy. *J. natn. Cancer Inst.*, **69**, 751–756.

Shamsuddin, A. K. M. and Trump, B. F., 1981, Colon epithelium. III. *In vitro* studies of colon carcinogenesis in Fischer 344 rats. *N*-Methyl-*N*'-nitro-*N*-nitroso-guanidine-induced changes in colon epithelium in explant culture. *J. natn. Cancer Inst.*, **66**, 403–411.

Trifillis, A. L., Regec, A. L. and Trump, B. F., 1985, Isolation, culture and characterization of human renal tubular cells. *J. Urol.*, **133**, 324–329.

Trump, B. F. and Harris, C. C., 1979, Human tissues in biomedical research. *Human Path.*, **10**, 245–248.

Trump, B. F., Valigorsky, J. M., Jones, R. T., Mergner, W. J., Garcia, J. H. and Cowley, R. A., 1975, The application of electron microscopy and cellular biochemistry to the autopsy. *Human Path.*, **6**, 499–516.

Trump, B. F., Mergner, W. J. Jones, R. T. and Cowley, R. A., 1978, The use and application of autopsy in research. *Am. J. Clin. Path.*, (Suppl.) **69**, 230–234.

Trump, B. F., Berezesky, I. K. and Phelps, P. C., 1981, The role of altered sodium and calcium regulation and the cytoskeleton in the pathogenesis of human disease. *J. clin. Electron Microsc.*, **14**, 366–369.

Trump, B. F., Berezesky, I. K., Sato, T., Laiho, K. U., Phelps, P. C. and Declaris, N., 1984, Cell calcium, cell injury and cell death. *Envirn. Hlth Perspect.*, **57**, 281–287.

Valerio, M. G., Fineman, E. L., Bowman, R. L., Harris, C. C., Trump, B. F., Hillman, E. A. and Heatfield, B. M., 1982, Preliminary studies of normal untreated and/or carcinogen-treated adult human breast, prostate, and esophagus as xenografts in nude mice. In *Proceedings of the Third International Workshop on Nude Mice*, edited by N. Reed (New York: Gustav Fischer), pp. 283, 296.

Vocci, M. J., Combs, J. W., Hillman, E. A., Resau, J. H. and Trump, B. F., 1983, The cell kinetics of the adaptation of the human esophagus to organ culture. *In Vitro*, **19**, 881–889.

Yoakum, G. H., Lechner, J. F., Gabrielson, E. W., Korba, B. E., Malan-Shibley, L., Willey, J. C., Valerio, M. G., Shamsuddin, A. M., Trump, B. F. and Harris, C. C., 1985, Transformation of human bronchial epithelial cells transfected by Harvey ras oncogene. *Science*, **227**, 1174–1178.

Problems and prospects in inter-species extrapolation

Thomas B. Starr

Department of Epidemiology, Chemical Industry Institute of Toxicology, Research Triangle Park, NC 27709, USA

Current risk assessment practice

Given the intense political pressures on regulatory agencies to act quickly on public health issues and the limited resources available to them, it is not surprising that a generic, empirical and cookbook-like approach to the problem of human carcinogenic risk assessment has evolved and is now finding increasingly widespread use (US Environmental Protection Agency, 1984). With few exceptions, this approach treats all chemicals alike, irrespective of potentially significant differences in species susceptibility, target sites, tumour types, and, most importantly, mechanisms of action. It culminates with the estimation of a single quantity, termed the carcinogenic potency, from the database regarding a chemical's toxicity. This derived measure is presumed to be representative of the cancer risk to humans from a life-time of exposure to the chemical at a constant unit daily dosage level.

Importantly, very few data are needed to produce this potency estimate. In fact, tumour-incidence data from a single chronic laboratory animal study that is positive for cancer in one sex of one species are sufficient. Even a completely negative chronic study can be used to construct an approximate upper confidence limit on this potency measure, although in such cases the estimated upper bound reflects little more than the limited size of the bioassay treatment groups.

This approach to carcinogenic risk assessment requires many assumptions, which are usually invoked in the absence of any specific scientific evidence that bears on their validity. Four of these assumptions are especially critical. The first is that at low doses the linearized version of the Armitage–Doll multistage model of carcinogenesis provides a valid description of the actual relationship between the probability of a carcinogenic response and the true underlying causal variable, namely, the amount or concentration of the biologically active form of a chemical that reaches specific target-tissue macromolecules. This internal and well-localized measure of exposure has been termed the 'effective' or delivered dose. Second, it is assumed that the dose administered to animals during a chronic study, which is a well-controlled but external measure of exposure such as mg/kg/day in food, or p.p.m. in air or drinking water, is a valid linear proxy for the delivered dose in all tissues and over the entire dose spectrum from infinitesimally small to nearly lethal doses. Taken together, these two assumptions permit one to estimate, from bioassay tumour data alone, the cancer risk to a test animal at low administered doses, provided that the temporal pattern of exposure for which risk estimates are desired, for example, six hours/day, five days/week, is the same as the one employed in the chronic study.

The third assumption deals with the problem of extrapolating cancer risk across different temporal patterns of exposure. It is simply that all exposure regimens which produce the same life-time average daily dose will also pose exactly the same carcinogenic risk. For example, exposure for the same number of days to 4 p.p.m. for 6 h/d, or 1 p.p.m. for 24 h/d, or 24 p.p.m. for 1 h/d, are all presumed to pose the same carcinogenic risk. And fourth, in order to extrapolate risk across species, there is an inter-species scaling assumption. For gavage, feeding and drinking water studies, it is usually assumed that all doses equivalent on a per unit surface area or body weight basis will yield the same carcinogenic risk, while for inhalation exposures the unadjusted airborne concentration is customarily taken to be the relevant exposure measure irrespective of the species.

Does this extrapolation approach work between rodent species?

Crouch & Wilson have explored, in a strictly empirical fashion, the question of whether or not inter-species extrapolation of such cookbook-derived potency estimates is actually possible (Crouch & Wilson, 1979; Crouch 1983). They utilized selected tumour incidence data for both sexes of rats and mice as obtained in the series of 187 carcinogenesis bioassays conducted by the National Cancer Institute (NCI) in the late-1970s (NCI, 1976–80). Doses used in gavage, feeding and drinking water studies were converted to life-time average daily doses per unit body weight, expressed in mg/kg/day. Next, the tumour incidence data versus dose for each chemical compound were used to estimate species- and sex-specific parameters α and β of the one-hit (or one-stage) dose–response model:

$$P(d) = 1 - (1 - \alpha)\exp(-\beta d/(1 - \alpha)).$$

At very low doses, this response model reduces to a straight line with intercept α (approximately the control group tumour incidence) and slope β:

$$P(d) \simeq \alpha + \beta d, \qquad d \simeq 0.$$

The low-dose slope β was selected as the index of carcinogenic potency.

Comparisons of estimated potencies were made between sexes within species and also between species. For the latter comparison, geometric means of the male and female potency estimates for each species were employed. Representative results for Osborne–Mendel (OM) rats and B6C3F1 mice are displayed in Table 1. Immediately apparent is the enormous range of variation, roughly four orders of magnitude, in potency estimates for different chemicals within each species-sex group. In addition, correlations between the potency estimates (on a logarithmic scale) across sex and across species are surprisingly large. Taken at face value, these results would suggest that inter-species extrapolation of such potency estimates, at least among rodent species, is indeed quite feasible.

Subsequently, Zeise *et al.* (1984) observed that there was a very strong negative correlation (again on a logarithmic scale) between the estimated carcinogenic potency, β, and a simple measure of acute toxicity, the LD_{50}, that single dose which will most likely kill 50% of a population. For the Osborne–Mendel rat, this correlation was found to be -0.93, while for the B6C3F1 mouse and the Fischer-344 rat it was -0.89 and -0.59, respectively. These unexpectedly strong relationships, coupled with the large correlations observed between potency estimates across rodent species, led these investigators to suggest that one could produce a reasonably accurate estimate of the carcinogenic potency of chemicals, even if bioassay data were *not* available. Such an estimate could be obtained simply by taking the reciprocal of the LD_{50}!

Recently, Bernstein *et al.* (1985) have re-examined in somewhat greater detail the question of whether or not inter-species extrapolation of carcinogenic potency estimates is feasible. Although they utilized essentially the same database as Crouch & Wilson (1979), their analysis focused on potency

Table 1. Potency estimates for OM rats and B6C3F1 mice.†

Species	Sex	Minimum β	Maximum β
OM	Male	0·00007	0·9
OM	Female	0·00010	0·7
	Correlation of $\log_{10} \beta = 0.93$ ($n = 22$)		
B6C3F1	Male	0·00010	0·6
B6C3F1	Female	0·00009	0·3
	Correlation of $\log_{10} \beta = 0.95$ ($n = 19$)		
OM	Combined	0·00014	0·14
B6C3F1	Combined	0·00009	0·4
	Correlation of $\log_{10} \beta = 0.72$ ($n = 17$)		

† Calculated with data from Crouch & Wilson (1979).

estimates only for female rats and female mice. A slightly different formulation of the one-hit (or one-stage) model was employed:

$$P(d) = 1 - \exp(-(a + bd)),$$

and the parameter b, sometimes referred to as the 'extra' risk per unit dose, was taken as the estimate of carcinogenic potency. At low doses, this response model reduces to:

$$P(d) \simeq (1 - \exp(-a)) + \exp(-a)bd, \qquad bd \simeq 0.$$

Thus, the relationships between the intercept (α) and potency (β) estimates of Crouch & Wilson (1979) and the parameters a and b of Bernstein *et al.*'s (1985) formulation of the one-hit model are given by:

$$\alpha = 1 - \exp(-a),$$

$$\beta = \exp(-a)b.$$

Across 49 different compounds that yielded statistically significant estimates of potency for female rats and female mice, Bernstein *et al.*, (1985) found the correlation between potency estimates to be $0 \cdot 86$ (on a logarithmic scale), that is, very large, and consistent with Crouch & Wilson's (1979) previous findings. Bernstein *et al.* (1985) also noted that an even stronger correlation ($0 \cdot 91$, $n = 186$, logarithmic scale) existed between the female rat and female mouse maximum doses tested in the NCI studies, irrespective of whether or not the compounds were carcinogenic. This is an extraordinarily high correlation considering the fact that across chemical compounds, the maximum doses tested spanned about seven orders of magnitude. Furthermore, Bernstein *et al.* (1985) suggested that the high correlation between rat and mouse potency estimates was due entirely to the even higher correlation between the maximum doses tested with rats and mice.

To understand why this strong connection between estimated potency and maximum dose tested exists, it is helpful to consider a hypothetical two-group bioassay with n_0 control and n_1 treated animals, respectively. Let c_0 and c_1 represent the number of animals that develop tumours in each group, and q_0 and q_1 represent the proportion remaining free of tumours, $q_0 = 1 - c_0/n_0$, while $q_1 = 1 - c_1/n_1$. Then it may be shown that the maximum likelihood estimates of the one-hit model parameters a and b are given by:

$$a = -\log(q_0),$$

$$b = \log(q_0/q_1)/d.$$

The equation for b shows that the potency estimate is the ratio of two terms. Thus, there are two sources of possible variation between species in the potency estimates. First, the doses for the different species may be different, but, as was noted earlier, for rats and mice these are very highly correlated. Second, the quantity $\log(q_0/q_1)$ may differ between rats and mice as a result of differences in the control and/or treated-group tumour incidences. However, as is discussed below, the range of possible variation in this quantity is highly restricted by the limited number of animals employed in the typical bioassay.

Table 2 shows some of the values of $\log(q_0/q_1)$ (and upper bounds on their 95% confidence intervals) that could be obtained in a bioassay with 50 animals in the treated group and an infinite number in the control group, for which the tumour incidence is arbitrarily taken to be 10%. The smallest value of $\log(q_0/q_1)$ that is still significantly greater than zero ($P < 0.025$, one-sided) is 0.118, which corresponds to $c_1 = 10$, that is a 20% incidence of tumours in the treated group, twice the control group incidence. The largest finite value (3.807) corresponds to $c_1 = 49$, that is 98% tumour incidence in the treated group. Thus, if we consider only statistically significant and finite values of $\log(q_0/q_1)$, no two can possibly differ by more than a factor of about 32, that is, $3.807/0.118$.

This result implies that statistically significant potency estimates for rats and mice tested at the same dose can differ at most by this same factor. Thus, a strong correlation between rat and mouse potency estimates across chemical compounds is not unexpected. Indeed, Bernstein *et al.* (1985) showed that if one independently and randomly assigned admissible values of $\log(q_0/q_1)$ to the studies of 49 compounds that had yielded statistically significant potency estimates in both female rats and female mice, the expected value of the inter-species correlation was 0.90, very close to the observed value of 0.86. Thus,

Table 2. Results from an ideal two-group experiment.

c_1	q_1	$\log(q_0/q_1)$	$\log(q_0/q_1)^u$†
5	0·90	0·	0·141
6	0·88	0·022	0·173
10	0·80	0·118	0·306
25	0·50	0·588	0·930
40	0·20	1·504	2·194
49	0·02	3·807	7·484
50	0·00	∞	∞

Adapted from Bernstein *et al.* (1985).
Parameter values: $q_0 = 0.9$, $n_0 = \infty$, $d = 1$.
† $\log(q_0/q_1)^u$ is the upper limit on the 95% confidence interval.

the strong correlation between rat and mouse potency estimates is not due at all to similarities in the pattern of tumour incidence in the two species. For such correlations to appear, all that is required is that the treated group incidence be statistically significant (and not 100%) relative to the control group incidence in both species.

It is also important to recognize that for any given species- and sex-specific group, all possible statistically significant and finite potency estimates must lie between the values $0 \cdot 118/d$ and $3 \cdot 807/d$. This implies that potency estimates across chemicals will be very highly correlated with the reciprocals of the maximum doses tested, since these reciprocals (and the doses themselves) range over about seven orders of magnitude. Thus, if one takes an objective but critical view of these findings, it would appear that the cookbook-like approach to inter-species extrapolation currently in use by the regulatory agencies yields little more than imprecise estimates of the reciprocals of maximum doses tested, no matter what the actual tumour incidence data are! Do such estimates really reflect the true risk at low exposure levels that humans are likely to encounter? The answer to this question seems to be a clear and resounding 'No'. Bioassay data by themselves, no matter how they are analysed, are simply inadequate to the task of accurately and quantitatively predicting human cancer risk. At best, they permit an identification of those chemical compounds that are carcinogenic in test species under the specific conditions of the studies.

Improving inter-species extrapolation with mechanistic data

It is of critical importance in assessing the potential carcinogenic effects of chemical exposure in humans to make the most effective use possible of toxicity data above and beyond that obtained in carcinogenesis bioassays. As noted earlier, a critical assumption in the present regulatory approach to extrapolation is that the relationship between administered and delivered doses is one of direct linear proportionality. However, the actual quantitative relationship between administered and delivered doses is a reflection of the entire spectrum of biological responses to exposure, ranging from physiological responses of the whole organism to intra-cellular biochemical responses in target tissues. Thus, the administered dose provides at best an indirect surrogate measure of the delivered dose, and the relationship between these two measures of exposure need not be a simple linear one. Indeed, given the marvellous complexity of living organisms, it is altogether reasonable to expect that the intricate processes of distribution and disposition of compounds which operate during and following exposures *in vivo* would exhibit some form of non-linear dependence on the administered dose.

This observation is especially important for two reasons. First, the various mathematical models of carcinogenesis are conceptualized and formulated in terms of interactions between the biologically active forms of chemical agents, i.e., the delivered dose, and cellular macromolecules in target tissues (Brown, 1976; Cornfield, 1977; Crump, 1979; Hoel *et al.*, 1983). These models lack the structure necessary to characterize the many physiological and pharmaco-kinetic factors that determine the actual relationship between administered and delivered doses. They characterize only the dependence of the carcino-genic process on the delivered dose.

Second, it is now known that low-dose risk extrapolations based upon the linear proportionality assumption will yield risk estimates that are either excessively conservative (too high) or anti-conservative (too low) when the true administered/delivered dose relationship is non-linear (Hoel *et al.*, 1983). This finding implies that risk estimates obtained with the administered dose as the measure of exposure will be biased, no matter what inter-species scaling assumptions are used, whenever the linear proportionality assumption is not valid.

Thus, when data regarding delivered dose are available, they can and should be used, at the very least, to provide a check on the validity of this critical assumption. Should these data demonstrate that the relationship between ad-ministered and delivered doses is non-linear, then risk assessment models will generate unbiased estimates of risk only when the delivered dose is utilized as the measure of exposure. A comparison of risks estimated with both exposure measures can also be made, and in this way the extent of the bias introduced by incorrectly assuming linearity can be determined.

Research conducted at the Chemical Industry Institute of Toxicology (CIIT) on formaldehyde provides an excellent illustration of the utility of mechanistic data to the extrapolation problem. Mechanistic studies have demonstrated that exposure of rodents to formaldehyde via inhalation of high, but not low, airborne concentrations induces the respiratory depression reflex (Chang *et al.*, 1983), inhibition of mucociliary clearance (Morgan, 1983; Morgan *et al.*, 1983), inhibition of intra-cellular metabolism of formaldehyde (Casanova-Schmitz & Heck, 1985) and stimulation of cell proliferation (Chang *et al.*, 1983; Swenberg *et al.*, 1983). Since each of these phenomena appears to be an impor-tant controlling factor in the relationship between administered and delivered formaldehyde doses (Starr & Gibson 1985), a non-linear relationship between administered and delivered doses would be expected to result.

The respiratory depression reflex, which is induced in rodents by exposure to irritant gases, mediates the inhaled dose. However, the extent of induction of this reflex is both species- and concentration-dependent. Mice reduce their respiration much more dramatically than rats at an airborne concentration of 15 p.p.m. formaldehyde (Chang *et al.*, 1983). As a result, after adjustment for differences in nasal cavity surface area, mice receive only about one half the dose that rats receive when they are identically exposed to 15 p.p.m. formal-dehyde for six hours/day. This inter-species difference in inhaled dose per unit nasal cavity surface area can account for the remarkable difference in the high-dose tumour incidence (50% in rats, 1% in mice) observed in the CIIT for-maldehyde bioassay (Kerns *et al.*, 1983). Parenthetically, it should be noted that mice are not more sensitive than rats to all inhaled irritant gases. For example, rats are more sensitive than mice to acrylic acid (Barrow *et al.*, 1986). As a consequence, rats receive only about one half the dose that mice receive when they are identically exposed to 75 p.p.m. acrylic acid for six hours/day. Thus, the extent of induction of the respiratory depression reflex is also chemical-specific.

Mucociliary clearance mediates the fraction of the inhaled formaldehyde dose that penetrates the mucus layer covering underlying epithelial cells in the nasal cavity. Intra-cellular metabolism mediates the fraction of formaldehyde entering these cells that remains free to bind with cellular macromolecules, in-cluding DNA. Important in this regard is the fact that formaldehyde is an essential biochemical that is normally present in all living cells. It is thus not surprising that efficient metabolic pathways exist for its detoxication, at least at low airborne formaldehyde concentrations. Finally, the rate of cell repli-cation mediates that fraction of DNA that is single-stranded, and it is known that formaldehyde can bind covalently only to single-stranded DNA (von Hippel & Wong, 1971; Lukashin *et al.*, 1976).

Additional biochemical studies have produced the first direct evidence that the formaldehyde dose delivered to the DNA of replicating cells in the rat nasal cavity is non-linearly related to airborne concentration (Casanova-Schmitz *et al.*, 1984; Casanova-Schmitz & Heck, 1985). Specifically, significantly less binding was observed to occur at airborne formaldehyde concentrations of 2 p.p.m. or below than would be predicted by linear extrapolation from the amounts of binding observed at concentrations of 6 p.p.m. and above. This discrepancy with the linear proportionality assumption is depicted graphically in Figure 1. At 2 p.p.m. the ratio of the predicted level of binding (assuming linearity) to the observed level is approximately $3 \cdot 5$. At $0 \cdot 3$ p.p.m., this ratio is even larger, being approximately $5 \cdot 6$. These ratios represent the factors by which the delivered dose in target tissue is overestimated when strict linear pro-portionality between the administered and delivered doses is assumed.

At first glance, an overestimation of the delivered dose by less than a factor of 10 might seem of little consequence. However, nearly all of the mathematical models that are employed for risk extrapolation purposes relate the probability of a tumour response to the measure of exposure in a non-linear manner. For example, with the multi-stage model that is currently favoured by regulatory agencies, the maximum likelihood estimate of the probability of a tumour response at low doses is approximately proportional to the measure of exposure raised to some integer power. If a three-stage model is employed to describe the squamous cell carcinoma incidence among rats in the CIIT bioassay, the resulting low-dose risk estimate is approximately cubic in the measure of exposure. Thus, if exposure is overestimated by a factor of 5, the risk of a tumour is overestimated by a factor of 125. Clearly,

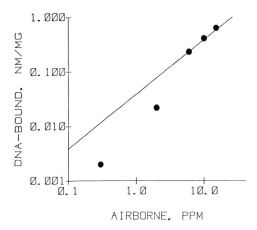

Figure 1. Plot of the concentration of formaldehyde covalently bound to Fischer-344 rat respiratory mucosal DNA (nm/mg) versus airborne formaldehyde concentration following two daily six-hour exposures. Observed values are denoted by dark circles. The straight line passes from the origin through the level of binding observed at 6 p.p.m., and represents predicted binding levels based on the assumption of linear proportionality between administered and delivered doses. Adapted from Starr (1985).

a comparatively small error in the specification of exposure level can produce rather large effects in the associated estimate of risk.

This phenomenon is displayed in more detail in Table 3, which presents maximum likelihood estimates of risk associated with exposure to $1 \cdot 0$ p.p.m. airborne formaldehyde, as determined with four commonly used quantal response models that were fit to the CIIT formaldehyde bioassay data for Fischer-344 rats (Starr & Buck, 1984). The first row shows results obtained by using administered dose − airborne formaldehyde concentration − as the measure of exposure. The second row shows corresponding estimates obtained by using the covalent binding data displayed in Figure 1 as a measure of the

Table 3. Maximum likelihood risk estimates† for $1 \cdot 0$ p.p.m. airborne formaldehyde.‡

Dose measure	Probit	Logit	Weibull	Multi-stage
Administered	$2 \cdot 6 \times 10^{-5}$	$2 \cdot 9$	$5 \cdot 9$	$251 \cdot$
Delivered	$4 \cdot 0 \times 10^{-14}$	$0 \cdot 02$	$0 \cdot 07$	$4 \cdot 7$
Reduction factor	$6 \cdot 6 \times 10^8$	$133 \cdot$	$83 \cdot 4$	$53 \cdot 4$

† Predicted excess nasal cancer risk in rats exposed to 1 p.p.m. formaldehyde, six hours/day, five days/week, for 24 months, expressed as number of cases per million rats.
‡ Adapted from Starr & Buck (1984).

delivered dose in target tissues. Finally, the third row provides the ratios of t
administered dose-based risk estimates to the corresponding delivered do:
based risk estimates.

It is readily apparent that use of delivered dose as the measure of exposu
resulted in a unilateral reduction in the estimates of cancer risk, irrespecti
of which dose–response model was employed. The largest difference occurr'
with the probit model, where the reduction factor was greater than 6×10
while the smallest difference, a factor of about 53, occurred with the mul
stage model. These results suggest that administered dose-based estimates
cancer risk from formaldehyde exposure such as those employed by tl
regulatory agencies are likely to be too high.

Critical assumptions still need validation

It is important to recognize that while the covalent binding data contradict tl
linear proportionality assumption, their use as measures of exposure for ri:
extrapolation rests on two other critical assumptions. First, covalent bindii
to target-tissue DNA was measured following just two six-hour exposures
airborne formaldehyde. Therefore, it must be assumed that these observatioi
are representative of events throughout the course of a long-term bioassa
Since formaldehyde is a very highly reactive chemical, there is no obvioi
reason to suppose that this is not the case, but on the other hand, there is r
direct evidence that the steady-state is achieved after just two days (
exposure. The assumption of steady-state distribution and pharmacokineti'
can only be tested with additional laboratory experiments that cover mo:
extended periods of exposure.

Second, it must be assumed that the covalent binding of formaldehyde 1
target-tissue DNA plays an important role in nasal tumour induction. Th
assumption is not implausible, since formaldehyde has been shown to hav
genotoxic activity in a variety of test systems. Furthermore, Hoel *et al.* (198:
have argued convincingly that it is likely to be "biologically more meaningfi
to relate tumor response to concentrations of specific DNA adducts in tl
target tissue than it is to relate tumor response to the administered dose of
chemical". Again, however, the assumption that covalent binding to DNA
directly relevant to nasal tumour induction remains to be validated in tl
laboratory.

Finally, it should be clear that differences between species in any of th
diverse factors that determine the quantitative relationship between ac
ministered and delivered doses can produce corresponding differences in th
delivered dose, and the attendant cancer risk, even when the different specic
are identically exposed to the same administered dose. This was well illustrate
by the remarkable disparity in tumour incidence among rats and mice expose
to $14 \cdot 3$ p.p.m. formaldehyde in the CIIT bioassay which can be explained b

the corresponding inter-species difference in inhaled dose (Chang *et al.*, 1983). Again, however, comparative studies in this research area with species that are more similar to humans than rodents, such as subhuman primates, are necessary to establish whether additional and substantial inter-species differences in delivered dose exist.

Summary

In conclusion, it should be apparent that the methods currently employed by regulatory agencies to estimate human cancer risk from chemical exposure fall well short of providing scientifically defensible answers to this extremely important problem. In essence, such estimates, derived as they are almost exclusively from laboratory animal bioassay findings, and based on many conservative and typically unverified assumptions, provide little more than an imprecise measure of the reciprocal of the maximum dose tested in those studies! In contrast, the delivered dose concept has great potential for improving both the scientific credibility and accuracy of quantitative estimates of human risk from chemical exposure. Nevertheless, this concept has yet to be fully elucidated for any chemical agent, including formaldehyde. Such knowledge cannot be acquired from bioassay data alone, but requires many detailed mechanistic studies of the distribution and biochemical disposition of chemical agents in whole animals, including humans if at all possible.

In the case of formaldehyde, mechanistically oriented studies have already identified several biological responses that appear to be important determinants of the dose delivered to target tissues in the rodent nasal cavity. These include respiratory depression in response to sensory irritation; localized inhibition of mucociliary clearance; intra-cellular metabolic detoxication and macromolecular binding in target tissues; and the cell proliferation response to cytotoxicity. The delivered dose concept provides a mechanism whereby these biological observations can be incorporated directly into the risk extrapolation process in a meaningful way. While further research must be undertaken to specify accurately the relationships between delivered and administered doses for humans and laboratory animals, careful study and elaboration of this concept should lead to more accurate and scientifically defensible assessments of human risk from chemical exposure than are presently available.

References

Barrow, C. S., Buckley, L. A., James, R. A., Steinhagen, W. H. and Chang, J. C. F., 1986, Sensory irritation: studies on correlation to pathology, structure-activity, tolerance development, and prediction of species differences to nasal injury. In *Toxicology of the Nasal Passages*, edited by C. S. Barrow (Washington, DC: Hemisphere), pp. 101–122.

Bernstein, L., Gold, L. S., Ames, B. N., Pike, M. C. and Hoel, D. G., 1985, Some tautologous aspects of the comparison of carcinogenic potency in rats and mice. *Fund appl. Tox.*, **5**, 79–86.

Brown, C. C., 1976, Mathematical aspects of dose-response studies in carcinogenesis – the concept of thresholds. *Oncology*, **33**, 62–65.

Casanova-Schmitz, M. and Heck, H. d'A., 1985, DNA–protein crosslinking induced by formaldehyde (FA) in the rat respiratory mucosa: dependence on FA concentration in normal rats and in rats depleted of glutathione (GSH). *Toxicologist*, **5**, 128.

Casanova-Schmitz, M., Starr, T. B. and Heck, H. d'A., 1984, Differentiation between metabolic incorporation and covalent binding in the labeling of macromolecules in the rat nasal mucosa and bone marrow by inhaled [^{14}C]- and [^{3}H]-formaldehyde. *Toxic. appl. Pharmac.*, **76**, 26–44.

Chang, J. C. F., Gross, E. A., Swenberg, J. A. and Barrow, C. S., 1983, Nasal cavity deposition, histopathology, and cell proliferation after single or repeated formaldehyde exposure in B6C3F$_1$ mice and F-344 rats. *Toxic. appl. Pharmac.*, **68**, 161–176.

Cornfield, J., 1977, Carcinogenic risk assessment. *Science*, **198**, 693–699.

Crouch, E. A. C., 1983, Uncertainties in interspecies extrapolation of carcinogenicity. *Envir. Hlth. Perspect.*, **50**, 321–327.

Crouch, E. and Wilson, R., 1979, Interspecies comparison of carcinogenic potency. *J. Tox. envir. Hlth.*, **5**, 1095–1118.

Crump, K. S., 1979, Dose response problems in carcinogenesis. *Biometrics*, **35**, 157–167.

EPA, 1984, Proposed guidelines for carcinogen risk assessment. *Fed. Reg.*, **49**, 46294–46301.

Hoel, D. G., Kaplan, N. L. and Anderson, M. W., 1983, Implication of nonlinear kinetics on risk estimation in carcinogenesis. *Science*, **219**, 1032–1037.

Kerns, W. D., Pavkov, K. L., Donofrio, D. J., Gralla, E. J. and Swenberg, J. A., 1983, Carcinogenicity of formaldehyde in rats and mice after long-term inhalation exposure. *Cancer Res.*, **43**, 4382–4392.

Lukashin, A. V., Vologodskii, A. V., Frank-Kamenetskii, M. D. and Lyubchenko, Y. L., 1976, Fluctuational opening of the double helix as revealed by theoretical and experimental study of DNA interaction with formaldehyde. *J. molec. Biol.*, **108**, 665–682.

Morgan, K. T., 1983, Localization of areas of inhibition of nasal mucociliary function in rats following *in vivo* exposure to formaldehyde. *Am. Rev. resp. Dis.*, **127**, 166.

Morgan, K. T., Patterson, D. L. and Gross, E. A., 1983, Formaldehyde and the nasal mucociliary apparatus. In *Formaldehyde: Toxicology, Epidemiology, Mechanisms*, edited by J. J. Clary, J. E. Gibson and R. S. Waritz (New York: Marcel Dekker), pp. 193–210.

NCI (1976–80). Carcinogenesis Technical Report Series (Bethesda, MD: National Cancer Institute).

Starr, T. B., 1985, The role of mechanistic data in dose-response modeling. In *Assessment of Risk from Low-Level Exposure to Radiation and Chemicals*, edited by A. D. Woodhead, C. J. Shellabarger, V. Pond and A. Hollander (New York: Plenum), pp. 101–124.

Starr, T. B. and Buck, R. D., 1984, The importance of delivered dose in estimating low-dose cancer risk from inhalation exposure to formaldehyde. *Fund. appl. Tox.*, **4**, 740–753.

Starr, T. B. and Gibson, J. E., 1985, The mechanistic toxicology of formaldehyde and its implications for quantitative risk estimation. *Ann. Rev. Pharmac. Tox.*, **25**, 745–767.

Swenberg, J. S., Gross, E. A., Randall, H. W. and Barrow, C. S., 1983, The effect of formalehyde exposure on cytotoxicity and cell profileration. In *Formaldehyde: Toxicology, Epidemiology, Mechanisms*, edited by J. J. Clary, J. E. Gibson and R. S. Waritz, (New York: Dekker), pp. 225–236.

von Hippel, P. H. and Wong, K. Y., 1971, Dynamic aspects of native DNA structure: kinetics of the formaldehyde reaction with calf thymus DNA. *J. molec. Biol.*, **61**, 587–613.

Zeise, L., Wilson, R. and Crouch, E., 1984, Use of acute toxicity to estimate carcinogenic risk. *Risk Analysis*, **4**, 187–199.

Summary

Selection and Extrapolation – the task of implementation

Ronald W. Hart and Angelo Turturro

Office of the Director, National Center for Toxicological Research, Jefferson, AR 72079, USA

Introduction

The task of selecting the most appropriate species, strain or test system for predicting health effects in humans is not an easy one. There are a number of scientific, statutory and sociological difficulties, including scientific uncertainty, statutory inflexibility and lack of confidence in public health policy.

Scientific uncertainty

Much as been heard about inter-species, inter-strain and individual differences and similarities that would affect extrapolation of data from laboratory animals to humans, techniques to assist in the definition of parameters to improve this extrapolation, and studies suggesting that new or improved state-of-the-science techniques are now available to aid selection of either species or strain in testing or extrapolation. As the discussions have suggested, there are problems in naively assigning any one strain or species the role of ultimate predictor.

Science has made great strides in clarifying the questions involved in extrapolating risk among species. Indeed, much of the present ferment surrounding the process of risk assessment comes from the realization that the scientific bases underlying risk assessment are open to experimental attack. Where previously questions were 'answered' by appeal to global theories, it is now appreciated that more specific answers may be possible. Related to this, certain practical considerations need to be emphasized.

1. No matter what animal is considered to be the best sentinel for a particular human health effect, it is known for endpoints in chronic studies that only three rodent species (the rat, mouse and hamster) appear to meet the requirements that the animals (*a*) are readily available; (*b*) have a lifespan long enough to see chronic toxic effects but short enough to allow a chronic test to be economically feasible; (*c*) can be handled with relative ease in the

laboratory environment; (*d*) are sensitive to a number of toxic effects; and (*e*) their biological response is similar in some respects to the human response. For the metabolic studies and other shorter term endpoints, other systems have been developed, for example, using dogs or rabbits, but the costs of such systems are slowly making them too expensive for routine use.

2. Whether to use outbred or inbred strains is a complicated question. The outbreds are relatively difficult to keep, while inbreds, especially inbred albinos, are probably more susceptible to unique spontaneous lesions. Layered upon these considerations is the problem that most of the present inbred strains were selected and are maintained as homogeneous for one or more genetic disease. Attempts to mimic the genetically heterogeneous human population with a homogeneous inbred strain encounter basic difficulties. However, how much is gained by maintaining a very limited number of variegated animals in a test as opposed to a larger number of homogeneous ones is not clear.

3. There exists a large and growing database for a few strains of animals. Introducing new or exotic strains must be done in this context, in order to make the best use of the information already available in these databases. At the very least, comparative studies among existing test strains and any new ones should be done in order to enable use of present databases.

4. It is not clear that a strain which is useful for predicting the human toxic response for any single endpoint or chemical would also be the one most useful for predicting other toxic effects for other chemicals. Strains vary in many parameters, so whereas one chemical may be processed similarly to that in humans another chemical may be processed differently. An example illustrating this is the guinea-pig. As a model for asbestosis, the guinea-pig is very useful at mimicking a number of responses seen in humans. However, it does not *N*-hydroxylate acetyl amino fluorene and, thus, is refractory to the carcinogenic action of this very potent agent.

5. As discussed in these papers, pharmacokinetics has made rapid progress over the last few years. However, there are over 200 separate 'tissues' in the body, each with its own 'cellular compartments'. Obtaining information on as many parameters as necessary to predict local concentrations of toxic substances and their metabolites under various physiological and nutritional conditions is still beyond current resources and abilities. The difficulties in representing reality in any pharmacokinetic model should not be under-estimated, especially since the actual chemical species which induces the toxic effect is often unknown for many compounds. General models for even relatively simple processes such as skin absorption have yet to be satisfactorily developed, although available information suggests that major advances are now being made in this area.

6. Although it is assumed that imposing conditions on a model similar to those seen in humans will improve prediction of the human toxic response, this is not necessarily true. Useful predictive tests may use fairly exotic endpoints

and species. An example is the Ames *Salmonella* test, where the organism is a prokaryote, with a genome significantly different than that of the eukaryotic mammal; the metabolism is vastly different; and the endpoint, mutagenesis, is evaluated in a locus which appears totally unrelated to any process related to carcinogenesis. However, the test is presently one of the best predictors of rodent carcinogenicity.

For this test, an attempt to mimic human response sometimes distorts test results, as evidenced by some carcinogenic compounds which are positive with totally non-mammalian enzyme activation, yet are negative when a rat liver microsome activation system is used. It is the presumption of identical mechanisms in rodent and man which is the basis for the effort to approximate the human exposure conditions for rodents. Reason for caution can be illustrated by results found in the investigation of 2-naphthylamine carcinogenesis. The rat does not hold urine long enough, or at conditions acidic enough, to reactivate conjugates in the urine which result in bladder carcinogenesis. Comparative pharmocokinetics in the rat and man, not allied to understanding this mechanism, would have been deceptive in this instance, since target organ local blood concentrations of the 'active' metabolite are irrelevant to the carcinogenic action on the bladder, which is exposed through the urine.

The scientific and practical problems in selecting species, thus, are not trivial. Uncertainties in the application of animal data to humans is one of the greatest sources of uncertainty in using animal tests in risk assessment. However, with the identification of problems, solutions are being generated. One key appears to be the step-by-step elucidation of the extrapolation of each component part of the mechanisms of action of human carcinogens in the test species to similar effects in humans. Although there are encouraging developments, for instance the Andersen model which attempts to characterize distribution in terms of physical parameters in a comparative sense, the application to human carcinogens and relating the effects of mechanisms of action are presently rudimentary. Elucidation of the general principles of each step in carcinogen action, for instance, would perhaps be specific to particular chemical classes or types. However, breaking the problem down to its component parts is likely to be fruitful. At NCTR work is performed with this perspective in mind, using biomarkers as indicators of result at different steps. An example is measuring a DNA adduct produced by the human carcinogens, 4-aminobiphenyl and 2-naphthylamine, as the integration of the uptake, disposition, metabolism, and DNA exposure in a particular tissue.

Regulatory inflexibility

Regulatory inflexibility is characteristic of some regulations, especially the older legislation. If we consider a material to be carcinogenic, that is an actual threat to humans under practical conditions of use and exposure, because it produces an effect in one species in a single experiment under some fairly exotic conditions, this beggars the question of extrapolation. However, some statutes require this risk calculus. The question of extrapolation is intimately involved in applying weight-of-evidence and exposure in estimating risk, where judgement and reason are applied to characterize the presence of real risk. In the presence of so much uncertainty in the process of extrapolation, this appears a better guide than arbitrary time-limited definitions of what constitutes a threat. Also, some present legislation actually demands that no risk be permitted, a situation that is clearly impossible in a world where we can measure a few thousand molecules of material. In practice, these impossible criteria become criteria based on technical feasibility. The price paid is that the question of the actual risk associated with the feasibility levels becomes moot, although the rapid pace of our technical proficiency brings it to the centre of attention. Regulatory flexibility is encouraged directly by legislation which suggests that the determination of safety be made in light of scientific consensus and the best science available at the time of the decision.

Other legislation which would be useful would clearly state that decisions which were made with the best knowledge available at a particular time, when new studies later show them to be wrong, would not be the basis of legal action against the government. This legislation would permit government regulators to apply the best current science, without demanding prescience or transcience. In the absence of such legislation, regulators are forced into a position of what appears to be ultraconservatism. This position hurts industrial development and erodes confidence in the government's ability to judge and shows action in the face of real risk.

Finally, legislation which encourages the improvement of risk assessment and programmes which result in the reduction of the uncertainty in risk assessment are the best long-term solution because it gets to the root of many of the problems involved.

Lack of confidence in public health policy

In implementing the rational selection of species, it should be recognized that confidence in the choice is an important question of public health policy which should involve all segments of the society.

An important part of having confidence in the selection is educating the public to the true nature of the risks involved. As set forth in the recent Department of Health and Human Services, Committee to Coordinate Environmental and Related Programs document on risk assessment and risk management, the degree of voluntary acceptance of the risk, its perception and its acceptibility are all components which should be clearly delineated. With these considerations set forth, the risk, could better be placed in perspective with the other risks which exist. The nature of the animal–man extrapolation as a component in estimating this risk should be explicated as much as possible. Failure to do so has led to statements such as (*a*) "such a test is equivalent to drinking over a hundred bottles a day", etc. (one might as well say about a substance assayed in an Ames Test that the test is relevant only if a great deal of the material is put in saline and added to one's culture media); and (*b*) "one molecule of this substance will give you cancer and should be banned" (although the substance is an essential nutrient). Such unfortunate statements are injudicious when applied to tests which use a small number of animals to test for a population of over a quarter billion, and whose results have to be evaluated carefully.

Confidence in the ability of government to distinguish risks will also grow with the adoption of a problem-solving approach to risk assessment, which seeks to resolve the problems resulting from exposure to a compound with some toxic effects. A consensus in the extrapolation from animal to man becomes more possible if the public is convinced that the primary purpose of governmental regulation is not to punish offenders or to permit illness, but to work to preserve the positive aspects of a substance (in which some company may have staked its economic future) while protecting the public health. With this attitude, the question of animal–man extrapolation, and its attendant uncertainties becomes a problem to be addressed in assessing risk from a particular compound. Consensus building in extrapolation, for example, by Consensus Workshops, is one approach.

Finally, it is clear that peer review at all steps in the process of selecting species will be a giant step towards instilling public confidence in the risks determined by an assay.

Conclusion

There is little prospect of getting epidemiological data on more than a tiny number of the 60 000 man-made chemicals and untold thousands of natural chemicals we, as a population, will be exposed to this year. Even if we could, these data would be limited by the conditions of the study in which they were obtained, for example, a particular cohort, certain confounding variables, and so on. Animal and short-term tests offer a chance to investigate many chemicals, their interactions, and to better understand their effects. Utilization of this invaluable resource should be consistent with best current science. In effecting this, there needs to be resolution of the problems related to the scientific uncertainties in the process, the regulatory inflexibilities, and the lack of confidence in public health policy. Since there is a conducive atmosphere towards solving the problems produced by the toxic effects of compounds, this resolve will quicken the implementation of the best science by choosing the optimal test systems.

Index